hematology

Middle East Edition

طبعة الشرق الأوسط

The National Medical Series for Independent Study

hematology

Emmanuel C. Besa, M.D.

Associate Professor of Medicine
Medical College of Pennsylvania
Philadelphia, Pennsylvania

Patricia M. Catalano, M.D.

Associate Professor of Medicine
Medical College of Pennsylvania
Philadelphia, Pennsylvania

Jeffrey A. Kant, M.D., Ph.D.

Associate Professor of Pathology and Laboratory Medicine
University of Pennsylvania School of Medicine
Director, Hematology and Molecular Diagnosis, William Pepper Laboratories
Hospital of the University of Pennsylvania
Philadelphia, Pennsylvania

Leigh C. Jefferies, M.D.

Assistant Professor of Pathology and Laboratory Medicine
University of Pennsylvania School of Medicine
Assistant Director, Transfusion Medicine Section, Blood Bank
Hospital of the University of Pennsylvania
Philadelphia, Pennsylvania

SANS TACHE NMS

National Medical Series from Williams & Wilkins
Baltimore, Hong Kong, London, Sydney

Harwal Publishing Company, Malvern, Pennsylvania

Mass Publishing Co. 9 Al-Tahrir St., Dokki, Giza, Egypt

Williams
& Wilkins

Middle East Edition طبعة الشرق الأوسط

MASS PUBLISHING CO.: 9 AL Tahrir St., Dokki, Giza, Egypt.
Tel: (202) 361 3012 Fax: (202) 361 3011

ISBN 977 - 269 - 046 - 2
Legal deposit No:4582 /93

Printed in Egypt by Elias Modern Press

Dedication

All of us thank our families for their support and patience during the long period of writing and rewriting this book.

I would like to dedicate this book to my parents, Drs. Augusto and Solita Besa, for inspiring me to pursue the educational aspects of medicine, and to Dr. Frank Gardener and Dr. Allen Caviles for introducing me to the mysteries of hematology.

Contents

Preface

Hematology has long been a leading discipline in research on basic mechanisms of human disease, due to the relative ease with which blood is obtained for study. This tradition has been accelerated in the last 15 years by modern tools of molecular biology. Today, mysteries of the human blood system are unraveling at a rapid rate, making hematology one of the fastest moving disciplines in medicine. As authors of NMS *Hematology,* our challenge has been to capture the essence of this rapidly evolving field in a book for physicians-in-training.

Using the outline format that is unique to the National Medical Series, we have presented basic principles underlying normal and abnormal hematologic phenomena, emphasizing the mechanisms of major hematologic disorders in the context of specific structural or functional features of the blood system. Although in a traditional curriculum, students typically study biochemistry, physiology, and immunology prior to hematology, we have included fundamental elements of these other disciplines since they are integral to understanding blood disorders. Thus, as students read NMS *Hematology,* they will refresh their memory of basic science principles while discovering the clinical relevance of those sciences. The outline format allows the reader to gain a quick overview of broad areas in hematology as well as review key features of pathophysiology, clinical behavior, and therapeutic options in specific hematologic disorders.

We feel four chapters warrant special attention. Chapter 10, "Approach to Patients with Red Cell Disorders," and Chapter 16, "Approach to Patients with Coagulation Disorders," are particularly useful because they integrate information from several chapters, focusing thinking and allowing the reader to work through everyday practical diagnostic issues. The presentation of information on hematologic neoplasia in a single chapter (Chapter 12) we believe facilitates the understanding of interrelationships among these disorders and highlights common points of clinical and laboratory differential diagnosis. Finally, a separate chapter on blood products in transfusion medicine (Chapter 17) has been included. Transfusion medicine is important to all practicing physicians and is fast becoming a separate specialty.

Conceptualized drawings are provided where necessary to clarify complex structural, functional, and pathophysiologic relationships, and algorithms are used to simplify the differential diagnostic approach to red cell and bleeding disorders. We suggest that the reader supplement NMS *Hematology* with a good atlas, since review of actual slides of blood smears is important to learning hematology.

The book also contains Board-type questions and explanations at the end of each chapter and in a comprehensive examination at the end of the text. The questions are intended to help the reader test and reinforce comprehension of important principles set forth in the book. The explanations serve to clarify concepts that may have been misunderstood by the reader.

We believe that NMS *Hematology* will be especially useful for medical students and house-staff during preclinical course work and again on the wards. Physicians in other specialties also may find it a valuable source of essential information on hematology.

Emmanual C. Besa
Patricia M. Catalano
Jeffrey A. Kant
Leigh C. Jefferies

Acknowledgments

We would like to acknowledge Matt Harris for getting this book started and Debra Dreger, Jane Velker, Donna Siegfried, and the rest of the staff at Harwal Publishing Company for editing the chapters and finally getting it through the finish line.

To the Reader

Since 1984, the National Medical Series for Independent Study has been helping medical students meet the challenge of education and clinical training. In today's climate of burgeoning information and complex clinical issues, a medical career is more demanding than ever. Increasingly, medical training must prepare physicians to seek and synthesize necessary information and to apply that information successfully.

The National Medical Series is designed to provide a logical framework for organizing, learning, reviewing, and applying the conceptual and factual information covered in basic and clinical sciences. Each book includes a comprehensive outline of the essential content of a discipline, with up to 500 study questions. The combination of an outlined text and tools for self-evaluation allows easy retrieval of salient information.

All study questions are accompanied by the correct answer, a paragraph-length explanation, and specific reference to the text where the topic is discussed. Study questions that follow each chapter use the current National Board format to reinforce the chapter content. Study questions appearing at the end of the text in the Comprehensive Exam vary in format depending on the book. Wherever possible, Comprehensive Exam questions are presented as clinical cases or scenarios intended to simulate real-life application of medical knowledge. The goal of this exam is to challenge the student to draw from information presented throughout the book.

All of the books in the National Medical Series are constantly being updated and revised. The authors and editors devote considerable time and effort to ensure that the information required by all medical school curricula is included. Strict editorial attention is given to accuracy, organization, and consistency. Further shaping of the series occurs in response to biannual discussions held with a panel of medical student advisors drawn from schools throughout the United States. At these meetings, the editorial staff considers the needs of medical students to learn how the National Medical Series can serve them better. In this regard, the Harwal staff welcomes all comments and suggestions.

1
Introduction and Principles of Hematologic Diagnosis

Emmanuel C. Besa

I. COMPOSITION OF THE BLOOD. Hematology is the study of the blood-forming tissues and circulating blood components. Normally, the functions of the blood are to deliver nutrients, hormones, and oxygen to tissues; to collect and dispose of the wastes from cellular metabolism; to deliver specialized cells to tissues for protection against the external environment; and to prevent leakage by closing holes in blood vessels. The circulating blood accounts for 5%–7% of the total body weight and is composed of two major elements.

A. Cellular elements

1. **Red blood cells** (RBCs, erythrocytes) are the cells responsible for carrying oxygen and carbon dioxide between the lungs and the tissues via the hemoglobin content in their cytoplasm. The name of the red blood cell reflects the bright red color of the cell that occurs when oxygen is attached to the hemoglobin. The cell is disk-shaped and biconcave. Because **the cell does not have a nucleus,** its life span is limited by its energy supply.

2. **White blood cells** (WBCs, leukocytes) are colorless **nucleated** cells whose primary function is protection against invading organisms. The white blood cell performs its function in one of two ways.
   a. **Phagocytes engulf,** or phagocytize, the pathogenic organism or foreign particle. These cells have the capacity to move from the bloodstream into the tissues where they are needed. Phagocytes can be identified by the histologic staining of their **granules** (**granulocytes,** such as neutrophils, basophils, eosinophils) or by their **nuclear characteristics** (**mononuclear cells** in the circulation are monocytes, in tissue are macrophages).
   b. **Immunocytes** are associated with humoral and cell-mediated reactions of the **immune system**. **B** and **T lymphocytes** are immunocytes in the blood; **plasma cells** are found in the bone marrow.

3. **Platelets** (thrombocytes) are anucleated, disk-shaped cytoplasmic fragments of megakaryocytes, the precursor cells in the bone marrow. Platelets are released into the circulation to prevent leakage or bleeding caused by inherent or acquired defects in blood vessel walls. The cells have a life span of about 1 week.

B. Fluid elements. Plasma is the fluid portion of the blood in which the cellular elements are suspended and circulated throughout the body. (**Serum** is the clear fluid that separates from the blood upon coagulation, when all cellular elements are removed.) Plasma has three main components.

1. **Water** is the main component of blood. Almost 70% of the body is water, most of which is contained in and around cells. The blood plasma maintains the water content of cells in the tissues.

2. **Electrolytes** in the plasma are essential to cellular function. The important plasma electrolytes are sodium, potassium, chloride, hydrogen, magnesium, and calcium.

3. **Proteins** are abundant in the plasma. Although highly varied in structure, plasma proteins can be divided into three main functional classes.
   a. **Coagulation proteins** are primarily involved in keeping the vascular system intact. Proteins that form clots (**procoagulants**) include components of the extrinsic and intrinsic pathways of the coagulation cascade and fibrinogen. Proteins that break down excessive coagulation (**anticoagulants**) are components of the fibrinolytic system. The procoagulants and anticoagulants maintain a balance of clot formation and clot dissolution.

b. **Proteins with immunologic functions** include **antibodies** (immunoglobulins) and the components of the complement system. These plasma proteins are involved in defending the body against infections caused by invading organisms and against the presence of foreign antigens.

c. **Transport proteins** serve several functions.

(1) **Osmotic pressure is maintained** in the intravascular space by **albumin,** which prevents excessive leakage of blood fluid extracellularly. This enables the circulation of blood within the vessels and prevents edema.

(2) **Binding and transporting** substances to the tissues and **removal of waste products and toxins** in the circulation are also functions of transport proteins.

(a) **Transferrin** is a plasma protein that binds and transports iron to the bone marrow for production of red blood cells.

(b) **Transcobalamin** is the carrier protein for vitamin B_{12}.

(c) **Haptoglobin** protects tissue cells from noxious substances by binding the byproducts of hemoglobin released from senescent or prematurely destroyed red blood cells and transporting the byproducts to the liver for disposal.

(3) **Transportation of lipids, cholesterol, and triglycerides** is carried out by the **lipoproteins.**

II. PRINCIPLES OF HEMATOLOGIC DIAGNOSIS.

Peripheral blood examination is a routine part of patient evaluation by most physicians, regardless of speciality. Because of its accessibility and close proximity to all tissues, the blood often provides the earliest evidence of changes in the state of health and the development of illness. An understanding of the mechanisms of blood alterations is very important and, together with information collected from a thorough medical history and physical examination, provides for accurate diagnosis and correct therapeutic choices.

A. History and physical examination.

Information about the patient's present and past health, genetic makeup, and environmental influences as well as specific details regarding the signs and symptoms of the present illness form the basis for further diagnostic evaluation.

1. History

a. **Medical history**

(1) The **present illness** should be the focus of the medical history, with an emphasis on the following:

(a) Bleeding

(b) Infections or symptoms related to enlargement of lymph nodes, the liver, or the spleen

(c) Nonspecific symptoms related to anemia (e.g., malaise, weakness, headache, weight loss)

(2) Any **exposure to drugs or chemicals** should be determined since such agents may cause or worsen many hematologic disorders (e.g., hemolysis, neutropenia, thrombocytopenia, myeloproliferative disorders).

(3) A **review of systems** (including the nervous system) is necessary, since blood dyscrasia affects many, if not all, organ systems.

b. **Family history.** Information about the health of family members as well as the ethnic background of the patient is important in certain inherited hematologic conditions, notably sickle cell anemia and the thalassemias.

2. Physical examination

a. Thorough physical examination of the hematologic patient is important and should focus closely on the skin and nails, mouth, mucous membranes, and eyes. Jaundice, pallor, cyanosis, petechiae and ecchymoses, excoriations, and ulcers are common findings.

b. Hepatomegaly, splenomegaly, enlarged or tender lymph nodes, soreness over the ribs or sternum, and a variety of neurologic abnormalities are common in hematologic disorders.

B. Peripheral blood measurements.

Information about the number of cellular components and about the concentration of plasma components is extremely useful to all clinicians.

1. **Principles and methods of blood cell counting.** Changes in the number of formed elements are investigated by performing a blood cell count. Automated blood counting is a more accurate method than manual (visual) counting.

a. Principles

(1) Accurate dilution is critical to precise quantitation of the cells under study. The measured volume of diluent varies with the cells being counted, with more required to count cells that are more numerous (e.g., red cells). Also, the chosen diluent must contain substances that lyse the other cells, enabling selective counting of the cells under study.

(2) Precise sampling of the diluted sample, with even distribution of the cells, is important regardless of the counting method.

(3) Reproducibility (i.e., the ability of a test to produce consistent results on repeated, independent trials) is required for useful quantitative data; all appropriate cells must be counted.

b. Manual counting

(1) Method. Manual counting is performed visually under a brightfield or phase-contrast microscope. A counting chamber with a grid inscribed at the bottom allows examination of a precise volume of diluted blood. Care and the skill of the technician are important for accurate manual counting.

(2) Reliability. The manual counting technique has limited accuracy, precision, and reproducibility. Inherent errors are those of dilution, of obtaining an even distribution of cells in the sample, and of accurately enumerating cells that may be superimposed on one another or that may vary in shape and size.

c. Automated counting has enabled laboratories to cope with increased routine blood testing, allowing greater efficiency and reliability than manual techniques while decreasing costs and sources of errors. The techniques currently used in automated blood counting are flow cytometry and image analysis (Figure 1-1).

(1) Flow cytometry

(a) Flow cytometry is an automated counting method that enables analysis of an extremely high number of cells within a very short period of time. Cells can be sorted out according to their physical characteristics, permitting retrieval of certain groups of cells from the blood for further examination.

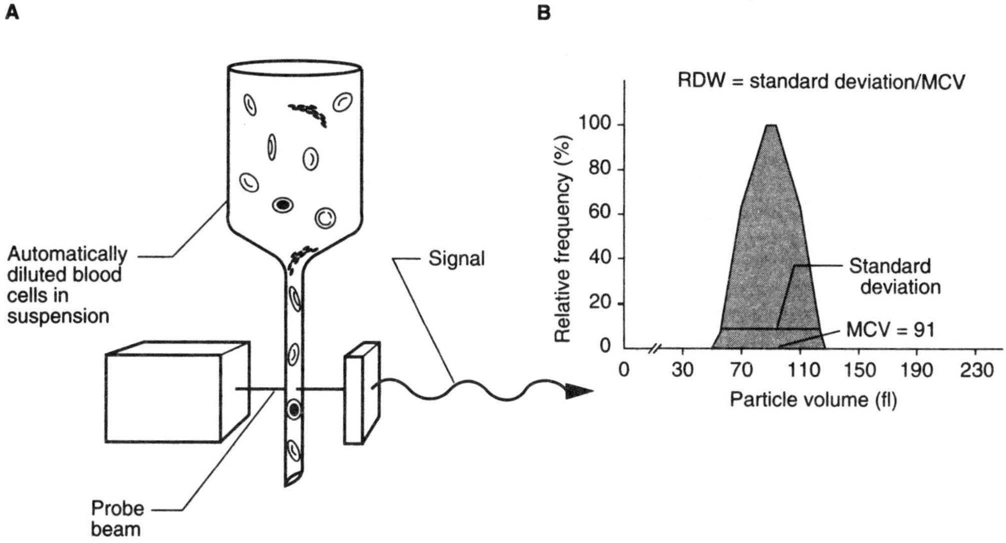

Figure 1-1. (*A*) Flow cytometry is accomplished in an automated cell counter by passing a single file of cells suspended in a stream of fluid past a probe beam. The probe beam is composed of either laser light or electric current that is directed through the stream of cells and measured by a detector. The beam is altered by the passage of each cell, and the occurrence and magnitude of this change is sensed by the detector and converted into a signal that is proportional to the magnitude of the cell variable being detected (e.g., cell size, fluorescence). (*B*) The data from 10,000 cells are rapidly collected and displayed as a histogram or scattergram that depicts the distribution of red cell sizes and shapes in the sample analyzed. A normal histogram with a normal variation in cell size and shape is shown. The standard deviation of the histogram (width of histogram) as well as the mean corpuscular volume (*MCV*), from which the red cell distribution width (*RDW*) is derived, are identified. (Adapted from Bessman JD: *Automated Blood Counts and Differentials.* Baltimore, Johns Hopkins University Press, 1986, p 2.)

(b) A serious limitation of flow cytometry is its inability to distinguish abnormal (nucleated) red cells from white blood cells (which are nucleated) because the method uses the nucleus as the distinguishing factor.

(2) **Image analysis**

(a) This method offers high-speed analysis of cells fixed on a slide according to programmed criteria for differential cell counting. Image analyzers can relocate and display cells as requested for visual confirmation.

(b) Reliance on fixed slides makes image analysis slower than flow cytometry.

(3) **Other uses of automated counting systems**

(a) **Histograms,** or graphic depictions of the distribution curve of blood cells, are automatically generated by the new counting systems.

(i) The histograms are scatter diagrams of 10,000 individual red cells showing the distribution (i.e., degree of heterogeneity) of the cells according to size.

(ii) These data provide clues to red cell abnormalities of size. This, however, does not reveal the specific abnormality, and examination of the peripheral blood smear is still necessary.

(iii) However, access to this information is limited because of logistics in transmitting the data from the laboratory to the patient's record or to the physician.

(b) **Red cell distribution width (RDW),** the numerical equivalent of the histogram, is also calculated by most automated systems. The RDW is reported to the physician.

(i) The RDW, or **coefficient of variation,** represents the ratio of standard deviation (i.e., width of the histogram) to the mean corpuscular volume (MCV) [see Figure 1-1B].

(ii) The degree of heterogeneity of the red cell population is represented as an increase in the RDW (normal = 12.5 ± 1.5).

2. Peripheral blood counts and measurements

a. **Red cell count and hematocrit (Hct).** The hematocrit is the proportion of the blood occupied by red cells. It can be measured manually or by electronic instruments.

(1) The hematocrit is determined manually by centrifuging a volume of anticoagulated blood in a 3-mm tube (macro scale) or a capillary tube (micro scale) and measuring the volume of packed red cells at the bottom of the tube. The hematocrit is expressed as a percentage.

(2) Automated systems derive the hematocrit by counting red cells and multiplying the total by the **MCV** [see II B 2 c (1)]. This value will be different from the manually determined hematocrit, since it does not include the space between red cells.

b. **Hemoglobin concentration** is most accurately estimated by measuring the light absorbance of cyanmethemoglobin—a stable derivative of hemoglobin—derived by colorimetric methods.

(1) Manual and automated measurements of cyanmethemoglobin concentration provide comparable estimates of hemoglobin concentration.

(2) The red cell volume is approximated by the hemoglobin concentration and hematocrit level, and each should be used as a check of the other to avoid laboratory error. However, since the method for measuring hemoglobin is more precise and the hemoglobin concentration is measured directly in contrast to the hematocrit, which is calculated indirectly from the MCV, the hemoglobin concentration is the preferred laboratory parameter for evaluating changes in red cells.

c. **Red cell indices** are measurements that indicate the size and hemoglobin content of red cells. These values can be calculated quantitatively from the hemoglobin concentration, red cell counts, and packed red cell volume. The accuracy of red cell indices has increased with the availability of more sophisticated measurement techniques; some electronic counting devices automatically calculate them.

(1) **Mean corpuscular volume** refers to the average volume of the individual red cells. The MCV is expressed in cubic micrometers (μm^3) per red cell, or femtoliters (fl), and is calculated as follows:

$$\text{MCV} = \frac{\text{packed red cell volume/1000 ml blood}}{\text{red cell count (millions/mm}^3\text{)}}$$

(2) **Mean corpuscular hemoglobin (MCH)** refers to the hemoglobin content per red cell. The MCH is expressed in picograms (pg) per red cell and is calculated as follows:

$$\text{MCH} = \frac{\text{hemoglobin (g/1000 ml blood)}}{\text{red cell count (millions/mm}^3)}$$

(3) **Mean corpuscular hemoglobin concentration (MCHC)** refers to the hemoglobin concentration of the red cells. The MCHC is expressed in grams per decaliter of red cells and is calculated as follows:

$$\text{MCHC} = \frac{\text{hemoglobin (g/1000 ml blood)} \times 100}{\text{packed red cell volume (\%)}}$$

d. White cell counts

(1) **White cell counts** are performed manually as well as electronically on blood samples that have been diluted appropriately to cause red cell lysis. Electronic counters differentiate white cells by the size of their nuclei; the cells are incubated in a suspension that collapses the cytoplasm, enabling the machine to distinguish each cell type. White cell counts may be falsely elevated due to the presence of nucleated red cells.

(2) The **differential white cell count** is an enumeration of the distinct morphologic subsets of leukocytes, most commonly segmented neutrophils, band neutrophils, metamyelocytes, promyelocytes, blasts, basophils, eosinophils, lymphocytes, and monocytes.

(a) Manual techniques can vary widely as a result of observer imprecision.

(b) Image analysis, in which several hundred cells are measured using programmed criteria, eliminates the variation inherent in the visual technique and is much more accurate than flow cytometry.

e. Platelet count. A rough count of platelets in a blood smear can be obtained manually or by machine.

(1) Platelets are anucleated and appear in the peripheral blood smear as small blue bodies with red or purple granules. A rough estimate of the platelet count from the blood smear (i.e., number per high-power field × 10,000) should confirm the need for or justify a request for a direct platelet count.

(2) A direct platelet count is performed manually using a phase-contrast microscope on an appropriately diluted blood sample after lysing both red and white cells.

(3) Automated systems count platelets and measure the **mean platelet volume (MPV)** accurately. However, because the normal values vary greatly, the MPV alone is not useful for detecting abnormalities or for indicating high platelet turnover. Correlation of the MPV with the platelet count may help to identify certain hematologic disorders [e.g., large platelets correlate with young or newly released platelets as seen in idiopathic thrombocytopenic purpura (ITP)].

3. Limitations of blood counts. Those measurements that represent ratios of blood cells to the plasma (e.g., hematocrit and hemoglobin concentrations) may be difficult to interpret or may even be misleading in some clinical conditions, since the values do not account for changes in plasma volume or for abnormalities that may affect cell number. Examples of such conditions include the following.

a. A **decrease in plasma volume** caused by dehydration will increase peripheral red cell values. Conversely, an increase in plasma volume resulting from the presence of abnormal proteins in multiple myeloma will exaggerate anemia. Red cell mass is more accurately evaluated by blood volume measurements (see II B 1).

b. Extramedullary red cell production in agnogenic myeloid metaplasia (AMM) and acute hemolysis will nullify the white cell count in automated methods.

C. Blood smear examination. Critical diagnostic information regarding the morphology of the cellular elements of the blood can be obtained through the examination of blood smears. Routinely, morphologic evaluation is performed using a fixed and stained sample of blood cells.

1. Wet preparation allows examination of fresh blood samples without the artifacts produced by fixation and staining. The use of hypertonic solutions may cause the formation of crenated cells. This method is particularly useful for demonstrating sickled red cells or spherocytes.

2. Supravital staining refers to the addition of stain to living cells before fixation. Certain tests are performed using this method.

a. **Reticulocyte staining**

(1) Immature red cells are identified by supravital staining of precipitated residual RNA with new methylene blue or brilliant cresyl blue; the cells containing the stained precipitate are counted and reported as a percentage of the red cells examined.

(2) The reticulocyte count is an effective means of assessing red cell production.

b. **Heinz body staining**

(1) Heinz bodies are precipitated denatured hemoglobin demonstrated by the supravital staining of red cells with crystal violet.

(2) This test is used to identify unstable hemoglobinopathies, hemolysis due to glucose-6-phosphate dehydrogenase (G6PD) deficiency, and hemoglobin H (Hb H) disease (an α thalassemia).

3. **Fixed blood smears.** Examination of a fixed peripheral blood smear stained with Wright's or Giemsa stain allows identification of various changes in blood cell morphology typical of certain diseases. This examination is used to target suspected disease and not as an indicator of general health.

a. **Blood cell morphology**

(1) **Red cell morphology** (Table 1-1). Red cells should be examined for size, shape, hemoglobin content, staining properties (e.g., polychromatophilia), distribution in the film (e.g., rouleau formation: the stacking of red cells like coins), and inclusion bodies.

(2) **White cell morphology.** The peripheral blood film also should be examined for the presence of immature white cells, a "shift to the left" (i.e., an increase in the number of band neutrophils), hypersegmentation or hyposegmentation of neutrophils, atypical lymphocytes, leukocyte inclusions (e.g., toxic granulations, Döhle bodies), and the presence of bacteria inside or outside granulocytes.

(3) **Platelet morphology.** The blood smear also can be evaluated for the presence of large platelets (young platelets are hypothesized to be larger than old ones), and the MPV (see II B 2 e) can be used to assess platelet production in a manner similar to the way in which the reticulocyte count is used to measure red cell production (i.e., low platelet counts caused by increased dysfunction as in ITP are associated with large platelets). However, certain blood disorders (e.g., myeloproliferative disorders) are associated with abnormally large platelets that are prominent on blood smear but do not correlate in number.

b. **Blood smear artifacts** often can confuse the examiner.

(1) **Red cell artifacts** (see Table 1-1) commonly seen include:

(a) **Vacuoles**, which are irregularly distributed in the red cell cytoplasm and result from the staining properties of an improperly dried blood smear

(b) **Target cells**, which are seen in a few areas of the film rather than being evenly distributed, as is characteristic of certain disorders

(c) **Red cells lacking the normal central pallor,** which also are unevenly distributed throughout the film

(d) **Red cells with distorted shapes,** which result from cells pressing on each other

(2) **White cell artifacts** include:

(a) **Crushed cells**, which result from the smear technique

(b) **Radial segmentation of nuclei,** which is caused by anticoagulants such as oxalate and ethylenediaminetetraacetic acid (EDTA)

(c) **"Pseudo" phagocytosis**, which is caused by a red cell (most often) overlying a neutrophil or monocyte that appears to be ingested

(d) **Endothelial cells**, which may exist in the first drop of blood drawn by phlebotomy and may be mistaken for abnormal white cells

(3) **Platelet artifacts** include:

(a) **Illusion of inclusion bodies**, which is caused by a platelet overlying a red cell and appearing to be an intracellular inclusion or parasite

(b) **Decreased number of platelets**, which results from platelets aggregating rather than appearing as individual cells

D. Other routine blood studies

1. **Blood volume measurements.** Direct measurement of the red cell mass is valuable for establishing a diagnosis of true (absolute) polycythemia.

a. **Total blood volume** is determined by labeling a patient's red cells with radioactive chromium, reinfusing the labeled cells, and resampling after enough time has elapsed for adequate body mixing (usually 30 minutes). The radioactivity of the injected cells and

Table 1-1. Red Cell Changes Observed on Blood Smear Examination

Red Cell Change	Description	Associated Conditions
Abnormal shape		
Acanthocytes	Few large spicules	Abetalipoproteinemia, cirrhosis, uremia, HUS
Echinocytes ("burr cells")*	Many tiny spicules	Abetalipoproteinemia, cirrhosis, uremia, HUS
Codocytes (target cells)	Target forms	Hb C or E, liver disease, obstructive jaundice, thalassemia, postsplenectomy
Dacrocytes	Teardrop shape	Myelofibrosis, Heinz body anemia, thalassemia, hemolytic anemia, myelophthisis
Drepanocytes	Sickle shape	Sickle cell disease (sickle cell trait after deoxygenation), other rare hemoglobinopathies
Schizocytes (schistocytes; "spur cells")	Helmet forms, red cell fragments	DIC, TTP, vascular or valvular prosthesis
Spherostomatocytes (spherocytes)	Spheroid shape	Hereditary or acquired hemolysis
Stomatocytes	Slitlike area of central pallor	Hereditary or acquired hemolysis
Abnormal distribution		
Rouleau formation	Cells arranged like coins in a stack	Multiple myeloma, Waldenström's macroglobulinemia
Inclusion bodies		
Nucleated red cells	Pyknotic nucleus	Acute bleeding, severe hemolysis, myelofibrosis, leukemia, myelophthisis, asplenia
Basophilic stippling	Punctate nucleus	Lead intoxication, sideroblastic anemia, severe hemolysis
Howell-Jolly bodies	Small round bodies	Megaloblastic anemia, asplenia, severe hemolysis
Cabot's ring bodies	Rings or figures of eight	Severe hemolysis

DIC = disseminated intravascular coagulation; Hb = hemoglobin; HUS = hemolytic uremic syndrome; TTP = thrombotic thrombocytopenic purpura.

*Synonymous terms are noted in parentheses.

withdrawn cells is measured in counts per minute (cpm), and total blood volume (in milliliters) is calculated from the following equation:

$$\text{Blood volume} = \frac{\text{cpm injected red cells}}{\text{cpm withdrawn red cells/ml blood withdrawn}}$$

b. Red cell mass (in milliliters) is calculated from the total blood volume using the hematocrit corrected for the difference between arterial and venous values:

$$\text{Red cell mass} = \text{blood volume (ml)} \times \text{hematocrit} \times 0.92$$

c. Plasma volume is calculated by subtracting the red cell mass from the total blood volume.

2. Further testing. In addition to the above procedures that are performed in routine hematologic evaluation, several other laboratory tests are used in hematology; these will be discussed in the context of the specific disorders for which they are relevant to patient evaluation, differential diagnosis, and quantification of the abnormality involved. For information regarding bone marrow examination, see Chapter 2 V.

STUDY QUESTIONS

Directions: Each of the numbered items or incomplete statements in this section is followed by answers or by completions of the statement. Select the **one** lettered answer or completion that is **best** in each case.

1. Several cellular elements of the blood are anucleated; these include all of the following EXCEPT

(A) erythrocytes
(B) reticulocytes
(C) thrombocytes
(D) leukocytes

2. Automated blood counting systems have advantages over manual counting methods in that they

(A) do not require an accurate set of dilution factors
(B) are not wholly dependent on technician skills
(C) do not rely on the examination of fixed slides
(D) require precise sampling of the diluted sample

Directions: The item below contains four suggested answers, of which **one or more** is correct. Choose the answer

A if **1, 2, and 3** are correct
B if **1 and 3** are correct
C if **2 and 4** are correct
D if **4** is correct
E if **1, 2, 3, and 4** are correct

3. Heinz bodies are found under conditions of

(1) α thalassemia
(2) glucose-6-phosphate dehydrogenase (G6PD) deficiency
(3) unstable hemoglobinopathy
(4) lead intoxication

Directions: The group of items in this section consists of lettered options followed by a set of numbered items. For each item, select the **one** lettered option that is most closely associated with it. Each lettered option may be selected once, more than once, or not at all.

Questions 4–8

For each function of transport proteins, select the associated protein.

(A) Albumin
(B) Transferrin
(C) Haptoglobin
(D) Transcobalamin
(E) None of the above

4. Iron transport
5. Vitamin B_{12} transport
6. Clot formation
7. Plasma osmotic pressure maintenance
8. Hemoglobin transport

1-D
2-B
3-A
4-B
5-D
6-E
7-A
8-C

ANSWERS AND EXPLANATIONS

1. The answer is D *[I A 1, 2].*
Leukocytes are among the cellular elements of the blood that retain their nuclei. The erythrocyte (red blood cell) is released from the marrow in its immature form (the reticulocyte) after the cell has extruded its pyknotic nucleus. However, in disease states resulting in severe hemolysis, immature nucleated red cells may be released into the circulation. The platelets (thrombocytes) in the circulation are fragments of the cytoplasm of the megakaryocyte, which is a large cell with a multilobulated nucleus. The megakaryocyte is confined to the bone marrow in normal states. All leukocytes (white blood cells) circulate in the blood with their nuclei intact.

2. The answer is B *[II B 1].*
The accuracy and reliability of automated counting systems are not wholly dependent on the skill of the technician; the accuracy of manual counting depends on the technician's skill at every step of the procedure. Automated blood counting methods are more accurate and precise, and have greater reproducibility of results, than manual counting methods. It is critical that samples be accurately diluted before either manual or automated counting methods are used. Automated image analysis is dependent on fixed slides, whereas flow cytometry is not.

3. The answer is A (1, 2, 3) *[II C 2 b].*
Heinz bodies are supravitally stained hemoglobin precipitates in the red cell and are found in conditions in which insoluble hemoglobin is present in the red cells. Such conditions include α thalassemia with precipitation of the unstable hemoglobin H (Hb H), glucose-6-phosphate dehydrogenase (G6PD) deficiency resulting in oxidative denaturation of hemoglobin into insoluble masses, and unstable hemoglobinopathy in which alpha- (α-) globin or beta- (β-) globin mutations result in the spontaneous formation of precipitates of hemoglobin. Lead intoxication does not affect the precipitation of hemoglobin in red cells but causes basophilic stippling.

4–8. The answers are: 4-B *[I B 3 c (2)]*, **5-D** *[I B 3 c (2)]*, **6-E** *[I B 3 a]*, **7-A** *[I B 3 c (1)]*, **8-C** *[I B 3 c (2)].*
The functions of transport proteins can be divided into three general classes: the control of diffusion into the tissues, the highly specific recognition of molecules, and the removal of toxins. Transferrin helps in transporting iron to storage and utilization sites in the bone marrow. The damage that free iron can cause to tissues other than the marrow is prevented when it is bound by transferrin. Transcobalamin binds vitamin B_{12} and prevents it from degrading while it is being transported to storage and utilization sites in tissues with high cellular turnover rates. Albumin is the main plasma protein responsible for the maintenance of serum osmotic pressure. Haptoglobin is a plasma protein that binds free hemoglobin in the blood and delivers it to the liver for recycling. The degree of intravascular hemolysis is determined by measuring the levels of depleted free forms of haptoglobin in the blood.

2
Normal Hematopoiesis and Evaluation of the Bone Marrow

Emmanuel C. Besa

I. INTRODUCTION

A. Definition. Hematopoiesis is the **proliferation** of progenitor cells, which are maintained by the stem cells, and their **differentiation** into all of the cellular components of blood.

B. Sites of hematopoiesis. The sites of hematopoiesis depend on the presence of disease and on the developmental state of the individual.

1. **Normal conditions.** Under normal conditions, all cellular components **originate in the bone marrow**. Some components (e.g., erythrocytes and platelets) complete their development at **medullary** (i.e., bone marrow) sites (see II B 4 a), whereas other components (e.g., T and B cells) complete their development at **extramedullary** sites (see II B 4 b).
   a. **Fetal sites of hematopoiesis.** In utero, hematopoiesis proceeds as follows.
      (1) Hematopoiesis can be detected first in the **blood islands,** groups of mesenchymal cells in the **yolk sac,** at 3–12 weeks gestation.
      (2) The **liver** is active in hematopoiesis from 5 or 6 weeks up to 6 months gestation and even as long as 2 weeks after birth.
      (3) The **spleen** is active at 4–8 months gestation.
      (4) **Bone marrow** becomes active at about 5 months gestation and becomes the **primary site** by 7 months. The bone marrow remains the principal site of hematopoiesis after birth.
   b. **Postnatal changes in the sites of hematopoiesis.** At birth, all bone marrow cavities are hematopoietic. As the individual ages, the loci of hematopoiesis shift.
      (1) The marrow cavities of **peripheral bones** stop producing blood cells.
      (2) The marrow cavities of the **axial skeleton** become more prominent until, after 20 years of age, blood production has become limited to the vertebrae, sternum, iliac bones, skull, and proximal ends of the long bones of the extremities.
      (3) **Gross morphologic changes** accompany the physiologic changes in marrow.
         (a) **Red marrow.** The hematopoietically active marrow retains its red color.
         (b) **Yellow marrow.** Fat cells begin replacing hematopoietic elements in inactive marrow, giving it the characteristic yellow color. This process is complete by 20 years of age.
2. **Disease.** In the presence of disease, extramedullary sites can serve as the primary sites of blood cell development.
   a. **Fetal hematopoietic sites** (liver and spleen) can assume the primary role in adults in disease states such as myeloproliferative disease.
   b. **Adult medullary sites** that are not normally hematopoietic in the adult can revert to an earlier condition, becoming hematopoietic to help meet the demand for increased blood cell production.

II. BONE MARROW.

The theory that the hematopoietic ability of the bone marrow depends on both its cellular and physical composition is supported by two findings. First, donor stem cells infused into the peripheral blood of a bone marrow transplant recipient home in on the bone marrow. Second, sites damaged by the irradiation of certain malignancies never regain their hematopoietic ability because of damage to the cells that support blood cell production.

A. Stem cells. The stem cells found within the bone marrow are the origin of all blood cells. Blood cells are formed by a process of differentiation from the least developed stem cell to a highly specialized blood cell (Figure 2-1).

1. **Pluripotential stem cells** are the earliest (least developed) stem cells. They are distinguished by their ability to generate pure and mixed colonies of progenitor cells on the spleens of irradiated mice; thus, they were first called **colony-forming units–spleen (CFU-S)**.
   a. CFU-S isolated from the lymphoid fraction of human peripheral blood have certain **identifying characteristics**.
      (1) They are **morphologically identical to small lymphocytes**.
      (2) They **do not form rosettes** on exposure to sheep red blood cells, indicating that they lack a typical antibody response to antigen.
   b. A cell with properties very similar to those of the CFU-S has been identified in human marrow cultures. These cells, which are referred to as **colony-forming units–blast (CFU-blast),** are thought to be the human pluripotential stem cells.

2. **Multipotential stem cells** develop from the differentiation of pluripotential stem cells. **Two cell lines can develop:**
   a. **Lymphoid multipotential stem cells,** which give rise to two lines of progenitor cells from which develop B and T cells
   b. **Myeloid multipotential stem cells**
      (1) These are the **earliest detectable stem cells** in bone marrow culture systems.
      (2) These **give rise to colonies** of erythroid, granulocytic, monocytic, and megakaryocytic progenitor cells, from which develop **precursor cells** and eventually mature red blood cells, platelets, monocytes, neutrophils, basophils, and eosinophils.

B. Microenvironment. The cellular, physical, and chemical properties of bone marrow that render it hematopoietic are collectively termed the microenvironment.

1. **Blood flow** closely correlates with cellular production.
   a. **Arterial circulation.** Blood is supplied by two sources:
      (1) **Nutrient artery,** which is the main source
      (2) **Cortical capillary system,** which drains from the muscular arteries
   b. **Venous circulation.** A **medullary sinus** drains the blood and forms a substrate on which blood cells develop and can be released into the circulation. The blood is collected by the **central vein**.
   c. **Marrow circulation.** The arterial blood coming from the arterial terminals flows into the marrow space, slowly percolates through the cords of hematopoietic tissue, and drains through fenestrations in the basement membrane and into the central venous sinuses and the radiating venous sinuses in a spokelike pattern.

2. **Hematopoietic tissue stroma** is composed of cells that provide the support on which the hematopoietic cells grow and divide. These cells provide growth factors and specific recognition and adhesion sites and control the size of the hematopoietic space by gaining or losing lipid globules.
   a. **Endothelial cells** line the inner wall of the basement membrane.
   b. **Fibroblasts and adventitial cells** are located on the outer side of the membrane in the interstitial spaces between sinusoids.
   c. A **central macrophage** (the **nurse cell**) provides the erythroblasts (red cell precursors) with iron.
   d. **Fat cells,** which contain the lipid globules, fill about half of the marrow cavity.

3. **Extracellular stromal matrix** also provides a framework on which differentiation can occur. Several matrix glycoproteins act as specific recognition sites and adhesion sites for the hematopoietic stem cells. These proteins include:
   a. Fibronectin
   b. Laminin
   c. Collagen
   d. Proteoglycan (acid mucopolysaccharide)

4. **Sites of precursor cell differentiation**
   a. The differentiation of **myeloid multipotential stem cells** continues at specific sites within the bone marrow microenvironment.

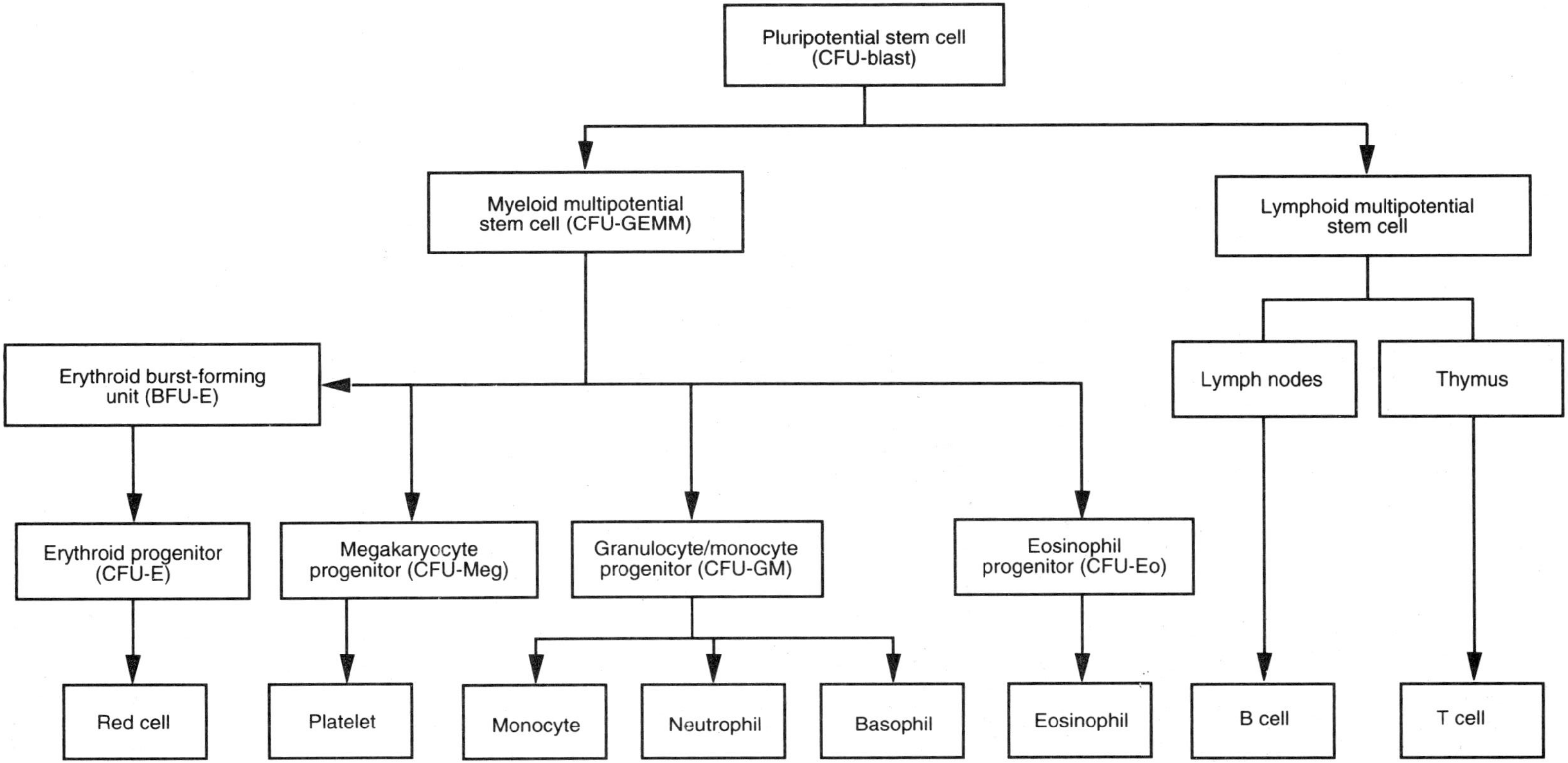

Figure 2-1. The hematopoietic stem cells and various pluripotential, multipotential, and committed cells are represented in the different stages during the formation of mature blood cells in bone marrow culture. The progenitor cells are represented by the type of colony formed. *CFU* = colony-forming unit; *BFU* = burst-forming unit; *GEMM* = mixed granulocyte/erythroid/monocyte/megakaryocyte; *E* = erythroid; *Meg* = megakaryocyte; *GM* = granulocyte/monocyte; *Eo* = eosinophil.

(1) **Megakaryocytes** are located along the outside surfaces of the vascular sinuses and release strings of cytoplasmic platelets through the fenestrations and directly into the circulation.
(2) **Erythroblasts** surround macrophages in distinctive erythroblastic islands near the sinus apertures. The maturing red cells squeeze through these apertures, leaving their pyknotic nuclei behind.
(3) The maturing and dividing **granulocytic/monocytic precursors** are located deep in the cords, and the mature cells become motile at the metamyelocyte stage.

b. **Lymphoid multipotential stem cells** leave the bone marrow and complete differentiation in the **lymph nodes (B cells)** and **thymus (T cells)**.

5. **Hematopoietic growth factors** are protein hormones that contribute to the microenvironment of bone marrow hematopoiesis; they also display extramedullary activity (Figure 2-2).
a. **General properties**
(1) They control the day-to-day **multiplication and differentiation of stem cells** into mature, circulating blood cells.
(2) They also affect the function of **mature cells,** such as leukocytes, in response to infection.
(3) Several are called **colony-stimulating factors (CSFs)** because they are necessary to the development of progenitor cell colonies from multipotential stem cells.
(4) They are produced by lymphocytes, monocytes, macrophages, endothelial cells, and fibroblasts.

b. **Classification**
(1) **Non–lineage-specific growth factors** act on pluripotential and multipotential stem cells to initiate self-renewal and differentiation.
(a) **Multi-colony-stimulating factor (multi-CSF),** also known as **interleukin-3 (IL-3),** induces the formation of colonies of granulocytes, macrophages, eosinophils, mast cells, erythroid cells, and megakaryocytes.
(b) **Granulocyte-macrophage colony-stimulating factor (GM-CSF),** induces the formation of granulocyte and monocyte colonies. (Note: Monocytes and macrophages are essentially interchangeable terms. Differentiating between the two is difficult. For the most part, monocytes are present in the circulation and macrophages are present in tissues.)
(2) **Lineage-specific growth factors** act on the committed progenitor cells and are involved in the differentiation and maturation of blood cells in the later stages of hematopoiesis. These factors include:
(a) Granulocyte colony-stimulating factor (G-CSF)
(b) Macrophage colony-stimulating factor (M-CSF)
(c) Eosinophil colony-stimulating factor (Eo-CSF)
(d) Erythropoietin
(e) Thrombopoietin
(3) **Lymphokines and monokines,** which are released by lymphocytes and monocytes (macrophages), respectively, have wide-ranging hematopoietic effects through an extensive network of interactions involving immune responses to infection and tumor invasion.
(a) **Interleukin-1 (IL-1),** an important monokine, is a glycoprotein produced by activated macrophages, endothelial cells, astrocytes, fibroblasts, and T cells.
(b) IL-1 is important because of its ability to stimulate marrow stromal cells to secrete CSF by acting as an **endogenous pyrogen**.

C. **Regulation of hematopoiesis.** Growth factors bound to the membranes of stem cells initiate two different mechanisms by which the signal to proliferate or differentiate is carried to the nucleus.

1. **Membrane phospholipid is hydrolyzed** by phosphatidylinositol 4,5-bisphosphate phosphodiesterase (PPDE).
a. This enzymatic activity initiates the release of two secondary messengers: **diacylglycerol (DAG),** which activates protein C kinase, and **inositol 1,4,5-triphosphate (IP_3),** which causes the intracellular release of calcium, thereby facilitating the activation of protein C kinase.
b. The action of PPDE is mediated by the formation of guanosine nucleotide-binding proteins **(G proteins),** which intervene between the membrane receptor and PPDE.

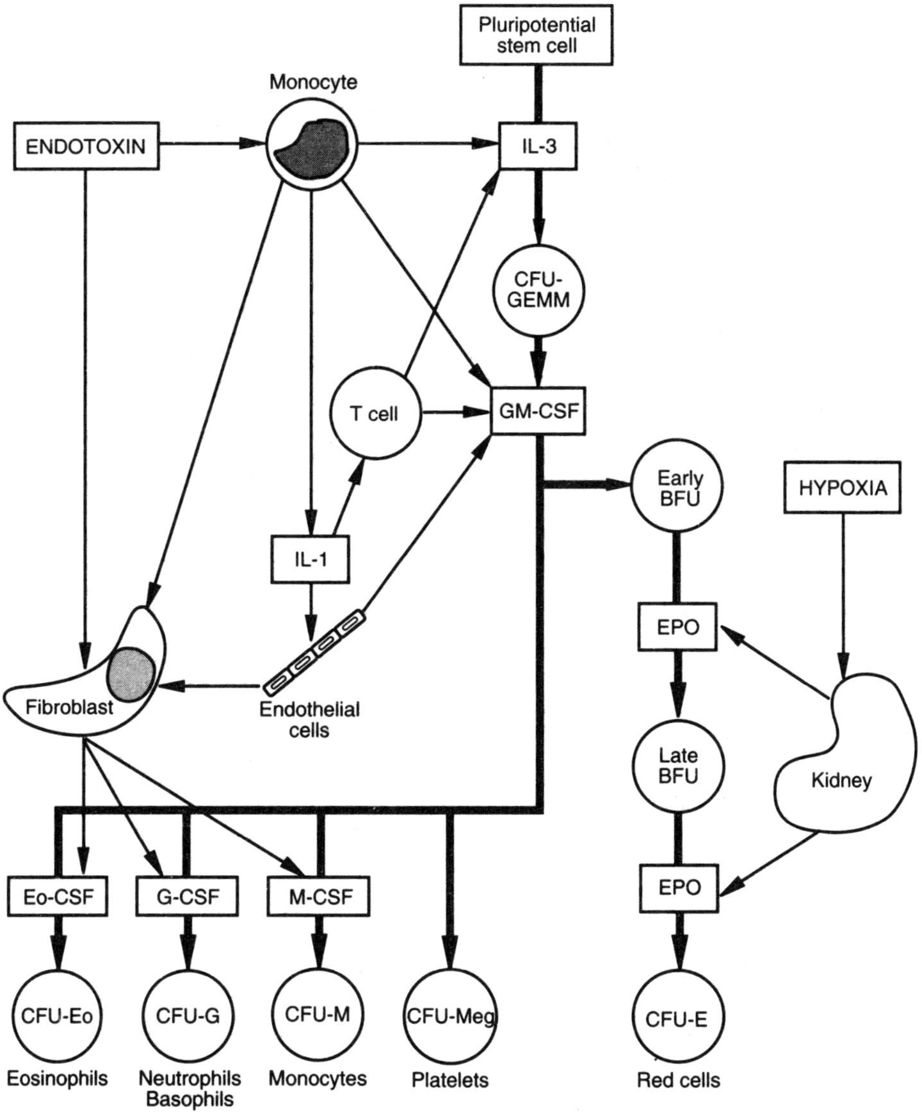

Figure 2-2. Schematic model of hematopoiesis, showing the cellular levels at which growth factors are active in regulating blood cell production. In granulopoiesis, endotoxin from infection stimulates the monocyte, which triggers release of interleukin-1 (IL-1), granulocyte-macrophage colony-stimulating factor (*GM-CSF*), interleukin-3 (IL-3; multi-CSF), and the lineage-specific colony-stimulating factors. (GM-CSF and IL-3 are active at the levels shown as well as in the later stages of differentiation to CFU-Eo, CFU-G, CFU-M, and CFU-Meg.) In contrast, erythropoiesis is stimulated by hypoxia and is mediated, via erythropoietin (*EPO*), by the kidneys.

2. **Adenylate cyclase in the membrane is activated,** increasing the intracellular level of cyclic adenosine monophosphate (cAMP) through the conversion of adenosine triphosphate (ATP), thereby increasing the cell response.

D. Interaction of growth factors and their receptors in malignancy. It has been theorized that the genes that regulate growth factors are responsible for the differentiation of normal cells into malignant cells (see also Ch 3 II B 3). This process, called the **autocrine mechanism** (Figure 2-3), is dependent upon the close relationship between viral genes and certain human genes. The primary participants in this process are **oncogenes** and **proto-oncogenes**.

1. **Oncogenes**
   a. These genes are found in **animal RNA tumor viruses**.

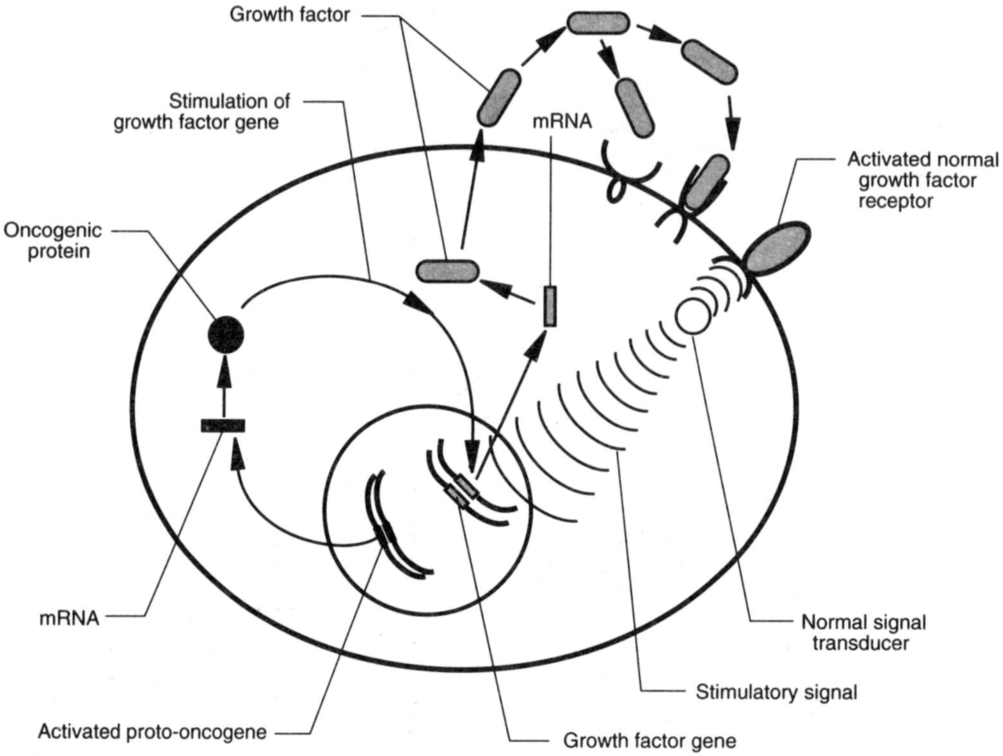

Figure 2-3. Proposed autocrine mechanism for malignant transformation of normal cells. It is theorized that proto-oncogenes, which are closely homologous to viral oncogenes, can be activated by the normal stimulatory signal to synthesize their own growth factors and stimulate cellular proliferation. (Adapted from Weinberg RA: Oncogenes and the mechanisms of carcinogenesis. In *Scientific American: Medicine.* New York, Scientific American, 1989, Section 12, subsection II, p 10.)

b. They are capable of transforming cells from a benign to a malignant phenotype by **activating proto-oncogenes**.

2. Proto-oncogenes

a. These genes are found in **human cells**.

b. They are closely **homologous to oncogenes** and can be **activated by oncogenes**.

c. When activated, they **code for the growth factors and receptor proteins** of cell differentiation or proliferation by generating a messenger RNA (mRNA). This mRNA produces a growth factor, or a receptor protein for a growth factor, that enables the cell to produce its own mechanism for proliferation, resulting in a malignant change in growth pattern.

d. Several proto-oncogenes have been identified.

(1) *c-sis* encodes for the β chain of platelet-derived growth factor.

(2) *c-erbB1* encodes for the epidermal growth factor receptor.

(3) *c-fms* encodes for the receptor for M-CSF.

(4) *c-abl, c-fes, c-ros, c-src,* and *c-yes* encode for protein tyrosine kinases.

(5) *c-mos* and *c-mil/raf* encode for protein serine-threonine kinases.

(6) *H-ras, K-ras,* and *N-ras* encode for guanosine triphosphate (GTP)–binding proteins.

(7) *c-myc, c-ets,* and *c-fos,* whose products are located in the nucleus, are closely involved with the induction of cell proliferation and differentiation. These proto-oncogenes are involved in the control of gene transcription; *c-myc* in DNA binding and *c-fos* in gene transcription and regulation. *c-ets* has not yet been well delineated. The mechanisms for how these proto-oncogenes work is still unknown.

III. SPLEEN. The spleen is the chief organ of the reticuloendothelial system (RES), which also includes the bone marrow, lymph nodes, liver, circulating monocytes, and fixed tissue macrophages. Its chief role in hematopoiesis occurs in utero; its postnatal participation is limited.

A. Functions. The functional capacity of the spleen is defined primarily by its ability to clear microorganisms by phagocytosis and filtering and its ability to synthesize antibodies and opsonizing proteins.

1. **The spleen participates in immunologic and phagocytic activities** that form the body's main defense against invading organisms.

2. **It destroys various intravascular cells and particles.**
   a. The spleen disposes of senescent or deformed red blood cells and processes the cellular components.
   b. It removes parts of red cells (a process called pitting) that are nonpliable, such as inclusion bodies and precipitated hemoglobin.
   c. It destroys infectious organisms.

3. **The spleen produces stem cells** capable of differentiating along hematopoietic, histiocytic, and fibroblastic cell lines.

4. **It plays a role in the autoantibody response.**
   a. The spleen is the major organ that **selectively removes or destroys red cells, granulocytes, or platelets** coated with autoantibody of the IgG type. Macrophages that contain a receptor for the Fc portion of IgG can adhere to the autoantibody on the cell surface during passage through the spleen and remove these cells from the circulation.
   b. There is evidence that the spleen **can be a site of autoantibody synthesis** early in the course of idiopathic thrombocytopenic purpura (ITP).

5. **The spleen plays a role in determining blood volume.** The splenic, portal, and intravascular volumes are closely interconnected. In cirrhosis with portal hypertension, a decrease in blood cell counts results from "dilution" caused by an expansion of the intravascular blood volume (from low serum albumin) and pooling of the cells in the portal circulation.

B. Structure

1. **The spleen consists of two regions.**
   a. **Red pulp** contains a tortuous system of sinuses and cordal tissue composed of reticular cells and mononuclear phagocytes.
   b. **White pulp** is composed of sheaths of lymphoid cells surrounding the arteries (periarterial lymphatic sheaths).

2. **Blood flow.** Blood from the splenic capsule flows through the arteries that support the white pulp and invests the red pulp in two ways.
   a. Arteries branch into a system of sinuses that drain the spleen.
   b. Other arteries drain into cordal tissue, where the sluggish flow allows the macrophages greater opportunity to interact with invading cells or organisms.

C. Pathophysiology

1. **Asplenia (absence of splenic function)**
   a. **Causes.** Asplenia can be the result of a congenital disorder, splenectomy, or a disease such as sickle cell anemia, in which multiple small infarctions of the spleen can lead to a state of atrophy and hypofunction known as **autosplenectomy** (Table 2-1).
   b. **Diagnosis.** Asplenia can usually be suspected if any of the following are found in a peripheral blood smear (see Table 1-1):
      (1) Nucleated red cells and red cell inclusions such as Howell-Jolly bodies (nuclear remnants) and Pappenheim bodies (iron granules)
      (2) Significant numbers of target cells and spiculated burr cells or acanthocytes ("thorny" red cells) among the erythrocytes
      (3) A marginal increase in the number of reticulocytes
      (4) A slight increase in the numbers of platelets and granulocytes
   c. **Postsplenectomy sepsis or pneumonia** is a consequence of asplenia that may occur days or years after splenectomy or infarction of the spleen. It has an abrupt onset and fulminant course that is associated with a high mortality rate (50%–80%). Although the incidence in adults is low, the presence of infection in a patient with asplenia should be treated immediately with systemic antibiotics and followed closely.

Table 2-1. Causes of Medical Asplenia or Hyposplenism

Atrophic spleen
Ulcerative colitis
Celiac disease, dermatitis herpetiformis
Thyrotoxicosis (Graves' disease)
Sézary syndrome
Graft-versus-host disease
Normal-size or large spleen
Sickle cell anemia
Sarcoidosis
Amyloidosis

2. **Splenomegaly and hypersplenism**
   a. The causes of **splenomegaly,** or enlargement of the spleen, are listed in Table 2-2.
   b. **Hypersplenism** is a term used to describe a condition of splenic hyperfunction that is associated with the following.
      (1) A reduction occurs in red cell, platelet, and granulocyte counts in the peripheral blood.
      (2) Hypersplenism is usually accompanied by splenomegaly, although the reverse is not necessarily true.
      (3) The bone marrow is cellular, indicating adequate blood production to compensate for the lowering of blood counts.
      (4) Correction of the blood counts follows removal of the spleen.
      (5) Small spleens are found in the hilum, the mesentery, the region of the tail of the pancreas; and elsewhere in 10% of individuals. These accessory spleens may enlarge and cause a recurrence of hypersplenism after splenectomy.

Table 2-2. Causes of Splenomegaly

Infections
Acute and subacute
Typhoid, abscess, infectious mononucleosis, subacute bacterial endocarditis
Chronic
Tuberculosis, syphilis, malaria, schistosomiasis, leishmaniasis, trypanosomiasis, histoplasmosis, echinococcosis
Inflammatory disorders
Rheumatoid arthritis (Felty's syndrome), sarcoidosis, systemic lupus erythematosus
Neoplasms
Leukemias (chronic myelogenous leukemia), lymphomas (Hodgkin's and non-Hodgkin's), chronic lymphocytic leukemia, hairy cell leukemia, polycythemia vera, agnogenic myeloid metaplasia (myelofibrosis), histiocytosis X, malignant reticuloendotheliosis, metastatic cancer
Hemolytic disorders
Hereditary
Thalassemia, hemoglobin C disease, spherocytosis, elliptocytosis
Acquired
Immune (idiopathic or drug-induced) hemolytic anemias
Deficiency disease
Severe iron deficiency, pernicious anemia
Storage disease
Gaucher's disease, Niemann-Pick disease, amyloidosis
Splenic vein hypertension
Cirrhosis, splenic and portal vein thrombosis, congestive splenomegaly
Idiopathic
With or without hypersplenism

IV. THYMUS AND LYMPH NODES

A. Thymus

1. **Function.** The thymus is the site of T cell maturation from progenitor cells. It is within the thymus that mature T cells develop the ability to recognize foreign antigens. These T cells then migrate to the peripheral lymphoid tissues for further differentiation.
2. **Structure.** The thymus is composed of numerous lobules that are divided into cortical and medullary regions.
   a. **Cortex.** The cortex contains **macrophages and immature T cells**. The T cells begin the process of maturation in the cortex and then migrate to the medulla.
   b. **Medulla.** The medulla contains **mature T cells** that have migrated from the cortex to complete their maturation. Most of the lymphocytes in the thymus are destroyed, but a few leave the medulla and travel to other organs.

B. Lymph nodes

1. **Function**
   a. The lymph nodes serve as **storage sites** for various lymphocytes that arrive from other organs and remain permanently (e.g., some B cells) or leave after a time to rejoin the blood (e.g., T cells).
   b. The lymph nodes are also a **locus of cellular activity,** where lymphocytes can interact with antigens and mount an immune response. Macrophages within the lymph nodes act as filters, phagocytizing antigen and particulate matter that has entered through the lymphatic capillaries.
2. **Structure.** The structure of the lymph node seems to help establish an immune response by enabling lymphocytes to better perform their individual functions.
   a. **Germinal centers** in the cortex concentrate immobile B cells.
   b. **Paracortical areas** are the loci of T cells traveling through the node.
   c. **Sinuses** receive lymph from the afferent vessels, exposing particulates in the lymph to macrophages that phagocytize the antigens and other foreign matter.
   d. **Reticular networks of dendritic cells** hold antigens, lengthening their exposure to lymphocytes.

V. EVALUATION OF THE BONE MARROW

A. Aspiration and biopsy are two techniques through which bone marrow can be examined. A thorough evaluation of the bone marrow should include both, since the tests complement each other.

1. **Indications for a bone marrow aspirate** include the following:
   a. **Evaluation of decreased numbers of cells from a single lineage** in patients who do not have clear evidence of increased cell destruction or blood loss, such as those with anemias with low reticulocyte counts (erythropoiesis), those with neutropenia (reduced granulocyte and monocyte production), and those with thrombocytopenia (reduced megakaryocyte and platelet production)
   b. **Evaluation of patients with decreased blood cell counts** in two cell lines (bicytopenia) or all three cell lines (pancytopenia) **and acute leukemias** (stem cell defects and disorders)
   c. **Evaluation of iron stores and abnormal iron in erythroid precursors** in patients with conditions such as anemia of chronic disease and sideroblastic anemias, unless the iron deficiency is obvious since other less invasive tests are available to establish the diagnosis
   d. **Diagnosis of tumor involvement** of the bone marrow for assessment of the patient's tumor stage (lymphomas, small cell lung carcinoma) and in evaluation for chemotherapy
   e. **Marrow aspiration to demonstrate possible infection by intracellular organisms,** such as malaria and kala-azar, and to demonstrate tuberculosis and histoplasmosis by culture of the marrow aspirates
   f. **Confirmation of infection** by a biopsy of caseating granulomas and demonstration of acid-fast organisms
   g. **Marrow aspiration to investigate an immunologic disorder,** such as a monoclonal increase of immunoglobulins in multiple myeloma, and to investigate lymphomas

h. Diagnosis of nonhematopoietic diseases (Table 2-3) in which the diagnosis can be made from the bone marrow

2. Bone marrow biopsy yields a core cut of the bone marrow with its architecture preserved.

a. The **differences between biopsy and aspirate examinations** are as follows.

(1) In biopsy, the **placement of cells in the microenvironment is preserved,** but overlap may make it difficult to identify individual cells or to assess their stage of development. **Morphology is best observed on an aspirate smear.**

(2) Biopsy material is excellent for providing a section of infiltrated, packed, or empty marrow for the **assessment of infiltrative processes;** most of these disorders prevent aspiration and result in a "dry" tap. Biopsy allows the examiner to:

(a) **Evaluate cellularity.** Cellularity is best observed when the architecture is preserved; aspirate smears are often subject to variations in technique that may alter the architectural appearance. Marrow aplasia, "packed" hypercellular marrows in acute leukemia, and myelofibrosis often lead to a "dry" or unsuccessful aspirate, and biopsy specimens may be the only specimens available for evaluation.

(b) **Evaluate tumors, granulomas, and infections.** These abnormalities are best demonstrated in the biopsy, since large clumps of cells tend to go to the edge of an aspirate smear and are often missed.

b. Indications for a bone marrow biopsy include the following:

(1) **Failure to obtain an adequate marrow aspirate** because of technical reasons or packed or dry marrow

(2) **Evaluation of pancytopenia or bicytopenia,** since accurate marrow cellularity is difficult to evaluate in the aspirate smear

(3) **Leukoerythroblastic findings in the peripheral blood smear** indicative of myelofibrosis or myelophthisis

(4) **Evaluation for hematologic malignancies** such as multiple myeloma

(5) **Evaluation of tumor staging** in lymphoma and small cell carcinoma of the lung

(6) The **need to define the endpoint of aplasia** in the treatment of acute leukemias

Table 2-3. Diagnosis and Findings of Nonhematopoietic Diseases in the Bone Marrow

Disease Type	Disease	Bone Marrow Findings
Bacterial	Tuberculosis	Aspiration shows acid-fast bacilli; biopsy shows epithelioid granulomas
Unknown	Sarcoidosis	Epithelioid granulomas (noncaseating)
Parasitic	Kala-azar (visceral leishmaniasis)	Organism-laden macrophages (Donovan bodies)
Fungal	Aspergillosis	Hyphae with areas of necrosis
Storage disorder		
Accumulation of glucocerebrosides	Gaucher's disease	Characteristic histiocytic cells with a fibrillar inclusion material that has an onion-skin pattern
Accumulation of sphingomyelin phospholipids	Niemann-Pick disease	Histiocytic cells with foamy cytoplasm containing lipids and sea-blue histiocytes
Metabolic	Cystinosis	Histiocytic cells laden with birefringent cystine crystals
Familial	Osteopetrosis (Albers-Schönberg or marble bone disease)	Compacted intramedullary osseous tissue with very little hematopoietic tissue
Immunoglobulin	Amyloidosis	Marrow replacement by pale acidophilic material that stains positive with Congo red

B. Bone marrow scans allow the assessment of function and quantity through the application of radioisotopes.

1. **Ferrokinetics.** In ferrokinetics, the uptake of radioiron 59 (^{59}Fe) and other isotopes by red cells in erythropoiesis is tracked. Ferrokinetics consists of three parts.
   a. **Plasma iron turnover rate** measures the clearance of transferrin-bound ^{59}Fe from the plasma and plasma iron content, which reflects the total amount taken up by the erythropoietic tissues, and includes both effective and ineffective red cell production. The normal clearance half-life of radioiron is 60–120 minutes.
   b. **Radioactive iron incorporation** into circulating red cells measures the effective portion of erythropoiesis, which reflects the iron incorporated into hemoglobin that reappears in the circulation. In normal iron incorporation, 70%–80% of the injected ^{59}Fe reappears in the circulating red cells in about 10–14 days.
   c. **Surface counting patterns** that scan for radioactivity over the sacrum, liver, spleen, and heart demonstrate medullary and extramedullary erythropoietic sites. Aplastic marrow displays no activity in the sacrum, and myelofibrosis patients show increased uptake at the liver and spleen.

2. **Bone marrow scan with indium 111 (^{111}In).** In bone marrow scan with ^{111}In, the uptake of isotope by erythroid precursors is similar to that which occurs in ferrokinetic techniques.

3. **Magnetic resonance imaging (MRI)** can be used to distinguish fat from the cellular elements in the bone marrow at active adult sites of hematopoiesis such as the sacrum and vertebrae.

STUDY QUESTIONS

Directions: Each of the numbered items or incomplete statements in this section is followed by answers or by completions of the statement. Select the **one** lettered answer or completion that is **best** in each case.

1. The major hematopoietic organ in the embryo is the

(A) bone marrow
(B) liver
(C) spleen
(D) lymph node
(E) yolk sac

2. The extracellular matrix or stromal matrix of the bone marrow supports hematopoiesis and consists of all of the following glycoproteins EXCEPT

(A) fibronectin
(B) laminin
(C) α_2-macroglobulin
(D) collagen
(E) proteoglycan

3. Which of the following hematopoietic growth factors is non–lineage-specific and would induce the formation of progenitor cells?

(A) Granulocyte colony-stimulating factor
(B) Macrophage colony-stimulating factor
(C) Granulocyte-macrophage colony-stimulating factor
(D) Erythropoietin
(E) Thrombopoietin

4. Interleukin-1 acts as an endogenous pyrogen and mediates the secretion of growth factors through all of the following activated cells EXCEPT

(A) B cells
(B) endothelial cells
(C) T cells
(D) macrophages
(E) fibroblasts

5. Asplenia is indicated in a peripheral blood smear by the presence of

(A) Döhle bodies
(B) hypersegmented neutrophils
(C) spherocytes
(D) Howell-Jolly bodies

6. The spleen performs all of the following functions EXCEPT

(A) destruction of infectious organisms
(B) disposal of old or deformed blood cells
(C) removal of nonpliable inclusion bodies from blood cells
(D) maturation of T cells
(E) production of hematopoietic stem cells

7. Hypersplenism results in all of the following EXCEPT

(A) hereditary spherocytosis and elliptocytosis
(B) immune hemolytic anemia
(C) thalassemia
(D) chronic myelogenous leukemia

1-E	4-A	7-D
2-C	5-D	
3-C	6-D	

Directions: Each item below contains four suggested answers, of which **one or more** is correct. Choose the answer

A if **1, 2, and 3** are correct
B if **1 and 3** are correct
C if **2 and 4** are correct
D if **4** is correct
E if **1, 2, 3, and 4** are correct

8. Bone marrow biopsy has advantages over bone marrow aspiration in the evaluation of

(1) marrow cellularity
(2) marrow iron stores
(3) infiltrative processes such as tumors, granulomas, and fibrosis
(4) megakaryocytes

9. Marrow aspiration is superior to biopsy in the

(1) assessment of bone marrow function
(2) evaluation of morphologic changes in the hematopoietic cells
(3) assessment of iron stores
(4) differential enumeration of the marrow cells

10. Hyposplenism or asplenia may occur from or in association with

(1) sickle cell anemia
(2) traumatic splenectomy
(3) ulcerative colitis
(4) graft-versus-host disease

11. A 58-year-old male alcoholic presents with an abnormal chest x-ray suggestive of miliary tuberculosis. Tests likely to demonstrate the pathogen include

(1) bone marrow biopsy and culture
(2) liver biopsy
(3) sputum
(4) gastric juice specimen

8-B
9-C
10-E
11-E

ANSWERS AND EXPLANATIONS

1. The answer is E *[I B 1 a].*
The sites of hematopoiesis change as the individual matures in utero and continue to change after birth until about 20 years of age. Hematopoiesis first occurs in the blood islands of the yolk sac, where it continues for up to 12 weeks gestation. The liver does not produce blood cells until the fifth week at the earliest. The spleen contributes to hematopoiesis by the fourth month. Bone marrow begins to produce blood cells by about the fifth month, and by the seventh month it is the primary hematopoietic organ. The marrow continues as such, under normal conditions, past birth, until by 20 years of age the sites of hematopoiesis have become limited to the marrow cavities of the axial skeleton.

2. The answer is C *[II B 3].*
The glycoproteins of the extracellular matrix or stromal matrix are important components of the microenvironment of the bone marrow, supporting hematopoiesis through their activity as specific recognition and adhesion sites for stem cells. The stromal matrix includes fibronectin, laminin, collagen, and proteoglycan but not α_2-macroglobulin, which is a serum antiprotease used to neutralize the toxic effects of activated enzymes released during inflammation and tissue injury.

3. The answer is C *[II B 5 b].*
Multi–colony-stimulating factor (multi-CSF, or IL-3) and granulocyte-macrophage colony-stimulating factor (GM-CSF) act on the pluripotential and multipotential stem cells to initiate self-renewal and differentiation, but only GM-CSF also acts on the committed cells, thereby identifying it as non–lineage-specific. Granulocyte colony-stimulating factor (G-CSF), erythropoietin, and thrombopoietin are active only at the level of the committed cells and thus are lineage-specific.

4. The answer is A *[II B 5 b (3)].*
Interleukin-1 (IL-1) is produced by activated macrophages, endothelial cells, astrocytes, fibroblasts, and T cells. They mediate the secretion of both lineage-specific and non–lineage-specific growth factors by these cells. B cells produce immunoglobulins and transform into plasma cells on activation; they are not involved in hematopoiesis.

5. The answer is D *[III C 1 b].*
Asplenia, or the absence of splenic function, can be expected if a peripheral blood smear demonstrates Howell-Jolly bodies, nucleated red blood cells, target cells, acanthocytes, or marginal increases in the numbers of reticulocytes, platelets, or granulocytes. Howell-Jolly bodies are nuclear remnants that the spleen removes from red cells as they pass through the organ. The presence of Döhle bodies in granulocytes is an indication of infection (activated granules). Hypersegmented neutrophils are present in folate and vitamin B_{12} deficiency. Spherocytes are demonstrated in immune hemolytic anemia or hereditary spherocytosis. The presence of Döhle bodies, hypersegmented neutrophils, and spherocytes usually indicates a hemolytic state.

6. The answer is D *[III A; IV A 1].*
The function of the spleen, which is the chief organ of the reticuloendothelial system (RES), is to destroy invading organisms with the help of antibodies, clear the old red cells and the unwanted parts of new ones, and provide a source for stem cells to help maintain hematopoiesis. The maturation of T cells occurs in the thymus as they move from the cortex to the medulla.

7. The answer is D *[III C 2].*
An increase in spleen size could be due to the chronic removal of deformed or abnormal red cells in hereditary spherocytosis or elliptocytosis, to the presence of abnormal hemoglobins in thalassemia, or to the presence of antibody-coated sensitized red cells in immune hemolytic anemia. Splenomegaly in chronic myelogenous leukemia (CML) is due to the extramedullary hematopoiesis and cellular infiltration that occurs in the liver and spleen. However, hypersplenism may occur in a markedly enlarged spleen at a later phase in CML.

8. The answer is B (1, 3) *[V A 2].*
Bone marrow aspiration does not preserve the normal marrow architecture as does biopsy, so that the cell distribution in the smear is subject to variation, making the estimation of cellularity vary widely. Infiltrative processes are best seen in the biopsy since the smear often misses these clumps of cells or they are mistaken for artifacts because of the distortion of the cells upon spreading on the slide. The evaluation of iron and megakaryocytes should be evident on both biopsy and aspiration studies.

9. The answer is C (2, 4) *[V A].*
Aspiration allows the study of the morphologic characteristics of the cells. In a core biopsy, the cells are not spread out, making it difficult to view them. The spreading of the cells enables the examiner to enumerate them at their different stages (differential) to detect abnormalities in maturation. Bone marrow function is best assessed in vivo by ferrokinetics. Iron stores can be evaluated in both aspirate and biopsy material.

10. The answer is E (all) *[III C 1; Table 2-1].*
Asplenia or hyposplenism can be due to surgical removal of the spleen (splenectomy) or to conditions that lead to medical hyposplenism (see Table 2-1), such as sickle cell anemia, in which multiple small infarcts in the spleen lead to replacement of splenic tissue with fibrosis. Hyposplenism occurs in 30%–50% of patients with inflammatory bowel disease; the mechanism involved is not known. Hyposplenism is found in ulcerative colitis and in graft-versus-host disease (GVHD), but the mechanism for this association also is still unknown.

11. The answer is E (all) *[V A 1 f].*
Bone marrow biopsy specimens, liver biopsy specimens, sputum samples, and gastric juice aspirates stained for acid-fast bacilli have a good chance of demonstrating the organisms responsible for miliary tuberculosis. Bone marrow aspiration is a good choice for making this determination, especially if the liver function in an alcoholic contraindicates liver biopsy because of abnormal coagulation. Note that it may be difficult to obtain a sample of sputum or gastric juice if the patient is uncooperative or very sick.

3
Stem Cell Disorders

Emmanuel C. Besa

I. INTRODUCTION. Disorders of the stem cells involve all of the myeloid (derived from the bone marrow) cell lines: red cells, white cells, and platelets. There are three main stem cell defects: decreased or damaged stem cells, maturation defects, and proliferation defects. Stem cell disorders are the result of bone marrow failure syndromes, myeloproliferative disorders, and myelodysplastic syndromes.

II. BONE MARROW FAILURE SYNDROMES

A. Aplastic anemia is characterized by an acellular or hypocellular marrow that causes bone marrow failure and a lower level of myeloid cell production, leading to pancytopenia.

1. **Description.** Aplastic anemia is a relatively uncommon disorder in the United States, with an incidence of about 1 in 200,000; it is more common in the Third World countries of Asia (although it is not seen in Japan). This disease is rare in patients younger than 1 year; its incidence increases to age 20, plateaus between 20 and 60 years of age, and increases again after age 60.

2. **Etiology.** The factors in the development of aplastic anemia are listed in Table 3-1 and can be summarized as follows.
   a. **Idiopathic aplastic anemia.** Half of the patients that present with aplastic anemia have no known cause for the disease.
   b. **Secondary aplastic anemia**
      (1) **Drugs and toxins**
         (a) Exposure to **chloramphenicol** is the most common drug-related cause of aplastic anemia. There are two mechanisms by which chloramphenicol suppresses hematopoiesis: a dose-dependent direct marrow suppression and a delayed idiosyncratic reaction that causes the aplastic anemia.
         (b) Other drugs that less frequently cause aplastic anemia are listed in Table 3-2.
         (c) Workplace exposure to a number of chemicals such as benzene and carbon tetrachloride and exposure to insecticides and fungicides have resulted in marrow toxicity.
         (d) Cancer chemotherapy and radiation exposure have also been implicated in the development of aplastic anemia.
      (2) **Infections**
         (a) **Viral hepatitis** (usually non-A, non-B hepatitis) is associated with a severe form of aplastic anemia that occurs a few weeks to 8 months after the onset of infection; an immunologic mechanism has been implicated in these cases. Similar associations have been observed with **infectious mononucleosis** and **cytomegalovirus (CMV) infections**.
         (b) A **direct marrow suppression** has been observed with **parvovirus** 19, which has been implicated in aplastic crises in patients with sickle cell anemia and other chronic hemolytic disorders.
      (3) **Thymoma and lymphoproliferative diseases** are usually limited to the erythroid cell line and present as a pure red cell aplasia (see Ch 4 II C) in patients with a thymoma or lymphoma (Hodgkin's and non-Hodgkin's) and in patients with chronic lymphocytic leukemia (CLL).

Table 3-1. Etiologic Factors in the Development of Aplastic Anemia

Idiopathic causes
Secondary causes
Drugs
Dose-dependent
Idiosyncratic
Toxins and chemicals
Radiation
Infection
Immunologic alterations
Viral hepatitis (non-A, non-B)
Infectious mononucleosis
Cytomegalovirus
Direct marrow injury (transient)
Parvovirus
Pregnancy
Lymphoproliferative disorders
Thymoma
Lymphoma
Chronic lymphocytic leukemia
Myelodysplastic syndromes and hypoplastic leukemias
Paroxysmal nocturnal hemoglobinuria
Genetic or constitutional causes
Fanconi's anemia
Familial aplastic anemia
Dyskeratosis congenita

(4) **Pregnancy.** The development of aplastic anemia during pregnancy, with remission after delivery, has been described. Relapses have also been observed during subsequent pregnancies. The mechanism for this association is unknown.

(5) **Paroxysmal nocturnal hemoglobinuria (PNH).** Aplastic anemia develops in 5%–10% of patients with PNH, and PNH develops in 25% of patients with aplastic anemia.

(6) **Preleukemic and leukemic conditions.** An association between myelodysplastic syndrome and hypoplastic leukemia has been described in patients with hypoplastic marrow; an increased number of blast cells or dyspoiesis in all three cell lines has been demonstrated.

(7) **Genetic or constitutional aplastic anemia** is a genetically transmitted predisposition to aplastic anemia that is expressed as one of the following.

(a) **Fanconi's anemia** is an autosomal recessive inherited condition of skeletal and renal defects, hyperpigmentation, small stature, and hypogonadism with chromosome abnormalities—breaks or gaps in chromosomes, endoreduplication, and chromatid exchanges—in the fibroblasts and lymphocytes.

(b) **Familial aplastic anemia** encompasses all other forms of aplastic anemia that occur in families but do not share all of the characteristics of Fanconi's anemia.

(c) **Dyskeratosis congenita** is an uncommon form of aplastic anemia associated with skin, nail, and hair abnormalities, as well as telangiectasia, alopecia, abnormal sweating, mental retardation, growth failure, and hypogonadism, which are observed without the chromosome abnormalities seen in Fanconi's anemia.

3. **Pathogenesis.** It is often difficult to identify a mechanism for the development of aplastic anemia in individual patients. Several pathologic mechanisms have been proposed.

a. **Quantitative or qualitative abnormalities of the pluripotential stem cell.** Stem cell injuries caused by viruses, toxins, chemicals, or an unstable genetic predisposition can lead to decreased numbers of stem cells or to mutations that result in stem cell clones with poor growth.

b. **Abnormal humoral or cellular control of hematopoiesis.** A deficiency in the substances that stimulate stem cells, such as interleukin-3 (IL-3) and granulocyte—macrophage colony-stimulating factor (GM-CSF), will result in a reduced number of blood cells. For example, a relationship has been noted between the amount by which levels of erythropoietin are elevated and the degree of anemia. Also, decreased helper T–cell functions were noted in patients with constitutional (congenital and familial) and acquired aplastic anemia.

Table 3-2. Drugs Associated with Aplastic Anemia

	Frequency of Association	
Class	**Common**	**Rare**
Antimicrobials	Chloramphenicol Quinacrine	Streptomycin Penicillins Tetracyclines Sulfonamides Amphotericin B
Anticonvulsants	Phenytoin Trimethadione	Ethosuximide Carbamazepine
Antithyroid agents		Carbimazole Methimazole Potassium perchlorate Propylthiouracil
Antidiabetic agents		Tolbutamide Chlorpropamide Carbutamide
Antihistamines		Tripelennamine
Analgesics	Phenylbutazone	Acetylsalicylic acid Indomethacin
Sedatives and tranquilizers		Meprobamate Chlordiazepoxide Phenothiazines Methyprylon
Miscellaneous	Gold compounds	Acetazolamide D-Penicillamine Cimetidine Thiocyanate Bismuth Metolazone

c. **Abnormal or "hostile" hematopoietic microenvironment.** The bone marrow microenvironment contains stromal cells that produce some of the growth factors that regulate hematopoiesis. Radiation therapy may damage these stromal cells, or the marrow may not be repopulated in areas that received enough radiation to destroy these stromal cells. The resultant loss of growth factors may result in aplastic anemia.

d. **Immunologic suppression of hematopoiesis.** Aplastic anemia may be the result of immunosuppression that is:
   (1) Humoral- or antibody-mediated
   (2) Cell-mediated or the result of T-cell abnormalities
   (3) Lymphokine-mediated

4. **Clinical manifestations** of aplastic anemia are the result of **pancytopenia**.
   a. **Presenting symptoms**
      (1) **Weakness, fatigue, congestive heart failure, stupor, and coma** result from reduced tissue oxygenation.
      (2) **Thrombocytopenia** results in certain bleeding disorders of the skin: petechia, ecchymosis, epistaxis, and gum bleeding. The bleeding tendency manifests itself when the platelet count falls below 20,000/μl. The degree of thrombocytopenia may be aggravated by a concomitant infection.
      (3) **Granulocytopenia** manifests itself as infections, usually in the upper respiratory tract, skin (cellulitis), urinary tract, and perirectal area.
   b. **Physical findings**
      (1) **Pallor**
      (2) **Purpura** and oral and nasal **mucosal bleeding**
      (3) **Organomegaly** of the liver, spleen, and lymph nodes, which is a rare finding

5. **Laboratory findings**
   a. **Peripheral blood counts** show varying degrees of pancytopenia.

(1) **Anemia** is always present and is usually normochromic or normocytic but may occasionally be macrocytic. The reticulocyte count is usually below 5%.
(2) **Low white blood cell count** is indicated by:
  (a) Granulocytopenia, in which the white cell count is below 1500/μl, and monocytopenia
  (b) A reduced helper or suppressor T-cell ratio
(3) **Thrombocytopenia** is evident. The severity varies, but the platelet count is below 150,000/μl.

b. Bone marrow findings are indicative of a low level of hematopoiesis.
(1) Aspiration is usually "dry" or scanty, showing few spicules.
(2) Biopsy smear displays hypocellularity, with a predominance of fat cells, lymphocytes, and plasma cells and residual erythroid, myeloid, and megakaryocytic cells. However, the marrow may contain small, isolated foci of hypercellularity; therefore, it is necessary to repeat these studies at other areas to confirm the overall hypocellularity.
(3) Magnetic resonance imaging (MRI) of the iliac bones, vertebrae, and sternum can reveal the increased fat content of the marrow, confirming the overall hypocellularity.

c. Other diagnostic tests
(1) **Coagulation tests are normal.**
(2) **Iron studies are usually normal,** but reduced utilization of iron by red cells may result in higher than normal levels of free iron. Occasionally, the iron stores may be low in patients with chronic bleeding owing to thrombocytopenia.
(3) **Serum erythropoietin is usually elevated** in proportion to the degree of anemia.

d. Fetal hemoglobin levels are elevated in some patients.

6. Course and prognosis

a. Survival patterns
(1) The survival curve is **biphasic:** One group of patients will die quickly, and a second group will survive from a few months to more than 1 year.
(2) The high initial mortality will claim 25% of all patients within the first 4 months, 25% will die within 4–12 months, and 35% will live for more than 1 year. About 10%–20% of the patients will recover spontaneously, either partially or completely.

b. Prognostic patterns
(1) The prognosis appears to be better when the cause of the anemia is known rather than when it is idiopathic.
(2) Aplastic anemia developing after viral hepatitis is associated with a poor prognosis.
(3) The **International Aplastic Anemia Study Group** devised the following criteria by which patients with severe disease could be separated from those with mild disease and thereby be considered as **candidates for bone marrow transplantation**. Patients who fulfill these criteria and do not undergo bone marrow transplantation have a median survival of 6 months, with only 20% surviving to 1 year.
  (a) Bone marrow cellularity of less than 25% or less than 50% if the majority of the cells are lymphoid or nonhematopoietic
  (b) Any two of the following:
    (i) Corrected reticulocyte counts of less than 1%
    (ii) Neutrophil counts lower than 500/μl
    (iii) Platelet counts lower than 20,000/μl

7. Management

a. Supportive therapy
(1) **Neutropenic precautions are advised** for patients with a total granulocyte count lower than 500/μl:
  (a) Avoidance of contact with other infected patients, relatives, or friends
  (b) Use of antiseptic soaps, electric razors, soft toothbrushes, and stool softeners
  (c) No intramuscular injections
  (d) Avoidance of fresh fruits and vegetables
  (e) Use of prophylactic antibiotics such as co-trimoxazole
(2) **Menstrual blood loss should be prevented** through the administration of an anovulatory agent or birth control pills.
(3) **Blood transfusions must be regulated.** Specific blood components such as packed red cells, platelets, and granulocytes can be given as required but should be avoided in

asymptomatic patients since serious complications such as iron overload, development of platelet antibodies, serum hepatitis, and acquired immune deficiency syndrome (AIDS) accompany multiple, long-term transfusions.

(a) **Packed red cell transfusions** should be given only when the patient becomes symptomatic (the hemoglobin level should be between 6 and 8 g/L). Iron overload may be avoided through the early subcutaneous administration of deferoxamine.

(b) **Platelet transfusions** are given when there is clinical bleeding or are administered prophylactically when the platelet count falls below 20,000/μl. Patients may become refractory to platelet transfusion through the development of antibodies; human leukocyte antigen–matched (HLA-matched) donor platelets can then be tried.

(c) **Granulocyte transfusions** are not used prophylactically but may be of benefit to patients with serious infections who are not responding to antibiotic therapy.

(4) **Antibiotic therapy.** Fever or any signs of infection should be treated with broad-spectrum antibiotics. After the conclusion of appropriate culture studies, an antibiotic specific for the infecting organism can be started.

b. **Marrow stimulants. Androgens** stimulate erythroid and myeloid proliferation as well as erythropoietin production. Hirsutism is more apparent in women and children and has been reported in fewer than half the patients treated. Androgen therapy is reserved for patients who are not candidates for bone marrow transplantation or for whom antithymocyte globulin (ATG) therapy has failed.

c. **Immunosuppression** from the administration of cyclophosphamide and from the preparation of patients for bone marrow transplantation may cause the recovery of the patients' bone marrow. Several therapies are available to attempt to restore bone marrow function, but the adverse effects of increased infection must be weighed against the potential for therapeutic benefit.

(1) **ATG** administration has a response rate of 50% and is assumed to work primarily through the elimination of activated suppressor T cells. **Antithymocyte gamma globulin (ATGAM)** is administered in a 20 mg/kg/day intravenous infusion in 9% saline over 4 to 6 hours for 8 days; **prednisone** is administered concurrently in a dosage of 40 mg/m^2 over 2 weeks with gradual tapering to relieve the patient of the effects of serum sickness. Patients are premedicated with acetaminophen and diphenhydramine to prevent fever, chills, rash, arthralgia, anaphylaxis, and serum sickness.

(2) **Corticosteroids. Cyclosporine** may be administered if an immunologic mechanism is implicated.

d. **Bone marrow transplantation** is an attempt to replace the defective stem cells in aplastic anemia.

(1) This is the **treatment of choice** in patients with severe disease who are younger than 40 years and have an HLA-identical sibling donor or who are any age and have an identical twin donor. Patients older than 40 years are at higher risk for graft-versus-host disease (GVHD), and the procedure is usually not undertaken in patients older than 50 years.

(2) **Long-term survival is 80%.**

(3) **Transfusion is avoided** as much as possible before transplantation since long-term survival is only 60%–75% in transfused patients who undergo allogeneic bone marrow transplantation.

e. **Splenectomy** is not indicated unless hypersplenism is a major contributor to the pancytopenia.

B. **Congenital dyserythropoietic anemias (CDAs)** are rare autosomal recessive diseases characterized clinically by anemia with jaundice from ineffective erythropoiesis, shortened red cell survival, and morphologically abnormal red cell precursors in the bone marrow. The anemia is often macrocytic, with reticulocyte counts that are increased but still relatively low for the degree of anemia. The disease is divided into three main groups according to the appearance of the bone marrow.

1. **CDA I** has megaloblastic changes with prominent intranuclear chromatin bridges.

2. **CDA II** is also known as hereditary erythroblastic multinuclearity associated with positive acidified serum.

3. **CDA III** is characterized by multinuclearity and large erythroblasts with karyorrhexis.

C. Other causes of bone marrow failure

1. **Immune cytopenias.** Immune-mediated precursor cell destruction has been observed to be associated with collagen vascular diseases and lymphoproliferative disorders and is seen in patients without obvious autoimmune disorders. Pure red cell aplasia (see Ch 4 II C) is an example of immune-mediated destruction of erythroblasts. Some immune thrombocytopenias resulting from antibodies against megakaryocytes and immune neutropenias are examples of these disorders. Absent precursor cells and no evidence of maturational defects are the hallmarks. Serum inhibitors may be demonstrated in marrow culture studies.

2. **Infiltrating lesions** in the bone marrow can **cause marrow failure and cytopenias**. There are three classifications of infiltrating lesions.
   a. **Myelophthisis** is the invasion of the marrow cavity and cellular elements by malignancies, infections such as granulomas, or abnormal storage macrophages as occurs in Gaucher's disease.
   b. **Secondary myelofibrosis,** resulting from carcinomas and lymphomas, may be due to the growth of fibroblasts and deposition of collagen and fibrin stimulated by platelet-derived growth factor (PDGF).
   c. **Myelosclerosis** (acute) is an aggressive form of myelofibrosis and is believed to be a type of acute megakaryoblastic leukemia (M7) [see Ch 12 II B 1 a (1) (e)].

III. MYELOPROLIFERATIVE DISORDERS

MYELOPROLIFERATIVE DISORDERS are a group of clonal stem cell disorders that lead to uncontrolled hematopoiesis. These related diseases can transform into each other as shown in Figure 3-1 and display marked increases in erythropoiesis (polycythemia vera; PV), granulopoiesis (chronic myelogenous leukemia; CML), thrombopoiesis (essential thrombocytosis), and numbers of fibroblasts (myelofibrosis or myeloid metaplasia).

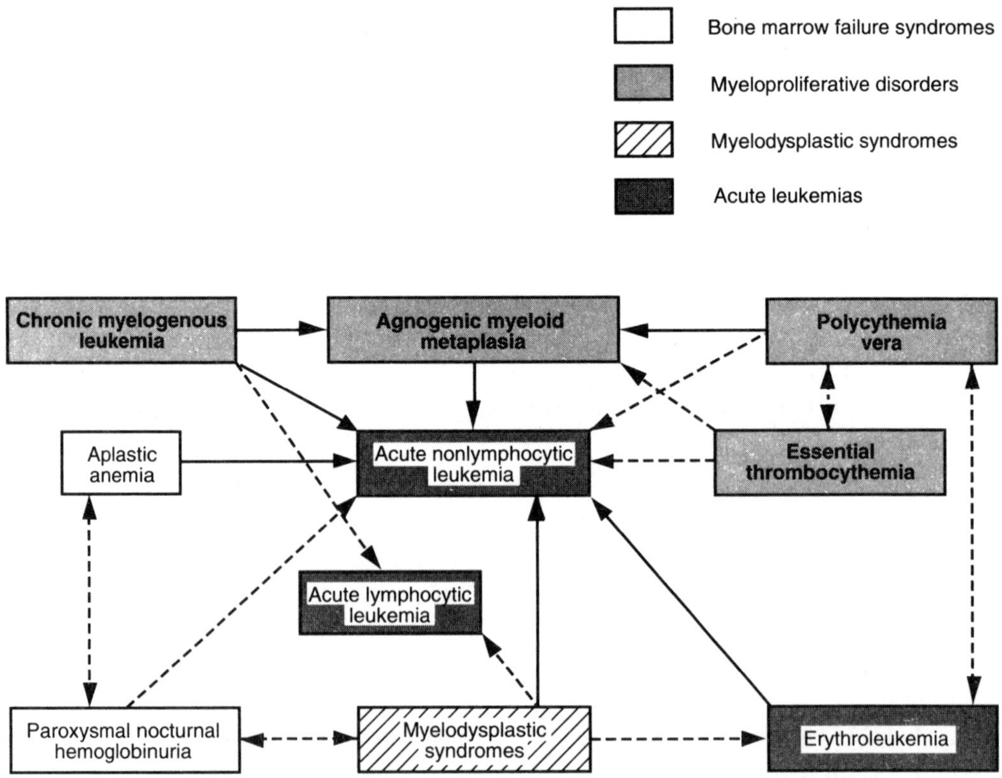

A. Polycythemia vera

1. **Description. Erythrocytosis** is a condition associated with increased red cell mass, and it can be primary or secondary (Table 3-3). **PV** is a more specific term for a condition associated with increased red cell mass that may be associated with increases in white cell and platelet counts. The normal red cell mass in individuals residing at sea level is 23–29 ml/kg for women and 26–32 ml/kg in men. Any increase above these levels is considered to be polycythemic.

2. **Incidence.** PV is an uncommon disease that is often diagnosed in patients between the ages of 50 and 60 years with equal sex distribution.

3. **Pathogenesis.** PV is a clonal disorder involving the hematopoietic stem cells; it leads to an autonomous proliferation of the erythroid, myeloid, and megakaryocytic cell lines. Increased erythroid proliferation is usually more prominent than that of the other cell lines and occurs independently of erythropoietin levels (which are usually very low in PV).

4. **Diagnosis and differential diagnosis.** High hematocrit and hemoglobin levels should raise the suspicion of PV. However, the possibility of a spurious elevation in hematocrit and hemoglobin concentration owing to a contracted plasma volume (**pseudopolycythemia**; see Ch 10 II B) is eliminated by performing red cell mass and plasma volume measurements. To establish a diagnosis of primary polycythemia, secondary causes of erythrocytosis must also be eliminated (see Table 3-3), and evidence of a myeloproliferative state should be obtained that satisfies the following criteria established by the **Polycythemia Vera Study Group** (Table 3-4).
   a. **Normal red cell mass.** The presence of a normal red cell mass should abort the extensive workup for PV. A determination of increased red cell mass made using ^{51}Cr-labeled red cells will rule out spurious polycythemia or pseudopolycythemia.
   b. **Normal arterial blood gases.** Normal concentrations of oxygen in arterial blood will eliminate tissue hypoxia and distinguish it from pulmonary and cardiovascular abnormalities as a cause of PV.

Table 3-3. Classification of Polycythemia

- Primary
  - Polycythemia vera
  - Pure erythrocytosis
- Secondary
  - Physiologic erythrocytosis resulting from low tissue oxygenation that is caused by:
    - Elevated altitude (low oxygen pressure)
    - Chronic lung disease associated with alveolar hypoventilation (hypoxia)
    - Right to left shunts in the cardiovascular system (venous mixture on arterial side)
    - Hemoglobin–oxygen dissociation abnormalities
      - Hemoglobinopathies associated with high oxygen affinity
      - Carboxyhemoglobin in "smoker's polycythemia"
      - Decreased red cell 2,3-diphosphoglycerate (DPG)
        - Hereditary increase in red cell adenosine triphosphate (ATP)
        - DPG mutase deficiency
  - Abnormal increases in erythropoietin with normal tissue oxygenation that are caused by:
    - Renal disease
      - Hypernephroma or renal cell carcinoma
      - Kidney cysts and hydronephrosis
      - Bartter's syndrome
      - Renal transplantation
    - Erythropoietin-producing tumors
      - Hepatoma
      - Uterine leiomyoma
      - Cerebellar hemangioblastoma
      - Other rare cases in ovarian carcinoma and pheochromocytoma
    - Production or administration of androgens
      - Adrenal cortical hypersecretion
      - Exogenous androgens
- Relative polycythemia (pseudopolycythemia or spurious polycythemia)
  - Stress polycythemia
  - Gaisböck's syndrome in hypertension

Table 3-4. Diagnostic Criteria for Polycythemia Vera

Category A
1. Total red cell mass
Male $\geq$ 36 ml/kg
Female $\geq$ 32 ml/kg
2. Arterial oxygen saturation $\geq$ 92%
3. Splenomegaly
Category B
1. Thrombocytosis (platelet count > 400 $\times$ $10^3/\mu l$)
2. Leukocytosis (white cell count > 12 $\times$ $10^3/\mu l$)
3. Increased leukocyte alkaline phosphatase (LAP) score
4. Serum B_{12} concentration > 900 pg/ml or B_{12} binding capacity > 2200 pg/ml
Polycythemia vera is established with:
A1 + A2 + A3
or
A1 + A2 + any two from category B

Source: Polycythemia Vera Study Group.

c. **Normal or low serum erythropoietin levels** will rule out the possibility that a tumor or other renal causes are producing erythropoietin or other erythropoietic substances or are causing increased levels of androgens, thereby stimulating erythropoietin production (see Table 3-3).

d. **Normal hemoglobin–oxygen ($Hb–O_2$) dissociation curve** (or P_{50}, the oxygen half-saturation pressure of hemoglobin, which is usually 27.5 mm Hg) will eliminate the possibility of abnormal hemoglobin concentrations with high oxygen affinity. A decreased P_{50} indicates a high oxygen affinity.

e. **Normal carboxyhemoglobin levels.** Carboxyhemoglobin levels would be elevated in smokers because of the higher affinity of hemoglobin for carbon monoxide compared with oxygen.

f. **Normal intravenous pyelogram** or renal ultrasound will rule out the presence of tumors or cysts, which can secrete erythropoietin.

g. **Normal liver scan.** Negative findings on liver scan will rule out hepatoma, which is another source of erythropoietin.

5. **Clinical manifestations** of PV are often nonspecific and insidious. The following symptoms are the consequences of the hyperviscosity that is caused by the increased concentrations of cellular elements in the blood, the abnormalities in blood cell function, and the increased turnover of the marrow hematopoietic cells:

   a. **Erythrocytosis and hyperviscosity,** leading to poor oxygenation and displaying symptoms of:
      (1) **Plethora**
      (2) **Poor central nervous system (CNS) circulation** (headaches, dizziness, vertigo, tinnitus, and visual disturbances) **or coronary circulation** (angina)
      (3) **Peripheral circulation intermittent claudication**

   b. **Abnormal platelet function** with or without thrombocytosis, causing:
      (1) Venous **thrombosis** or **thromboembolism**
      (2) **Hemorrhage** (epistaxis, gingival bleeding, ecchymoses, and gastrointestinal bleeding)

   c. **Increased myeloproliferation,** displaying symptoms of:
      (1) **Splenomegaly** in 75% of patients, which causes early satiety and hepatomegaly in 30% of these patients
      (2) **Pruritus** in 40% of patients, which is secondary to increased histamine release from the basophils and mast cells

6. **Laboratory findings**

   a. **Peripheral blood counts** show the following anomalies.
      (1) **Elevated hemoglobin concentrations and hematocrit** are verified by the increased total red cell mass.
      (2) **Increased leukocytosis and granulocytosis** occur in about 60% of patients, with a shift to the left and an increase in the numbers of basophils. The leukocyte alkaline phosphatase (LAP) score of the granulocytes is elevated in 70% of these patients.
      (3) **Thrombocytosis** is between 400,000/μl and 800,000/μl in 50% of patients.

b. **Bone marrow hyperplasia** is evident and involves mainly increases in the number of erythroid cells with small increases in the numbers of myeloid and megakaryocytic cells. A mild form of myelofibrosis may be present.
   (1) **Iron stores may be low or absent** in patients with a history of gastrointestinal blood loss.
   (2) Cytogenetic studies show an **abnormal stem cell clone** in about 30% of untreated patients and in 50% of patients treated with myelosuppressive therapy in the form of alkylating agents or radioactive phosphorus. Complex karyotypic abnormalities are associated with the transformation of PV to acute leukemia.

c. **Other abnormalities** may also be seen.
   (1) **Elevated serum histamine** is seen in 90% of patients.
   (2) **Increased serum B_{12} levels and B_{12} binding capacity** are observed in 75% of patients and result from an increase in transcobalamin III.
   (3) **Hyperuricemia** secondary to the high marrow cell turnover rate is seen in 40% of patients.

7. **Course and prognosis.** The survival of patients with **untreated** PV ranges from 1.5 to 3 years; effective management that utilizes various therapies can extend survival to a median of 10 years. The major causes of morbidity and mortality in PV are the following **complications**.
   a. **Thrombosis** has been reported in 15%–60% of patients and is the cause of death in 10%–40% of these patients. Venous as well as arterial thromboses have resulted in pulmonary emboli, renal failure (renal vein or artery thrombosis), intestinal ischemia or gangrene (mesenteric vein thrombosis), or peripheral arterial emboli.
   b. **Hemorrhagic complications** occur in 15%–35% of patients with PV and lead to death in 6%–30% of these patients. The bleeding is generally concurrent with thrombosis and is the consequence of vascular system compromise that results from ischemic changes. The complications may be due to hyperviscosity that is a consequence of erythrocytosis or to abnormal platelet function, but the risk for either bleeding or thrombosis does not correlate with platelet counts, bleeding time, or platelet function tests.
   c. **Peptic ulcer disease** has a reported incidence associated with PV that is threefold to fivefold higher than in the general population and that has been attributed to the **increased serum histamine** levels.
   d. **Pancytopenia and myelofibrosis** that develop in 3%–10% of patients with PV are considered to be indicative of the "spent" phase of PV, but the incidences of these conditions may increase as the therapy for other complications increases patient survival.
   e. **Acute leukemic transformations** occur in approximately 1% of PV patients who undergo management with phlebotomy alone. The risk for transformation increases to 13.5% within 5 years of diagnosis in those patients treated with chlorambucil, and the risks increase to 10.2% within 6–10 years in patients treated with radioactive phosphorus (^{32}P).

8. **Management**
   a. **Reduction of hyperviscosity.** Initial management should be directed at relieving the patient's hyperviscosity that has been caused by erythrocytosis. A hematocrit of less than 47% should be attained through **phlebotomy**. The **volume and frequency** of phlebotomy should be tailored to the individual patient to reduce the risks of thrombosis and transformation to leukemia.
      (1) **Patients younger than 50 years** with no history of thrombosis can undergo phlebotomy in which 1 U of blood (450 ml) is withdrawn as often as every other day. The hematocrit can be maintained by varying the intervals between phlebotomies according to myeloproliferative activity. Careful control of the phlebotomy interval is preferred to the administration of myelosuppressive agents, which increase the risks for leukemia or secondary malignancies.
      (2) **Patients older than 70 years** with underlying cardiovascular abnormalities may only be able to withstand phlebotomy of 250–300 ml twice weekly and will require additional myelosuppressive therapy. The patient with a history of thrombosis should not be maintained by phlebotomy alone. Severe iron deficiency should be avoided since microcytic red cells contribute to hyperviscosity and tissue depletion leads to symptoms of fatigue and low energy in most patients.
   b. **Control of myeloproliferation.** Evidence of increases in white cell and platelet counts and of organomegaly indicate that myeloproliferative activity is not being controlled by phlebotomy and that **myelosuppressive agents** may be required.
      (1) **Administration of ^{32}P** in patients older than 70 years can effectively decrease the risks

of thrombosis, and the effects of ^{32}P last 6–24 months. The increased risk of leukemia resulting from the use of ^{32}P should be balanced against the average life span of the elderly since the risk does not increase until 6–10 years after administration.

(2) **Administration of hydroxyurea,** an inhibitor of ribonuclease reductase, in patients younger than 70 years of age is effective in controlling PV without increasing the risk of leukemia. However, it is necessary to monitor blood counts as frequently as every month or every 3 months.

(3) **Administration of alkylating agents** such as chlorambucil and melphalan has fallen out of favor because of the increased incidence of leukemia and secondary malignancies within 3–5 years of their use. Busulfan is still in use, but because of its prolonged myelosuppressive effects and the associated increased incidence of pulmonary fibrosis and hyperpigmentation, this agent is not desirable for long-term therapy in this chronic disease.

B. Agnogenic myeloid metaplasia

1. **Description.** Agnogenic myeloid metaplasia (AMM, or idiopathic myelofibrosis) is a myeloproliferative disorder **characterized by** hypocellular and fibrotic bone marrow. **Extramedullary hematopoiesis** arises usually in the liver or spleen.

2. **Etiology of AMM is not known.** It is considered to be a stem cell abnormality that is caused by the increased proliferation of hematopoietic cells outside the bone marrow and that results in fibrosis of the bone marrow. The fibrosis is believed to be a reaction to a malignant or abnormal stem cell clone.

3. **Pathogenesis.** The **initiating cause of AMM is unknown,** but its origin from a single stem cell implies that **it is an acquired genetic disease similar to leukemia and cancer**. The chromosome abnormalities involving chromosome 13 (13q-) and translocations involving chromosomes 1 and 13 [t(1;13)] have been described frequently in this disorder. It has been suggested that PDGF is released inappropriately by the platelets, stimulating proliferation of marrow fibroblasts, leading to the fibrotic process.

4. **Diagnosis and differential diagnosis.** Focal fibrosis of the bone marrow can be part of an inflammatory disease (tuberculosis) or of metastatic cancer (breast and prostatic carcinoma) and mimic AMM. These causes of secondary fibrosis rarely lead to extramedullary hematopoiesis in the liver and spleen.

5. **Clinical manifestations.** The following symptoms of AMM are related to the effects of **organomegaly,** which can be massive, and **hypermetabolism,** which causes an increased cellular turnover:
   a. **Weight loss** caused by poor gastric filling because of an enlarged spleen
   b. **Abdominal pain** from capsular stretching to accommodate an enlarging liver and spleen
   c. **Weakness, fatigue, night sweats, and fever,** which are common
   d. **Bone pain,** which may be due to the rapid proliferation (ineffective hematopoiesis) and fibrosis in the marrow

6. **Laboratory findings**
   a. **Peripheral blood findings. Leukoerythroblastic blood** is evident in this disorder, with circulating immature forms of the marrow cells.
      (1) **Anemia** is common.
      (2) **Anisocytosis and poikilocytosis** are characteristic. The red cells display the classic teardrop shape (dacryocytes), and nucleated red cells and normoblasts circulate in the blood.
      (3) **Leukocytosis** is common, with counts similar to those seen in chronic myelogenous leukemia (CML); however, the LAP score is generally normal to high, compared with the very low LAP score in CML, and the Philadelphia (Ph) chromosome (see III C 2) is not found. Immature blood cell forms ranging from myeloblasts to myelocytes may be seen in the peripheral blood, again confirming the leukoerythroblastic blood picture. Neutropenia may be found in advanced cases.
      (4) **Abnormal platelets** (large and agranular), with platelet counts ranging from high to low levels, are seen. Abnormal bleeding times and platelet aggregation may be associated with a high incidence of bleeding or thrombosis in this disorder.
   b. **Bone marrow**
      (1) **Aspirate** is usually dry or unobtainable.

(2) **Biopsy** will often show a hypercellular marrow with increased reticulin fibers and variable collagen deposition. Increased numbers of megakaryocytes are frequently seen with increased bone density.

c. **Other laboratory findings** include:

(1) Increased serum B_{12} binding capacity and high levels of serum B_{12}

(2) High serum uric acid and lactate dehydrogenase (LDH) levels, which reflect the increased but ineffective turnover of the hematopoietic cells

7. **Course and prognosis**

a. The usual course of AMM consists of **an asymptomatic phase of 2 years duration, with progression at the onset of the symptoms and signs**. A previous myeloproliferative disorder such as PV or essential thrombocythemia (ET) can be established in about 30% of patients, and progression to acute leukemia is seen in 10% of patients.

b. **Acute myelofibrosis is a rare disease** and is now considered to be a form of acute megakaryoblastic leukemia.

(1) Fatigue, weight loss, and severe cytopenia with very little organomegaly may develop suddenly.

(2) The bone marrow is usually hypocellular with atypical megakaryocytes and abnormal megakaryoblasts.

8. **Management** primarily addresses symptoms and includes:

a. **Transfusion of packed red cells** for anemia **or platelets** for thrombocytopenia with bleeding

b. **Androgen administration** in some patients to alleviate cytopenia (but this usually does not prevent the progressive organomegaly)

c. **Chemotherapy with hydroxyurea or alkylating agents** such as busulfan to lower the high white cell and platelet counts in some patients

d. **Splenic irradiation or splenectomy,** which is useful in a minority of patients who have symptoms from massive splenomegaly, hypersplenism, and increasing transfusion requirements

e. **Allopurinol administration** to prevent urate nephropathy and the development of gout from the high uric acid concentration as a consequence of the high marrow cell turnover rate

C. Chronic myelogenous leukemia

1. **Description.** CML (or chronic granulocytic leukemia) is a myeloproliferative disorder characterized by **increased proliferation of granulocytes** without loss of their capacity to differentiate and evidence of **myeloproliferation** involving the liver and spleen.

a. CML accounts for 20% of all leukemias affecting patients in middle age, when it appears in its chronic stable clinical phase.

b. It progresses to a more aggressive acute leukemic form after a variable time period.

2. **Etiology.** CML is an acquired abnormality that involves the hematopoietic stem cell and is characterized by a specific **chromosome translocation** between the long arms of chromosomes 22 and 9, which is called the **Ph chromosome**. The chromosome has been found in all myeloid cells as well as in lymphoid cells, indicating the involvement of the pluripotential stem cell. Although the initiating factor is still unknown, exposure to irradiation (as observed in patients from Hiroshima and Nagasaki, Japan) or to organic solvents such as benzene has been implicated as a cause of the disease.

3. **Pathogenesis.** The molecular biology of CML is one of the most studied among the neoplastic disorders.

a. The **key event** in the translocation that creates the Ph chromosome is the **movement of an oncogene (c-*abl*) from chromosome 9 to chromosome 22** (Figure 3-2), where it is placed in an area called the *bcr* cluster gene. The *bcr* and c-*abl* genes fuse, and that fusion product has a greater tyrosine kinase activity and stimulates cell division to a much greater degree than does the normal c-*abl* gene product.

b. The role of oncogenes in the transformation of CML and the type of acute leukemia that develops are related to the type or manner of the translocation and the *bcr* protein produced.

4. **Diagnosis and differential diagnosis**

a. Secondary causes of granulocytosis, such as the leukemoid reaction, must be eliminated.

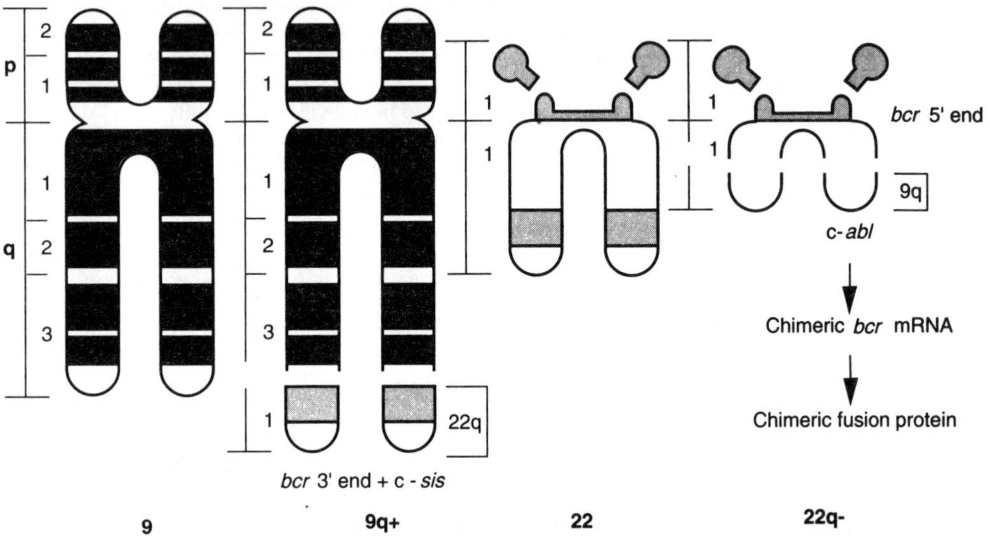

Figure 3-2. The Philadelphia (Ph) chromosome is the product of the reciprocal translocation between the G-banded chromosomes 9 and 22. The cellular oncogene c-*abl,* which codes for a tyrosine protein kinase, is translocated to a specific breakpoint cluster region (*bcr*) of chromosome 22. The 5′ end of the *bcr* region remains with chromosome 22, and the 3′ end moves to chromosome 9 along with the oncogene c-*sis,* which codes for a protein that is homologous to platelet-derived growth factor (PDGF). The translocation produces a chimeric *bcr*–c-*abl* messenger RNA (mRNA) that codes for a mutation protein with much greater tyrosine activity than the normal protein. (Reprinted from Hoffbrand AV, Pettit JE: *Clinical Hematology,* London, Gower, 1988, p 162.)

b. Overlap of the myeloproliferative disorders often makes differentiation difficult, since high granulocyte counts are often seen in PV, ET, and AMM, and myelofibrosis often accompanies CML.

c. However, **the specificity of the chromosome abnormality in CML often decides the diagnosis** by the presence of the Ph chromosome and the low-to-absent LAP score in the mature-appearing neutrophils.

5. **Clinical manifestations** of CML may be insidious; they may be accidentally discovered by routine examination or may be symptoms caused by the enlarged spleen.
   a. **Nonspecific symptoms** of weakness, weight loss, and fatigue may be experienced.
   b. **An enlarged spleen, liver, or both** may cause left upper quadrant pain or discomfort.
   c. **Quantitative or qualitative abnormalities of the platelets** may cause bleeding manifestations: petechiae, ecchymoses, purpura, and bleeding from mucous membranes.
   d. **Hypermetabolism** may be the cause of fever and sweating.

6. **Laboratory findings**
   a. **Peripheral blood**
      (1) A moderate-to-marked **elevation of the white blood cell count** (WBC) from 50,000/μl to 300,000/μl is evident and due mainly to granulocytosis. Occasional early granulocytic precursors that show all stages of maturation are present in the blood. Mild elevation in percentages of basophils and eosinophils is described and may increase as the disease progresses.
      (2) There is a **very low-to-absent LAP score** since polymorphonuclear leukocytes do not stain for alkaline phosphatase.
      (3) **Platelet counts may be normal or markedly increased** (over 1 million in some cases) or may be low at the later stages.
      (4) A **mild-to-moderate anemia** is often found.
   b. **Bone marrow is hypercellular,** with an increased number of myeloid elements that are in all stages of maturation. Increased numbers of megakaryocytes, eosinophils, and basophils may be noted. Mild fibrosis of the marrow may be seen in 10%–15% of patients, which is often related to thrombocytosis and increased numbers of megakaryocytes. A false depletion of iron stores may be due to masking by the hypercellular myeloid elements.
      (1) Chromosome studies show the typical Ph chromosome in 90% of patients.

(2) Patients who lack the Ph chromosome may either have a chronic myelomonocytic leukemia (CMML; see IV D 5) or a true CML with an inapparent translocation, since the arms seem to be equivalent in length; however, the *bcr–c-abl* protein is still detectable. In actuality, this subgroup of CML, which reportedly has a shorter chronic phase and is less responsive to therapy, may be CMML.

c. **Other laboratory findings** in CML are:

(1) **Hyperuricemia**

(2) **Elevated B_{12} binding capacity** (owing to increased levels of transcobalamin I, a B_{12}-binding protein) and high levels of serum B_{12}

7. **Course and prognosis.** The clinical course of CML may be described as having three phases, although patients may present to the physician in any of them. They progress as follows.

a. The **chronic stable phase** lasts from 1 to 5 years and is characterized by **mild anemia** with a mild-to-moderate elevation of the white blood cell count (WBC) and **organomegaly,** which usually responds to intermittent administration of oral myelosuppressive chemotherapy. A short chronic phase has been noted to be associated with advanced age (>60 years), male sex, persistent anemia, thrombocytopenia or thrombocytosis, and increasing numbers of basophils and blasts in the peripheral blood smears.

b. The **accelerated or transformation phase** evolves gradually from the stable chronic phase after unsuccessful myelosuppressive therapy. It is accompanied by the following changes:

(1) An increasing degree of anemia

(2) Thrombocytopenia or progressive thrombocytosis

(3) Increasing numbers of blast cells

c. **Blast crisis** occurs when the criterion for acute leukemia is fulfilled (≥ 30% blast cells in the bone marrow) and may occur abruptly or gradually over weeks. The acute leukemia is usually myelogenous in type but may be lymphocytic in 20%–30% of cases with a pre–B cell type and is positive for terminal deoxynucleotidyl transferase (TdT) and common acute lymphoblastic leukemia antigen (CALLA). Chromosomal changes such as an additional Ph chromosome (double Ph^+) and trisomy 8, 9, 19, or 21, isochromosome 17, or deletion of Y chromosomes are associated with transformation or blastic crisis in CML.

8. **Management.** Traditional and investigational forms of treatment are used in the management of CML.

a. **Traditional therapy.** Symptoms are treated by **controlling the myeloproliferative process.** None of these measures offer prolonged survival or can alter the clinical course of the disease (i.e., progression to acute leukemia). Traditional chemotherapy for blast crisis is associated with a complete remission rate of less than 10%, and the duration of remission is short (<3 months). The poor results of traditional chemotherapy have brought about major changes in the treatment philosophy of CML. Traditional therapies include the following.

(1) **Hydroxyurea,** an inhibitor of deoxynucleotide synthesis, is preferred in the control of myeloproliferation because of its low toxicity, shorter duration of myelosuppressive effects, and fewer associated secondary malignancies, since it is not an alkylating agent. It is also effective in lowering the marked elevation of platelet count in some patients. The usual oral dose is 1000–1500 mg/day or 30 mg/kg/day; the effects should be monitored within 2–6 weeks.

(2) **Busulfan** is an alkylating agent that can be given intermittently to keep the WBC around 15,000/μl. The effects of the current dose are not observed until 4–6 weeks, and prolonged myelosuppression lasting up to 6 months may be disastrous if the patient becomes pancytopenic from therapy. Long-term therapy is also associated with hyperpigmentation and pulmonary fibrosis. The usual oral daily dose is 6–8 mg until the WBC decreases to 50% of its pretreatment level. If there is evidence of progression after therapy is discontinued, a daily maintenance dose of 2–4 mg may be given with careful monitoring of blood counts.

(3) **Splenic radiation and splenectomy** are other, less effective, forms of therapy.

b. **Myelosuppression and leukapheresis.** In rare cases, the increasing WBC (>300,000/μl) may impair the cerebral circulation because of hyperviscosity; myelosuppressive drugs and leukapheresis may be employed to lower the count and decrease organomegaly.

c. **Investigational therapies** have resulted in the disappearance of the Ph chromosome and in cures in a small number of patients, offering promise in the near future. These forms of therapy include the following.

(1) **Bone marrow transplantation,** in which intensive chemotherapy and total body irradiation are followed by the transplantation of allogeneic bone marrow from an human

leukocyte antigen (HLA)–identical sibling, has been shown to cure certain patients with CML and lead to a 60% disease-free survival rate at 3 years. Bone marrow transplantation is successful in patients in the chronic stable phase, less successful in those in transformation, and not successful in patients with blast crisis.

(a) Use of this **therapy is limited to young patients (<35 years old) with an HLA-matched donor**. As techniques for the procedure improve, older patients with unrelated HLA-matched donors may become eligible.

(b) However, with the significant morbidity and mortality of the procedure and the unpredictability of the duration of the indolent stable phase, it is difficult to determine which patients should be identified for this treatment and when bone marrow transplantation should be done.

(2) **Alpha interferon** administration has recently been shown to decrease marrow cellularity; control WBC, platelet counts, and organomegaly; and progressively reduce the presence of the Ph clone, leading to its disappearance in 10%–20% of patients. Alpha interferon may be the only alternative to bone marrow transplantation for curing CML or altering its natural course.

(a) The **response rates** in CML vary from 20%–30% in heavily pretreated CML patients to 75%–80% in patients with previously untreated CML who received alpha interferon within 1 year of diagnosis.

(b) The **treatment regimen** is subcutaneous daily doses of 3–9 million units for 1 year followed by a maintenance dose schedule of three times a week.

(c) The **side effects** of alpha interferon therapy differ from those of chemotherapy: Acute flu-like symptoms that last from 2 to 4 weeks, a chronic fatigue syndrome, and occasional central nervous system (CNS) manifestations have been described.

D. Essential thrombocythemia

1. **Description.** ET is a myeloproliferative syndrome in which **thrombocytosis is present without a reactive cause** such as acute or chronic inflammatory conditions or malignancy. It is an **uncommon disorder** that is observed in men and women from 20 to 80 years of age (median age is 60 years). More than 90% of patients have platelet counts of at least 1,000,000/μl.

2. **Etiology.** ET is a **clonal disorder** involving the multipotential hematopoietic stem cell, similar to the other myeloproliferative disorders.

3. **Pathogenesis** of ET is similar to that of PV: There is an autonomous proliferation of the megakaryocytic cell lines.

4. **Diagnosis and differential diagnosis.** Although a platelet count higher than 600,000/μl establishes the presence of thrombocythemia, it is associated with several conditions other than ET, which must be eliminated in the differential diagnosis. Secondary causes of thrombocytosis must be eliminated (see Ch 13 IV B) and differentiated from the other myeloproliferative disorders. The criteria for the diagnosis of ET have been established by the Polycythemia Vera Study Group as follows.

   a. **A hemoglobin concentration** of less than 13 g/dl or a normal red cell mass (males <36 ml/kg, females <32 ml/kg) eliminates the possibility of PV.

   b. The **presence of stainable iron** in the marrow or the **failure of an iron therapy** trial to cause a rise in hemoglobin of more than 1 g/dl after 1 month eliminates iron deficiency as a reactive cause of thrombocytosis and eliminates the possibility that the iron deficiency is associated with PV.

   c. The **lack of a Ph chromosome** in the marrow cells rules out 90% of CML patients.

   d. The complete **absence of collagen fibrosis of the marrow** or the absence of fibrosis in more than half of the biopsy material eliminates AMM. In addition, splenomegaly or leukoerythroblastic peripheral blood must be absent to eliminate the diagnosis of AMM.

   e. The **absence of possible causes of reactive thrombocytosis,** such as iron deficiency, asplenia, neoplasm, and inflammatory and infectious diseases, is indicative of ET.

5. **Clinical manifestations.** The symptoms of ET are associated with thrombosis, bleeding, and symptoms referable to the CNS and peripheral vascular ischemia. These symptoms include:

   a. **Weakness** similar to that experienced in **transient ischemic attacks** in 38% of patients

   b. **Hemorrhage** in 35% of patients

   c. **Headaches**

   d. **Paresthesias**

   e. **Dizziness**

f. **Visual disturbances** (amaurosis fugax) in 19% of patients
g. **Peripheral vascular insufficiency** in 14% of patients
h. **Pruritus** in 14% of patients
i. Physical findings suggestive of **myeloproliferative disease:**
   (1) **Splenomegaly** in 40%–70% of patients at the time of diagnosis, with the spleen rarely extending more than 4 cm below the left costal margin
   (2) **Hepatomegaly** in 20%–40% of patients

6. **Laboratory findings**
   a. **Red cells are normal,** but there is **mild anemia,** with the hemoglobin concentration ranging from 10 to 13 g/dl.
   b. **Leukocytosis** is evident, with a WBC as high as 40,000/μl (median of 11,000/μl), but immature leukocytes are not present in the peripheral blood smear.
   c. The **LAP score is generally normal,** but in a minority of patients it is low and in 40% of patients it is elevated.
   d. The **platelet count is at least 1,000,000/μl** in 90% of patients and is associated with abnormal platelet aggregation in response to epinephrine but normal aggregation in response to adenosine diphosphate (ADP), collagen, and thrombin.

7. **Course and prognosis. ET in young people usually does not require treatment.** The incidences of hemorrhage and thrombotic complications increase with age. Transformations to AMM and acute leukemia have been described in a minority of patients.

8. **Management** of ET may vary from observation in the young asymptomatic patient to an aggressive therapy to lower and control bleeding or thrombosis by lowering the platelet count.
   a. **Plateletpheresis** is used during periods of acute bleeding as an emergency measure in symptomatic severe thrombocytosis.
   b. **Myelosuppressive therapy**
      (1) **Hydroxyurea is the drug of choice** for the control of ET over a long period of time since this agent has not been shown to be leukemogenic after 10 years of study by the Polycythemia Vera Study Group.
      (2) **^{32}P may be used in elderly patients,** but responses to it are often delayed and it is not useful in treating symptomatic patients.
      (3) **Melphalan, thiotepa, and busulfan** are alkylating agents that control the platelet count, but their use in prolonged maintenance therapy increases the risk of secondary leukemias and malignancies.

IV. MYELODYSPLASTIC SYNDROMES

A. Description. The myelodysplastic syndromes (MDSs, or preleukemia) are also known as subacute myelogenous leukemia, smoldering leukemia, refractory anemia, and refractory dysmyelopoietic anemia.

1. They are a heterogeneous group of closely related clonal hematopoietic disorders **characterized by dysmyelopoiesis** (a cellular marrow with impaired maturation) and **peripheral blood cytopenias** resulting from ineffective blood cell production.

2. A chromosome abnormality in bone marrow cells is present in 40%–50% of patients. The majority of these patients are elderly, with a median age of 65 years.

3. The clinical course of MDS is marked by morbidity and mortality from infections, hemorrhage, and the development of acute leukemia. About 25%–45% of patients progress to acute leukemia, and the rest develop infections from granulocytopenia and bleeding caused by thrombocytopenia or from associated diseases, since many patients are in older age groups.

B. Pathogenesis. MDS is a **clonal disorder** involving the pluripotential stem cell as evidenced by the presence of chromosome abnormalities and glucose-6-phosphate dehydrogenase (G6PD) enzyme variants in the peripheral blood cells.

1. Although the abnormal clone may replace the normal marrow stem cell, in some patients the clone and the normal cell can coexist. Progressive suppression of the normal cell manifests as stages of anemia, granulocytopenia, and thrombocytopenia.

2. In addition to the suppression of normal marrow stem cells is the appearance of abnormally maturing cells with impaired function that are often ineffective in maturing into functional cells in the peripheral blood circulation.

3. Whether these disorders are leukemic in nature and have been discovered in their early phases or whether they are a manifestation of a damaged stem cell pool that progresses to acute leukemia after the occurrence of a secondary event is still unresolved. However, some forms of acute leukemia demonstrate trilineage abnormalities suggestive of MDS that may or may not be preceded by a preleukemic phase.

C. **Etiology.** Exposure to **alkylating chemotherapy drugs** and **radiation therapy** can lead to the development of secondary MDS. Daily or monthly administration for over 2 years increases the risk for MDS. The cause of MDS in patients who have not undergone these therapies is not known.

D. **FAB classification** (see Ch 12 II B) is based on the criteria established by a panel of French, American, and British experts to **define the leukemias and MDSs**. This classification is **based on the presence of dysmyelopoiesis and the quantification of the myeloblasts** (type I blasts [myeloblasts] and type II blasts [promyeloblasts]) **or erythroblasts** (Figure 3-3).

1. **Refractory anemia (RA)** is characterized as anemia with dysplastic changes in the marrow and fewer than 5% blasts in the marrow, which can be hypercellular, normal, and even hypocellular. Sideroblasts may be present, but they usually number fewer than 15% of all nucleated cells.

2. **Refractory anemia with ringed sideroblasts (RARS)** is usually associated with an erythroid marrow that is dysplastic and with sideroblasts accounting for at least 15% of the cells seen in Prussian blue stains of the marrow. The total number of erythroblasts is lower than 30%, which distinguishes RARS from erythroleukemia.

3. **Refractory anemia with excess blasts (RAEB)** is a type of MDS in which the total number of type I and type II blasts is between 5% and 20%.

4. **Refractory anemia with excess blasts in transformation (RAEBIT)** is a worsening of RAEB in which the total number of type I and type II blasts is between 20% and 30%. RAEBIT is usually associated with a rapid transformation to acute leukemia (≥30% blasts).

5. **CMML** is a type of MDS associated with an elevated WBC, a persistent monocytosis of more than 1000/μl, and splenomegaly. CMML is often confused with CML, but the Ph chromosome is not found in CMML, and CMML is associated with a **trilineage dysplasia** (red cells, white cells, and platelets) that is not present in CML. **CMML may transform into acute leukemia** when the total number of blasts exceeds 20%, and **it may transform into acute nonlymphocytic leukemia (ANLL)** when the total number of blasts reaches 30% or more.

E. **Diagnosis.** The diagnosis of a MDS is based on laboratory findings of peripheral blood cytopenia and evidence of dysmyelopoiesis.

1. **Peripheral blood counts** indicate anemia, bicytopenia, or pancytopenia.
   a. The **anemia** is usually macrocytic with oval-shaped red cells, or it may be bimorphic with hypochromic microcytic red cells.

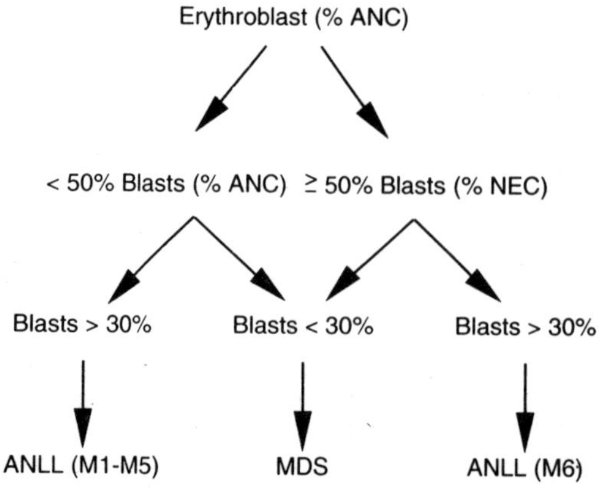

Figure 3-3. The FAB (French, American, and British) classification uses the percentages of blasts (i.e., all type I and type II myeloblasts or erythroblasts) to distinguish acute nonlymphocytic (myelocytic) leukemia (*ANLL*) from myelodysplastic syndrome (*MDS*). *ANC* = all nucleated cells; *NEC* = nonerythroid cells; *M1* = ANLL without differentiation; *M2* = ANLL with differentiation; *M3* = acute promyelocytic leukemia; *M4* = acute myelomonocytic leukemia; *M5* = acute monocytic leukemia; *M6* = erythroleukemia. (See Ch 12 II B for further discussion of the FAB classification.) [Reprinted from Bennett JM, Catovsky D, Daniel MT, et al: Proposed revised criteria for the classification of acute myeloid leukemia: a report of the French–American–British cooperative group. *Ann Intern Med* 103:626, 1985.]

b. **Bicytopenia** can be expressed as a combination of anemia with thrombocytopenia or neutropenia. However, occasionally there may be an increased WBC along with the presence of immature cells and monocytes.
c. **Pancytopenia** is a decrease in all three cell lines.

2. **Dyserythropoiesis** indicates the presence of abnormal erythroid precursors.
   a. Megaloblastoid maturation is similar to that found in the megaloblastic anemias but without the evidence of vitamin B_{12} or folate deficiency.
   b. Impaired nuclear maturation results in the creation of binucleate or multinucleate normoblasts with abnormal formation of hemoglobin.
   c. Ringed sideroblasts are present.

3. **Neutropenia** is associated with **morphologically abnormal granulocytes** that may be agranular or may contain granules with abnormal lobulations (round, bilobular, or hypersegmented). The finding of dysgranulopoiesis indicates that there is abnormal maturation of the myeloid elements.
   a. There is **hyperplasia of myeloid elements** with an increased number of granulocytes in the intermediate stages of maturation (myelocytes and metamyelocytes), in contrast to the maturation gap observed in acute leukemia. The identification of these cells is difficult because of the lack of coordination between maturation markers in the cytoplasm and in the nucleus.
   b. Abnormalities in granulocytes include hypogranulation, the pseudo–Pelger-Huët anomaly, and abnormal cell forms.
   c. The number of monocyte precursors is increased.
   d. Patients with the FAB (French, American, and British classification) subtype of chronic myelomonocytic leukemia (CMML) usually have an elevated WBC and monocytosis.

4. **Thrombocytopenia** may or may not be present, but abnormal platelets, such as giant hypogranular forms, are usually observed. Occasionally, patients may have an increased platelet count. The finding of dysthrombocytopoiesis indicates that there is abnormal maturation of megakaryocytes, such as micromegakaryocytes or mononuclear or bilobular megakaryocytes.

5. These **trilineage changes** in bone marrow are specific for MDS and can be used to differentiate it from the other causes of marrow failure and myeloproliferation.
   a. The marrow is usually hypercellular, indicating defects in both maturation and proliferation. A few patients, particularly those with refractory anemia (RA) and refractory anemia with ringed sideroblasts (RARS), may have normal or even hypocellular marrow.
   b. The identification of specific abnormalities such as ringed sideroblasts, multinuclear normoblasts, and abnormal megakaryocytes helps reinforce the findings in other cell lines.
   c. Bone marrow cells reveal nonrandom chromosome abnormalities, commonly a trisomy 8, deletion of the long arm of chromosome 5 (5q–), a missing chromosome 7, and various translocations.

F. **Clinical manifestations.** Patients with MDSs usually present with signs and symptoms related to the **peripheral blood count and degree of cytopenia**.

1. **Symptoms related to anemia** range from fatigue and malaise to congestive heart failure in patients with underlying cardiac problems.

2. **Recurrent localized or systemic infections** are associated with granulocytopenia and poor phagocytic functions of the circulating granulocytes.

3. **Bleeding manifestations** from petechiae to gross hemorrhage occur in thrombocytopenic patients with or without associated platelet dysfunction.

G. **Course and prognosis.** The clinical course of MDSs is heterogeneous and varies from a few weeks to 10 years.

1. Acute leukemic patients with **aggressive forms** of MDS **survive from a few weeks to 3 months,** as do patients in transformation.

2. Patients with the **intermediate forms** of RAEB and CMML with excess blasts **survive from 6 months to 1 year**.

3. Patients with the **indolent forms** of RA and RARS with no excess blasts **may survive as long as 6–10 years,** and patients will usually die of complications of their cytopenia rather than because of transformation to acute leukemia.

H. Management

1. **Supportive care is the main form of treatment** and includes packed red cell transfusion for anemia, platelet transfusion for thrombocytopenia and bleeding, and antibiotic administration for infections. The benefits derived from these types of therapies are temporary and limited.
2. **Aggressive cytotoxic (antileukemic) chemotherapy** that is available for younger patients in transformation or in the acute leukemic phase may be of benefit for a minority of MDS patients, but the recovery marrow usually remains dysplastic, and remission is short-lived.
3. **Experimental forms of therapy** range from bone marrow transplantation to the use of differentiating agents and recombinant growth factors such as GM-CSF, granulocyte colony-stimulating factor (G-CSF), and erythropoietin.

V. BONE MARROW TRANSPLANTATION is now an accepted form of treatment in aplastic anemia and acute leukemia and in certain immunodeficiency syndromes. Abnormal, malignant, or nonfunctioning marrow cells are replaced with normal marrow stem cells in a process made possible by developments in immunology and the cryopreservation of cells.

A. Types of bone marrow transplantation

1. **Allogeneic marrow transplantation.** Normal bone marrow cells are harvested for infusion into the patients after aggressive marrow ablative therapy. The success of bone marrow engraftment is compromised by the fact that the transplanted lymphocytes may react with the recipient's tissues. The class II antigens are responsible for the mixed lymphocyte reaction (MLR; patient and donor marrow are mixed to see if there is a rejection reaction). There are **three categories of donors**.
   a. An **identical twin donor** is the closest to an autologous marrow donor.
   b. There is a one in four chance of an **HLA-matched sibling**.
   c. An **HLA-matched nonrelated donor** may be located from a large pool of volunteer donors.
2. **Autologous marrow transplantation** is the process of harvesting, purging (treating for residual malignancy), and cryopreserving the patient's marrow cells for reinfusion after high-dose chemotherapy or total body irradiation. This procedure is limited by the toxicity of the high-dose anticancer therapy to organs other than the bone marrow and by the persistence of tumor cells in the bone marrow.

B. Indications and procedures

1. **Indications.** Hematopoietic stem cell transplantation is used to replace failed bone marrow and improve the cure rates in **aplastic anemia,** in **genetic diseases** such as Wiskott-Aldrich syndrome and severe combined immunodeficiency, and in **acute leukemia of the lymphocytic and nonlymphocytic types** either in first or later remission.
2. **Procedure**
   a. **Aspiration of donor marrow.** In order to supply the approximately 10 million nucleated bone marrow cells needed for infusion, 50–500 ml of bone marrow is aspirated from the donor's iliac crests.
   b. **Preparation of aspirate.** The donor's aspirates are anticoagulated and filtered through a steel mesh before infusion into the patient.
   c. **Preparation of the recipient.** The process by which the patient is prepared for infusion is called **conditioning,** and the exact procedure followed is contingent upon the disease and the antigenic compatibility of the donor and recipient. For example, **ablative treatment of the marrow** by high-dose chemotherapy, total body irradiation, or both, followed by varying degrees of immunosuppression, is required for an immunodeficient, aplastic anemic, or acute leukemic patient who is to receive marrow from an **HLA-identical and MLR-nonreactive sibling**.
   d. **Mechanism of action.** Donor hematopoietic cells infused into the recipient's peripheral blood will zero in on the bone marrow microenvironment (see Ch 2 II).
   e. **Recovery phase.** After 1–2 months, reticulocytes and nucleated red cells will reappear, and the rest of the peripheral blood counts will begin to rise. **Engraftment** can be substantiated through the analysis of genetic markers, such as sex chromosomes.

C. Complications in transplantation may occur early or late; 20%–50% of patients will experience one or more of the following.

1. **Chemotherapy and radiation toxicity,** expressed as:
   a. **Mucositis** of the gastrointestinal tract, respiratory tract, bladder, and other mucosal cell-lined tracts
   b. **Intrahepatic vascular occlusive disease** from centrilobular necrosis and collagen deposition, obliterating the central vein
   c. **Toxic pneumonitis**
   d. **CNS toxicity,** such as dementia or leukoencephalopathy
   e. **Endocrine dysfunction,** such as hypothyroidism, which will occur late
   f. **Cataracts,** which are common delayed complications in patients who survive more than 2 years

2. **Graft rejection or failure of engraftment,** which is usually due to:
   a. Degree of genetic disparity between donor and recipient
   b. Abnormal marrow microenvironment in the patient
   c. Immunocompetence of the recipient
   d. Type and intensity of posttransplant immunosuppressive treatment
   e. Sensitization of recipient to donor antigens because of earlier transfusions or pregnancy

3. **GVHD,** which can develop acutely (within 20–100 days) or chronically (after 6–12 months) and is due to engraftment of immunocompetent T cells that react against the recipient tissues
   a. GVHD occurs in 30%–60% of all allogeneic transplant patients, and there is an increased risk in older patients (70% in patients older than 40 years).
   b. GVHD is fatal in about half of affected individuals.

4. **Infections,** which are due to the resulting immunodeficiency and granulocytopenia and are mostly caused by opportunistic organisms:
   a. **Bacterial infections** by either gram-negative or gram-positive organisms
   b. **Fungal infections,** such as those caused by *Candida*
   c. **Viral infections,** such as herpes zoster and CMV
   d. **Parasitic infections** by such organisms as *Pneumocystis carinii*

5. **Interstitial pneumonitis,** which may be due to direct chemotherapy and radiation toxicity or to one of the above infections and which carries a high mortality rate of 50%–70%

STUDY QUESTIONS

Directions: Each of the numbered items or incomplete statements in this section is followed by answers or by completions of the statement. Select the **one** lettered answer or completion that is **best** in each case.

1. All of the following complications are associated with pancytopenia resulting from bone marrow failure EXCEPT

(A) sepsis
(B) fatigue and general malaise
(C) gum bleeding
(D) thrombosis
(E) pallor

2. Viral infections related to an "aplastic crisis" in a patient with an underlying hemolytic anemia are usually caused by

(A) varicella-zoster virus
(B) parvovirus
(C) non-A, non-B hepatitis virus
(D) cytomegalovirus (CMV)
(E) Epstein-Barr virus

3. Which of the following is a quick and inexpensive way to differentiate between chronic myelogenous leukemia (CML) and an elevated white cell count that is the result of an inflammatory process such as pneumonia, a necrotic tumor, or vasculitis (leukemoid reaction)?

(A) Bone marrow test
(B) CT scan of the abdomen and chest
(C) Leukocyte alkaline phosphatase (LAP) stain
(D) Ultrasound of the spleen

4. The first step in diagnosing polycythemia is to

(A) determine red cell mass and plasma volume
(B) determine erythropoietin serum level
(C) conduct intravenous pyelogram or renal ultrasound
(D) determine carboxyhemoglobin level
(E) determine arterial blood gas level

5. A patient is considered to have essential thrombocythemia (ET) if a platelet count persistently higher than 1 million is associated with

(A) absent iron stores in the bone marrow
(B) Philadelphia (Ph) chromosome in the bone marrow cells
(C) recent splenectomy
(D) fibrosis of more than one-third of the marrow
(E) none of the above

6. All patients with myelodysplastic syndromes (MDSs) display

(A) ringed sideroblasts
(B) a total number of blasts that exceed 5%
(C) nonrandom chromosome abnormalities
(D) transformation into acute leukemia
(E) dysplastic marrow changes in all cell lines

7. Bone marrow transplantation is indicated for all of the following conditions EXCEPT

(A) aplastic anemia
(B) severe combined immunodeficiency
(C) acute myelogenous leukemia (AML) in second remission
(D) thalassemia minor
(E) chronic myelogenous leukemia (CML)

8. A 57-year-old woman with multiple myeloma of 5 years' duration presents with transfusion-dependent anemia and neutropenia. She entered a stable phase after 2 years of treatment and has not received melphalan or prednisone for the past 2 years. There is no evidence of disease progression, and she displays stable M protein, renal function, and serum calcium levels. Bone marrow study reveals no increase of plasma cells above the levels in previous studies, but the appearance of ringed sideroblasts heralds the diagnosis of

(A) transfusion iron overload
(B) hemochromatosis
(C) a myelodysplastic syndrome (MDS)
(D) pyridoxine deficiency
(E) iron deficiency from occult bleeding

1-D
2-B
3-C
4-A
5-E
6-E
7-D
8-C

9. Which of the following FAB subtypes of the myelodysplastic syndrome (MDS) is associated with a good prognosis and a prolonged clinical course?

(A) RAEBIT
(B) CMML
(C) RA
(D) RAEB

9-C

ANSWERS AND EXPLANATIONS

1. The answer is D *[II A 4].*
The symptoms of pancytopenia are attributable to anemia, which causes the pallor and fatigue, thrombocytopenia, which can cause gum bleeding, and sepsis from granulocytopenia. Thrombosis is not due to pancytopenia but is commonly seen in the myeloproliferative syndromes that are associated with increases in cell counts.

2. The answer is B *[II A 2 b (2)].*
The virus implicated in the transient aplastic crisis in patients with sickle cell anemia or hereditary spherocytosis is the parvovirus. This virus appears to be directly toxic to erythroid precursor cells. Other viruses, such as the hepatitis virus (most frequently the non-A, non-B type), cytomegalovirus (CMV), and Epstein-Barr virus have been implicated in aplastic anemia in which there is a more prolonged or permanent bone marrow failure.

3. The answer is C *[III B 6 a (3), C 6 a (2)].*
Leukocyte alkaline phosphatase (LAP) is a special stain for alkaline phosphatase granules in the granulocytes. A fresh smear of the peripheral blood is stained, the positive cells are scored, and the number of cells is compared with that from normal blood. The patients with chronic myelogenous leukemia (CML) have more granulocytes that do not take up the stain than is found in normal blood, so that the score is low or absent. Pregnancy or the presence of infection will increase the number of granulocytes rich in alkaline phosphatase and will yield a high score. Although the bone marrow test, CT scan, and ultrasound may be helpful for determining the source of a leukemoid reaction, they are not cost-effective means of differentiating between the two conditions.

4. The answer is A *[III A 4].*
The most cost-effective method of diagnosing polycythemia is to rule out pseudopolycythemia, a condition in which the elevated hemoglobin level and hematocrit are due to a contracted plasma volume and not to an increase in red cell volume. If the patient does not have true polycythemia, then determinations of erythropoietin serum level, carboxyhemoglobin level, and arterial blood gas level and intravenous pyelogram or renal ultrasound are not necessary. However, hyperviscosity may still present problems in pseudopolycythemia and will require treatment in certain clinical situations.

5. The answer is E *[III D 4].*
Essential thrombocythemia (ET) is diagnosed by excluding secondary causes of thrombocytosis. These include iron deficiency or a recent splenectomy and other overlapping myeloproliferative disorders, such as chronic myelogenous leukemia (CML) or agnogenic myeloid metaplasia (AMM), or iron-deficient polycythemia vera (PV) in which red cell mass increases when the patient is given iron.

6. The answer is E *[IV E].*
The presence of trilineage dysplastic marrow changes (trilineage dysmyelopoiesis) is required in the FAB (French, American, and British) criteria for the diagnosis of myelodysplastic syndromes (MDSs). The findings of ringed sideroblasts, excess blasts, abnormal chromosomes, and transformation into acute leukemia are not present in all myelodysplastic patients.

7. The answer is D *[V B].*
Bone marrow transplantation is undertaken to replace hematopoietic stem cells in aplastic anemia, replace the immune system in severe combined immunodeficiency, increase the tolerance to high-dose chemotherapy and radiation in acute leukemias, and treat chronic myelogenous leukemia (CML). Recent cures of severe thalassemias have been effected by bone marrow transplantation; however, patients with mild hemoglobinopathies, such as thalassemia minor, do not need a bone marrow transplant.

8. The answer is C *[IV E].*
Prolonged exposure to alkylating agents such as melphalan risks the occurrence of a myelodysplastic syndrome (MDS) and secondary acute leukemia; the development of ringed sideroblasts as well as trilineage dysplasia heralds a preleukemic phase. Transfusion iron overload, iron deficiency, and hemochromatosis do not cause the formation of ringed sideroblasts. Sideroblasts from pyridoxine deficiency are usually due to the administration of drugs such as isoniazid for the treatment of tuberculosis.

9. The answer is C *[IV D].*
The FAB (French, American, and British) subtypes of myelodysplastic syndromes (MDSs) with good prognoses are those with fewer myeloblasts (<5%)—refractory anemia (RA) and refractory anemia with ringed sideroblasts (RARS)—as compared with the rest of the FAB subgroups, such as chronic myelomonocytic leukemia (CMML), refractory anemia with excess blasts (RAEB), and their corresponding forms in transition to acute leukemia (between 20% and 30% myeloblasts), such as refractory anemia with excess blasts in transformation (RAEBIT).

4
Erythropoiesis and Disorders of Hypoproliferative Marrow

Emmanuel C. Besa

I. ERYTHROPOIESIS is the process by which red blood cells are produced in the adult bone marrow. Erythropoiesis is closely regulated by physiologic mechanisms involving several **growth factors** that moderate the differentiation of **erythroid progenitor cells** (Figure 4-1). These committed progenitor cells are derived from the pluripotential and multipotential stem cells and respond in the bone marrow to the differentiating activity of these growth factors.

A. Erythropoietic growth factors. Hematopoietic growth factors are glycoproteins that participate in the self-renewal of stem cells and in the proliferation and differentiation of the various committed progenitor cells involved in hematopoiesis. The names of these growth factors were derived from the original description of their activity in bone marrow cultures. The following growth factors are important in erythropoiesis.

1. **Multi-colony-stimulating factor (multi-CSF),** which is now known as **interleukin-3 (IL-3),** is a glycoprotein with a molecular weight of about 20–30 kilodaltons.
   a. IL-3 is important in the production of all hematopoietic cell lines [see Ch 2 II B 5 b (1)]. It is required throughout the various stages of hematopoiesis, acting on early pluripotential stem cells for self-renewal as well as enhancing differentiation of the pluripotential cells into committed cells.
   b. IL-3 is essential for providing the bone marrow with cells that are responsive to erythropoietin.

2. **Erythropoietin** is a glycoprotein hormone that stimulates erythropoiesis by acting on bone marrow stem cells. In the absence of erythropoietin, red cell production ceases (see I C).
   a. Erythropoietin is **synthesized primarily in the kidneys** (90%) **and in the liver** (10%) and is released into the circulation **in response to hypoxia.**
   b. Patients with **severe renal failure** are unable to respond to anemia or hypoxia with increased erythropoietin synthesis and red cell production. A human recombinant preparation of erythropoietin is currently available for treatment of anemia in renal failure.

B. Erythroid progenitor cells in bone marrow. These cells are functionally classified by their ability to produce colonies of erythroid cells in different stages of maturation that are derived from human bone marrow in culture studies. True morphologic identification of the progenitors, however, is not possible. A more comprehensive discussion of stem cells and their differentiation is presented in Chapter 2 II A.

1. **Pluripotential stem cells** are early hematopoietic cells that can give rise to any of the differentiated blood cells, including red blood cells.

2. **Myeloid multipotential stem cells** are early precursors of myeloid cells, from which erythrocytic, granulocytic-monocytic, and thrombopoietic cells are derived.

3. **Erythroid-committed cells** are early precursor cells that can differentiate only into red blood cells. These cells are identified by their characteristic growth pattern in bone marrow culture studies.
   a. The **erythroid burst-forming unit (BFU-E)** is detected in bone marrow or peripheral blood cell cultures by **large clusters of erythropoietic cells** that bear characteristics of early red cells.

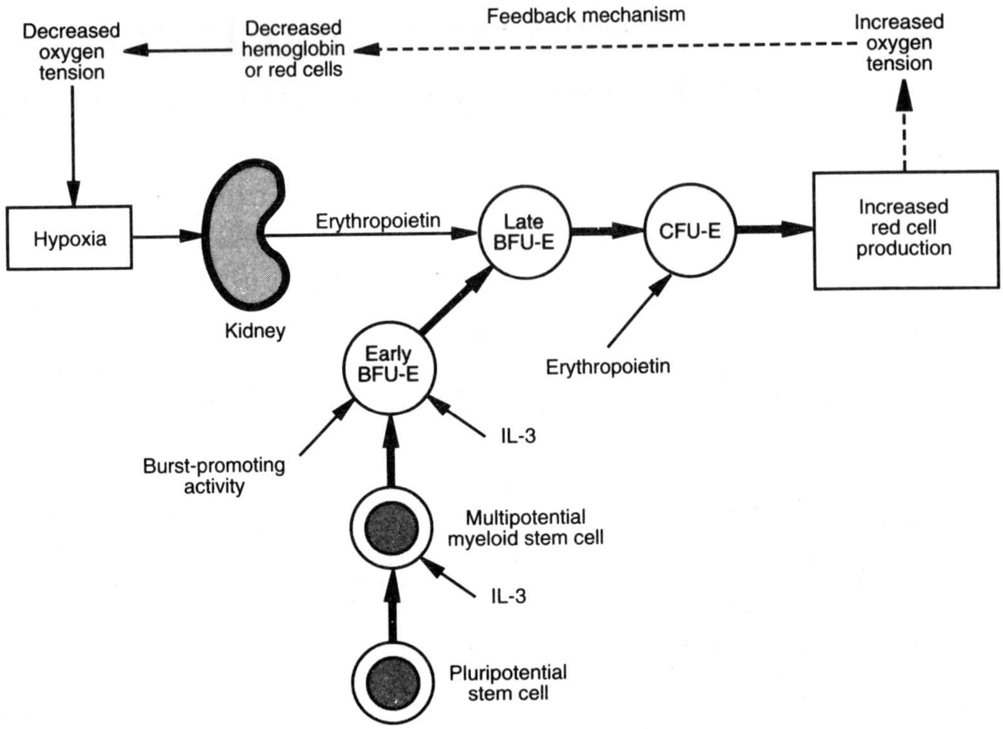

Figure 4-1. Schematic diagram showing the interrelationship between precursor cells and growth factors in erythropoiesis. Precursor cells in the bone marrow committed for erythroid differentiation are derived from the pluripotential and multipotential stem cells, which are regulated by interleukin-3 (*IL-3*). The important stimulus for red cell production is renal hypoxia, which signals the kidney to start producing the erythropoietic growth factor, erythropoietin. Erythropoietin is transported by the circulation to erythropoietic sites in the bone marrow, where it stimulates the proliferation and maturation of erythroid precursor cells, resulting in increased red cell production. Feedback control of erythropoietin production is provided by the increases in the number of red cells and increases in the amount of oxygen received by the kidney. *BFU-E* = erythroid burst-forming unit; *CFU-E* = erythroid colony-forming unit.

(1) BFU-E is **the most primitive functionally detectable red cell precursor** and has the capacity to generate thousands of erythroid precursor cells.

(2) The BFU-E is maintained in small numbers in the bone marrow and peripheral blood by **self-replication** and **migration** from the multipotential stem cell compartment.

(3) **Regulation** of BFU-E is accomplished through the action of an ill-defined growth factor, referred to as **burst-promoting activity (BPA),** which is generated by reticuloendothelial cells. It is now believed that this factor is IL-3, and that BFU-E is generally insensitive to erythropoietin and to changes in oxygen tension.

b. The **erythroid colony-forming unit (CFU-E)** is a more mature erythroid precursor cell generated from proliferative responses of BFU-E. It is identified in culture studies by its ability to **generate small clusters of erythroid cells** that eventually become mature red cells. Each CFU-E can produce four or five cell divisions and generate 16–32 red cell progeny.

(1) Cell division and viability of all CFU-E rely on erythropoietin. The number of CFU-E in vivo depends on tissue oxygen tension and erythropoietin titers.

(2) It is known that the in vitro development of erythropoietin-dependent erythroid colonies is enhanced by substances such as cyclic adenosine monophosphate (cAMP) and thyroid hormones; however, in vivo association is not clearly known.

C. Erythropoietic regulatory mechanisms. Erythropoietin maintains the number of circulating red cells within a narrow range through sensitive adjustments to the rate of red cell production.

1. Erythropoietin release. A decrease in tissue oxygen tension (e.g., hypoxia) in the kidney (see Figure 4-1) is the principal stimulus initiating erythropoietin production. Decreased oxygenation in the kidney triggers an increase in production of erythropoietin in the kidney and, thus, its release into the circulation. Erythropoietin circulates in the blood, stimulates production of new red cells, and is excreted in the urine. As the circulating number of red cells increases, erythropoietin activity decreases by increased oxygen tension in the kidney cells.

2. **Mechanism of erythropoietin activity.** Erythropoiesis is promoted in bone marrow through the stimulation of committed erythroid progenitor cells (i.e., CFU-E) by erythropoietin.

3. **Anemia related to erythropoietin.** Clinically, it is useful to determine whether an anemic condition is related to erythropoietin, since the recombinant form of this glycoprotein is a potent and effective agent for the treatment of some anemias. Thus, it is important to distinguish anemia caused by unresponsiveness of the marrow cells to erythropoietin from anemia caused by decreased erythropoietin levels (Table 4-1).

II. DISORDERS OF DECREASED ERYTHROPOIESIS.

Some disorders involve an isolated decrease in erythropoiesis that produces a **normocytic, normochromic anemia** (normal-sized red cells containing normal amounts of hemoglobin) but no change in white cell and platelet production. **Signs of decreased erythropoiesis** include a lower than expected reticulocyte count for the observed hematocrit and a decrease in red cell precursors. The following clinical conditions are associated with reduced red cell production.

A. **Anemia of chronic renal failure.** Anemia is the most common sequela of chronic renal failure. The degree of anemia is roughly proportional to the degree of uremia.

1. **Etiology and pathogenesis.** This type of anemia typically is **hypoproliferative and multifactorial,** with the following factors contributing to the anemia.
   a. **Renal excretory failure** may affect the degree of anemia through many **proposed mechanisms.**
      (1) A **lower hematocrit** may be caused by the increased plasma volume from hydremia.
      (2) **Reduced red cell survival** may be caused by uremia through either metabolic or mechanical means. Decreased activity of certain intracellular enzymes [i.e., transketolase and adenosine triphosphatase (ATPase)] has been observed; this is proportional to the degree of uremia.
      (3) **Direct marrow suppression** by uremic toxins has been implicated.
      (4) **Deficiencies of certain nutrients** (e.g., iron, folate) may occur in chronic dialysis patients.
      (5) **Impaired platelet function** with a resultant bleeding tendency has been observed in one-third of patients with chronic renal failure. Blood loss contributes greatly to anemia in these patients.
   b. **Renal endocrine failure** (i.e., decreased or absent production of erythropoietin) is **the primary cause of anemia** in chronic renal failure. Erythropoietin production appears to occur in the renal cortex. Anephric patients with total absence of renal erythropoietin demonstrate a very poor compensatory capacity in the bone marrow, with erythropoietic activity

Table 4-1. Disorders Associated with Reduced Erythropoiesis

Disorders that cause decreased erythropoietin levels
Renal disease
Endocrine deficiencies
Hypopituitarism
Hypothyroidism
Hypocorticoidism
Hypogonadism (testes)
Starvation (protein deficiency)
Anemia of chronic disease (ACD)
Chronic inflammation
Malignancy
Disorders that may cause marrow unresponsiveness to erythropoietin
Deficiency states
Iron deficiency
Folate or vitamin B_{12} deficiency
Sideroblastic anemias
Primary refractory anemia
Pure red cell aplasia

maintained at a subnormal level by the remaining 10% of erythropoietin from the liver. Clinical trials of recombinant human erythropoietin in these patients show that normal levels of hemoglobin can be achieved by administration of exogenous erythropoietin.

2. **Clinical features and laboratory findings** vary, depending on the underlying cause of chronic renal failure. Characteristic hematologic features include the following.
   a. The **anemia** typically is **normochromic and normocytic** and associated with a **normal or decreased reticulocyte count.**
   b. Typical **red cell deformities** seen on blood films include (see Table 1-1):
      (1) **Echinocytes,** or "burr cells" (i.e., cells with multiple tiny spicules and a decreased red cell volume)
      (2) **Acanthocytes** (i.e., cells with a few large spicules) and **schistocytes,** or "spur cells" (i.e., cells with irregular spiny projections), which are seen in the microcirculation in hemolytic-uremic syndrome (see Ch 15 III B)

3. **Therapy.** With the exception of red cell transfusions, **treatment varies with the severity of the anemia** and consists of addressing the various causes that contribute to the symptoms.
   a. **Correction of the uremia** by efficient dialysis may improve hemoglobin levels.
   b. **Replacement of folate** (which may be lost as a water-soluble vitamin) **and iron** (which is lost through capillary bleeding and through frequent blood testing) is important in dialysis patients.
   c. **Splenectomy** occasionally is performed in patients with shortened red cell survival.
   d. **Administration of androgens** (e.g., nandrolone decanoate) stimulates erythropoietin production but **causes undesirable side effects:** hirsutism, fluid retention, skin infections, and cholestasis. Androgens are not effective in anephric patients.
   e. **Recombinant human erythropoietin, the treatment of choice,** is now available for therapeutic use. Doses of 3000 units given subcutaneously three times per week is recommended. In recent tests, this hormone has produced normal or high hemoglobin levels in treated patients but has been associated with the development of hypertension. Therefore, erythropoietin replacement to a low-normal hemoglobin level is recommended.

B. Anemia of endocrine disorders. Erythropoiesis is affected by hormones other than erythropoietin. A deficiency of any of these hormones can lead to erythroid hypoplasia and anemia.

1. **Anemia of hypothyroidism**
   a. **Thyroid hormones** have a positive effect on erythropoiesis, possibly by controlling cellular oxygen requirements through their effects on the metabolic rates of the tissues.
   b. **Hypothyroidism causes a normocytic or a slightly macrocytic type of anemia.**
      (1) This anemia is a physiologic response of the bone marrow to the **decreased tissue oxygen consumption** that occurs in hypothyroidism. The marrow of these patients is normal but its rate of hematopoiesis is low because of the diminished release of erythropoietin from the kidneys.
      (2) **Macrocytosis is uncommon:** It may be seen in fewer than 10% of patients with hypothyroidism. This may be related to pernicious anemia (see Ch 6 III D 3) from cobalamin (vitamin B_{12}) deficiency in association with hypothyroidism from Hashimoto's disease, or it may be the result of poor dietary intake of folate.

2. **Anemia of hypopituitarism**
   a. **The pituitary gland affects erythropoiesis** both directly and indirectly through the action of several hormones.
      (1) **Androgens increase erythropoiesis** by exerting a direct effect on the marrow and by stimulating production of erythropoietin, making marrow cells more responsive to erythropoietin.
      (2) **Growth hormone has a trophic effect on the bone marrow.**
   b. **Hypopituitarism can lead to anemia** as a result of an associated decrease in thyroid function, low androgen levels (i.e., hypogonadism) in men, or low levels of adrenal cortical hormones and growth hormone. The **anemia of panhypopituitarism is normochromic, normocytic,** with a reduced reticulocyte count, low erythropoietin levels, and a somewhat hypocellular marrow.

3. **Anemia of hyperparathyroidism.** Primary hyperparathyroidism occasionally is associated with anemia that subsides after parathyroidectomy. **Parathyroid hormone may suppress**

erythropoiesis by renal calcification (with decreased erythropoietin formation) or by marrow sclerosis (with decreased proliferation of erythroid precursors).

4. **Therapy.** Treatment of the anemia of endocrine disorders is directed to **correction of the underlying endocrine disorder**.

C. **Pure red cell aplasia** is a rare disorder characterized by the **isolated loss of erythroid precursor cells**. The disorder occurs in an acute and a chronic form.

1. **Acute form**
   a. **Incidence and etiology**
      (1) Transient red cell aplasia (also known as **aplastic crisis**) most often occurs in the presence of **preexisting hemolytic disease** (e.g., sickle cell disease, hereditary spherocytosis, aquired hemolytic anemia), although it also has been reported in hematologically normal patients.
      (2) The cause of aplastic crisis is not clear; however, the episodes have been related to **certain viral infections** (e.g., primary atypical pneumonia, infectious mononucleosis, parvovirus infection) **and toxicity to certain drugs** (e.g., chlorpropamide, diphenylhydantoin). An **immunologic mechanism** has been implicated in cases associated with thymoma or lymphoma.
   b. **Clinical and laboratory features**
      (1) Typically, the acute incident is preceded by a **mild febrile illness,** which is followed by the rapid onset of **pallor and fatigue**. A rapid **drop in hemoglobin levels and reticulocyte count** is characteristic with an **absence of erythroid cells** in the bone marrow.
      (2) **Antibody** (usually IgG) has been demonstrated in the serum of patients, which suppresses the growth of erythroid precursors in culture.
   c. **Therapy depends on the clinical situation and the possible underlying cause** of the aplastic crisis. If possible, all drugs should be discontinued, and any related illness should be treated. Transfusion support may be necessary for the chronic hemolysis patient until the aplastic crisis remits.

2. **Chronic form**
   a. **Incidence and etiology.** Chronic pure red cell aplasia may be **inherited or acquired**.
      (1) The **inherited form** that occurs in young children is called **Diamond-Blackfan syndrome**. The cause is not certain, but a defective stem cell has been suggested.
      (2) The **adult form is acquired** and may be associated with autoimmune diseases, a thymoma, or lymphoproliferative disorders (e.g., chronic lymphocytic leukemia, lymphoma). In some cases, no associated disease or precipitating factor can be determined.
   b. **Clinical and laboratory features**
      (1) In children, **manifestations of anemia** (i.e., pallor and loss of appetite) may be evident as early as 2 weeks after birth and are followed by the development of **congestive heart failure, hepatomegaly, and splenomegaly;** transfusion may correct these problems. In adults, pallor may be the only manifestation.
      (2) A more gradual decrease in hemoglobin levels, reticulocyte count, and erythroid precursors in the bone marrow is seen in the chronic form than in the acute form in both adults and children.
   c. **Therapy**
      (1) The **congenital form is treated with androgens** to stimulate erythropoietin production and to render the bone marrow more responsive, thus increasing red cell production. Unfortunately, long-term androgen administration is associated with growth retardation and hirsutism in girls.
      (2) In adults, **thymectomy** is performed for patients with known or suspected thymoma; thymectomy also has been shown to be of some benefit in some idiopathic cases. Immunosuppressive agents (e.g., cyclophosphamide) and corticosteroids also have been tried, with variable success. Anecdotal responses have been reported using plasmapheresis and high doses of intravenous immunoglobulin.

STUDY QUESTIONS

Directions: Each of the numbered items or incomplete statements in this section is followed by answers or by completions of the statement. Select the **one** lettered answer or completion that is **best** in each case.

1. The primary factor that regulates erythropoietic activity is

(A) the kidney
(B) erythropoietin
(C) the erythroid colony-forming unit (CFU-E)
(D) oxygen
(E) bone marrow

2. Which of the following anemias is most likely to respond to the administration of erythropoietin?

(A) Iron deficiency anemia
(B) Pernicious anemia
(C) Sideroblastic anemia
(D) Pure red cell aplasia
(E) Anemia of renal disease

3. A 48-year-old woman with known hereditary spherocytosis who usually has a mild anemia (hemoglobin of 10 g/dl and reticulocyte count of 16%) comes to the emergency room complaining of extreme shortness of breath after having had a "bad cold" for a week. Hematologic testing reveals a hemoglobin concentration of 5 g/dl, a reticulocyte count of 1%, a white cell count of 6700/μl, and a platelet count of 200,000/μl. What is the best course of action for this patient?

(A) Plasmapheresis to remove autoantibody directed at erythroblasts plus supportive transfusions
(B) Surgical consultation for thymectomy after confirming a diagnosis of pure red cell aplasia
(C) Slow transfusion of packed red cells to avoid volume overload plus 1 mg/day of oral folate
(D) Administration of 60 mg of prednisone to suppress autoantibodies directed at erythroid precursor cells
(E) Bone marrow transplantation

1-D
2-E
3-C

ANSWERS AND EXPLANATIONS

1. The answer is D *[I C 1–2; Figure 4-1].*
The primary signal triggering erythropoiesis is a decrease in the oxygen tension (i.e., hypoxia) in the kidney. Tissue oxygen tension depends on the number of circulating red cells bearing functioning hemoglobin. A "sensor" thermostat in the kidney is activated by renal hypoxia to transmit a "message" to erythroid-committed precursor cells (erythroid colony-forming unit, or CFU-E) in the bone marrow. The message is the erythropoietic growth factor, erythropoietin, which the kidney produces and secretes into the circulation. Erythropoietin increases proliferation and maturation of the erythroid precursors and accelerates the release of new red blood cells. More red cells, then, carry higher amounts of oxygen, which increase tissue oxygen tension, which in turn cause the kidney to stop releasing erythropoietin. Thus, oxygen acts as the stimulus for starting and stopping the process and the "thermostat" for maintaining a normal level of red blood cells.

2. The answer is E *[II A 1 b, 3 e].*
The major cause of anemia in renal disease is decreased levels of erythropoietin, which is produced and secreted by the kidney. Clinical studies have shown that administration of exogenous erythropoietin produces normal hemoglobin levels in patients with this form of anemia. The other causes of anemia cited are associated with elevated, not decreased, erythropoietin levels. The anemia is caused by a lack of erythroid precursor cell response to erythropoietin because of either an absence of iron for the formation of hemoglobin (in iron deficiency), an absence of vitamin B_{12} for nuclear maturation (in pernicious anemia), a defect in porphyrin synthesis for hemoglobin production (in sideroblastic anemia), or immunologic damage to the early erythroid precursors (in pure red cell aplasia).

3. The answer is C *[II C 1 c].*
Patients with chronic hemolysis are at risk for having a transient episode of red cell aplasia, or an "aplastic crisis." The episode is characterized by an acute drop in hemoglobin because of the absence of erythroid compensation for the hemolysis, as shown by a low reticulocyte count. In most cases, the aplastic crisis occurs in association with a viral infection that is self-limited; thus, transfusion support through this period is all that is necessary. Immunosuppression is effected with corticosteroids when pure red cell aplasia is associated with an autoimmune disease; cytotoxic drugs are administered when the disorder is associated with a lymphoma. Thymectomy is indicated in cases of known or suspected thymoma and in some idiopathic cases in an attempt to remove the source of the autoantibody. Plasmapheresis is another treatment used to remove autoantibodies. Bone marrow transplantation is not indicated for pure red cell aplasia but would be used for aplastic anemia, a diagnosis that can be eliminated in this patient by her normal white cell and platelet counts.

5
Disorders of Heme Synthesis

Emmanuel C. Besa

I. INTRODUCTION. Hemoglobin, the oxygen-carrying component of red cells, is composed of globin and the iron-containing heme compound protoporphyrin. **A defective hemoglobin synthesis** that reduces hemoglobin production **can result in microcytic, hypochromic red cells** (smaller than normal and deficient in hemoglobin) **and eventually anemia** (a low total red cell production). In this chapter, a brief overview of heme and globin synthesis is followed by a discussion of the major defects that result in the microcytic, hypochromic type of anemias. A discussion of the structure and function of hemoglobin appears in Ch 9.

II. HEME

A. Composition. Porphyrins are compounds that contain the **porphin structure:** four pyrrole molecules connected by methine bridges (=CH=) in a ring conformation. The complex molecule **heme is composed of a porphin structure with an iron molecule at its center** (Figure 5-1).

B. Function. There are two main functions of heme.

1. **Heme is the oxygen-carrying component of hemoglobin.**
2. **Heme is an electron carrier** for a variety of enzymes that catalyze oxidation–reduction reactions.

C. Synthesis. The synthesis of heme is a multistep process (see VII), part of which, including the incorporation of iron, **occurs in the mitochondria of erythroid precursor cells** as they mature into red cells (Figure 5-2). Therefore, heme cannot be fully synthesized in mature cells that lack mitochondria, such as erythrocytes.

III. IRON METABOLISM. Iron in the body is used primarily for the synthesis of hemoglobin, and normal erythropoiesis requires 20–25 mg of iron per day.

A. Iron compartmentalization in the body. Most of the iron in the body is in the form of **hemoglobin** (2 g, or 67%); the rest is stored as **ferritin or hemosiderin** (1 g, or 27%), is found in **myoglobin** (0.1 g, or 3.5%), and is found in the **labile pool** or is in transport, **bound to transferrin** (0.09 g, or 3%).

B. Requirements for exogenous iron. The body conserves iron efficiently: Almost all iron required for red cell production is acquired through the recycling of iron extracted from senescent red cells. Only 5% of the iron needed for erythropoiesis, or 1 mg/day, is absorbed from the gastrointestinal tract to balance the losses from feces, urine, sweat, and desquamated skin.

C. Iron absorption

1. **Absorption sites.** The entire gastrointestinal tract is capable of absorbing iron, but maximal absorption occurs in the **duodenum and upper jejunum,** where the acidic gastric juice reduces insoluble ferric iron to its soluble ferrous state. The factors that affect iron absorption are shown in Table 5-1.
2. **Absorption regulation.** The intestinal mucosal cells are involved in a physiologic mechanism that regulates the body's intake of iron. The level of the body's iron stores is apparent by the cytoplasmic iron concentration.

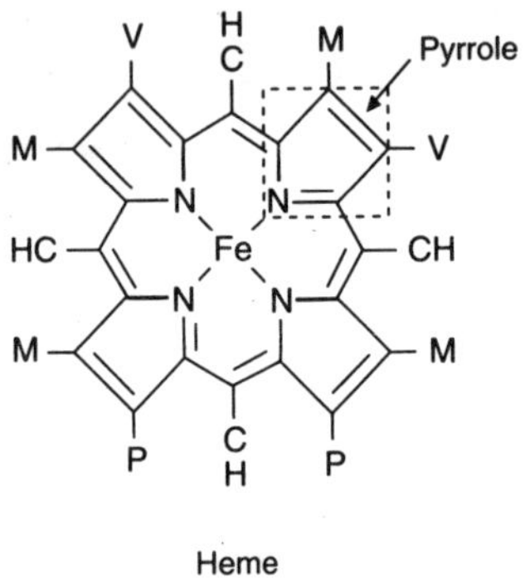

Figure 5-1. A heme molecule is composed of four molecules of pyrrole bound in a ring conformation that contains an atom of iron at its center. Various substituents attach to the periphery of the ring. *M* = CH_3; *V* = vinyl–CH=CH_2; *P* = propionyl–CH_2CH_2COOH; *N* = nitrogen.

a. **When the body's store of iron is high, mucosal cells:**
   (1) **Decrease absorption.** Mucosal cells prevent the absorption of excess iron by maintaining a high iron concentration in their cytoplasm that acts as a barrier to the passage of more iron from the intestinal lumen into the plasma.
   (2) **Increase excretion.** Mucosal cells, along with their iron store, are constantly being shed into the lumen to keep the mucosa in a state of renewal and aid in the excretion of excess iron.

b. **When the body's store of iron is low,** the low concentration of iron in the cytoplasm of the mucosal cell allows iron to pass from the intestinal lumen to the plasma. However, the mucosal cells continue to regulate the flow of this passage: The cytoplasmic concentration of recently ingested iron in the mucosa acts as a temporary barrier to the passage of iron. This effect lasts for several hours.

D. **Iron transport.** There are two mechanisms of iron transport.

1. **Pinocytosis.** Erythroid precursors absorb iron from the macrophage through the process of pinocytosis.

2. **Transferrin transport.** Transferrin, **the principal means for moving iron,** is a transport protein with two iron-binding sites. Transferrin picks up iron from the mucosal cells of the intestine and delivers it to receptors on the surfaces of nucleated erythroid cells and reticulocytes; these receptors are absent from mature red cells. Macrophages then transport the iron-free transferrin back to the plasma. The amount of transferrin in the serum is measured directly as the **total iron-binding capacity (TIBC).** The TIBC is the sum of the serum iron and the **unsaturated serum iron-binding capacity (UIBC).**

E. **Iron storage.** Iron is stored in two different configurations.

Table 5-1. Factors that Influence Iron Absorption

Increase Iron Absorption	Decrease Iron Absorption
Acids	Alkalis
Hydrochloric acid (HCl)	Antacids
Vitamin C	Pancreatic secretions
Inorganic iron	Organic iron
Ferrous iron (Fe^{2+})	Ferric iron (Fe^{3+})
Agents that solubilize iron	Agents that precipitate iron
Sugars	Phytates, tea
Amino acids	Phosphates
Iron deficiency	Excess iron
Increased demand	Decreased utilization
Pregnancy, infancy, adolescence	Infections
Hemolysis or bleeding	Inflammation
Primary hemochromatosis	Gastrectomy
	Achlorhydria
	Intestinal mucosal abnormalities

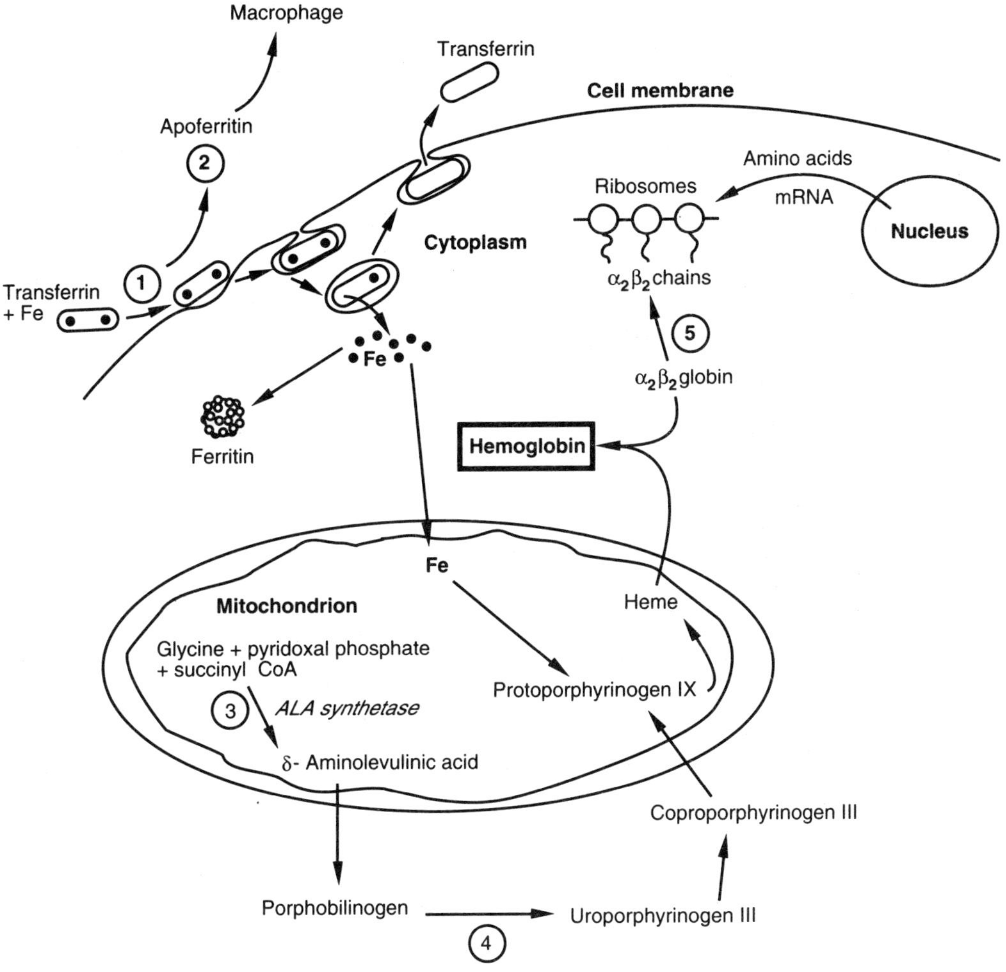

Figure 5-2. Hemoglobin is synthesized in the cytoplasm and mitochondria of erythroid precursor cells. Several important steps in synthesis occur in the mitochondria, including the δ-aminolevulinic acid synthetase (*ALA synthetase*) reaction. ALA synthetase is the rate-limiting enzyme in heme synthesis. Disruption at various points in the synthetic pathway result in (*1*) iron deficiency anemia, (*2*) anemia of chronic disease, (*3*) sideroblastic anemia, (*4*) porphyria and lead intoxication, and (*5*) thalassemia. (Adapted from Hoffbrand AV, Pettit JE: *Essential Haemotology,* 2nd edition. Oxford, Blackwell Scientific, 1984, p 9.)

1. **Ferritin** is a water-soluble micelle of iron, hydroxyl ions, and oxygen combined within a shell composed of the protein **apoferritin**. Each micelle can accommodate more than 4000 atoms of iron. Because macrophages trap iron in such a concentrated form, **macrophages facilitate the transfer of iron by endocytosis** from transferrin to erythroid precursor cells, the transferrin serving as a cytosolic transport protein.

2. **Hemosiderin** is an insoluble, amorphous **aggregate of ferritin molecules that have been stripped of apoferritin** and further compressed. Hemosiderin iron is less accessible for hemoglobin synthesis than iron stored in ferritin.

F. **Metabolic pathway of iron.** Iron metabolism is a highly efficient, closed loop in which little essential iron is lost and, consequently, little exogenous iron is required. The efficient salvage of iron proceeds as follows.

1. **Phagocytic macrophages** in the liver, spleen, and bone marrow **take up senescent red cells** that have completed their 120-day life span. **Hemoglobin is broken down** into its constituents, **and iron is stored** as ferritin and hemosiderin.

2. **Erythroid precursors** in the marrow develop around the macrophages and **take up the ferritin** from these nurse cells by phagocytosis. The most recently stored iron is exchanged first.

3. **Macrophages** in the marrow and spleen **remove excess ferritin and hemosiderin** from red cells.

4. **Transferrin mediates iron transport** from macrophages and intestinal mucosa **to immature erythroid cells and delivery for storage** in the liver and other parenchymal cells.

IV. IRON DEFICIENCY ANEMIA

A. **Etiology.** Iron deficiency anemia is **the most common anemia.** Its effects range from the simple depletion of iron stores to severe iron deficiency, and it can cause significant tissue changes. The causes of iron deficiency are listed in Table 5-2; the major causes (listed in decreasing order of frequency) are chronic blood loss, increased iron requirement, iron malabsorption, and inadequate dietary intake.

1. **Chronic blood loss.** The **most common causes of iron deficiency in adults** are occult bleeding from the gastrointestinal tract and blood loss caused by menstruation or pregnancy, including birth.
   a. **Gastrointestinal bleeding.** Occult blood loss from the gastrointestinal tract can be chronic without displaying any symptoms and may go undetected until the patient presents with symptoms of anemia. As a result, malignancy is often not discovered until the advanced stages; therefore, the finding of occult blood in the stools should immediately initiate an investigation for the cause of the blood loss. Gastrointestinal tract bleeding may also have benign causes (see Table 5-2).
   b. **Uterine bleeding.** Menstrual bleeding is the **most common cause of iron deficiency in women**. Although the amount of blood lost during each menstrual cycle varies markedly, the average is about 45 ml, which represents about **25 mg of iron lost each month**. Thus, the dietary iron requirement for menstruating women is about 1 mg/day higher than for men.
   c. **Other sources of bleeding.** Rarely, a patient may present with chronic blood loss that results from hematuria or hemoglobinuria or may expectorate bloody sputum as a result of pulmonary hemosiderosis.

2. **Increases in the physiologic requirement for iron.** Certain normal physiologic states are associated with marked increases in the requirements for iron that exceed the amounts of iron normally available in the diet. These requirements cause a negative iron balance unless the diet is supplemented.
   a. **Infancy.** In the infant, iron deficiency usually results from an unsupplemented diet of milk that is not capable of providing enough iron for erythropoiesis.
   b. **Adolescence.** In the adolescent, iron deficiency is apt to result from the increased demands during periods of increased growth. In female adolescents, iron deficiency can also result from the onset of menstruation.
   c. **Pregnancy and lactation.** Although menstruation ceases during pregnancy, there is an increased demand for iron because of fetal growth and an increased maternal red cell mass. During pregnancy, a mother requires 400 mg of iron to compensate for maternal red cell increment, fetal and placental growth demand another 400 mg of iron, and blood loss during delivery requires an additional 300 mg of iron, amounting to a total iron demand during pregnancy of 1100 mg. Another 30 mg of iron may be required during each month of lactation.

3. **Iron malabsorption.** Iron deficiency may result from two absorption deficiencies.
   a. **Malabsorption syndromes** such as adult celiac disease and tropical and nontropical sprue can interfere with iron absorption when the iron-absorbing mucosal cells of the duodenum are damaged.
   b. **Subtotal gastrectomy.** As a result of subtotal gastrectomy, gastric acid may not be available for converting insoluble dietary ferric iron to the soluble ferrous form that can be absorbed and transported rapidly through the duodenum.

4. **Inadequate iron intake.** In developed countries, it is quite uncommon for the intake of dietary iron to be deficient in adult men and postmenopausal women in the absence of other causative factors. However, the poor food quality and largely vegetarian diet in many underdeveloped

Table 5-2. Causes of Iron Deficiency

- **Chronic blood loss**
  - **Uterine blood loss:** menstrual losses and blood loss related to pregnancy and delivery
  - **Gastrointestinal blood loss**
    - **Benign conditions**
      - Peptic ulcers (gastric or duodenal)
      - Esophageal varices
      - Hiatal hernia
      - Colonic diverticula or polyps
      - Hemorrhoids
      - Chronic aspirin use
      - Long-distance running that induces mild diffuse gastrointestinal bleeding
      - Hereditary hemorrhagic telangiectasia
      - Parasites (e.g., hookworm)
    - **Malignancy**
      - Colon and colorectal carcinoma
      - Gastric carcinoma
      - Esophageal carcinoma
      - Small intestinal carcinoma
  - **Pulmonary**
    - Hemosiderosis
  - **Urinary tract**
    - Hypernephroma
    - Bladder and collecting system carcinoma
    - Paroxysmal nocturnal hemoglobinuria
- **Increased iron requirement**
  - **Periods of rapid growth**
    - Infancy
    - Adolescence
  - **Pregnancy and lactation**
- **Iron malabsorption**
  - **Intestinal mucosal disorders**
    - Celiac disease
    - Tropical and nontropical sprue
  - **Subtotal gastrectomy:** multiple mechanisms lead to iron deficiency
    - Rapid transit through the duodenum
    - Achlorhydria, absence of sufficient gastric acid to convert ferric iron to the ferrous form that is soluble and easier to absorb
    - Perioperative blood loss
    - Occult bleeding secondary to recurrent ulceration
    - Decreased iron in postgastrectomy diet
- **Poor diet**

countries may result in deficiency when the patient's condition is compounded by hookworm infestation, repeated pregnancy, and prolonged lactation.

B. Clinical manifestations

1. **Stages of iron deficiency**
   a. **Depletion of tissue iron.** A negative iron balance in an individual causes the mechanisms that preserve the levels of iron in the serum and red cells to progressively deplete tissue iron stores. This depletion is made evident by the following.
      (1) **Reduced levels of ferritin and hemosiderin in tissue macrophages.** These signal depleted tissue iron stores.
      (2) **Reduced levels of serum ferritin.** Serum ferritin is often a reliable reflection of the amount of iron in tissue macrophages, except in patients who have an underlying tumor or a damaged liver that secretes ferritin into the serum.

(3) **Reduced levels of iron in bone marrow macrophages.** Bone marrow aspirates or biopsy specimens stained with Prussian blue will not display as many of the characteristic blue granules as seen when iron stores in the reticuloendothelial macrophages are at normal levels.

b. **Certain changes in serum iron** are indicative of depleted iron stores.

(1) Serum iron levels are usually low **when tissue stores are depleted**. However, measurements of serum iron fluctuate depending on what the patient ate before the blood sample was drawn. Serum levels usually reflect the current absorption of iron from the gastrointestinal tract.

(2) **As the level of serum iron declines** and the amount of unsaturated transferrin increases, the TIBC increases.

c. **Progressive anemia.** If depletion of the iron stores continues, anemia predictably worsens.

(1) **Initially, normochromic, normocytic anemia develops.** The conversion of free protoporphyrin to heme ceases, which impairs hemoglobin synthesis. Therefore, the marrow conserves its dwindling iron store by producing fewer red cells, each with an adequate amount of hemoglobin.

(2) **Eventually, hypochromic, microcytic anemia results** from the reduced mean corpuscular hemoglobin (MCH) and reduced mean corpuscular volume (MCV) caused by the continued depletion of iron stores. Variations in red cell size and shape are usually present as is an increasing red cell distribution width (RDW).

(3) **Finally, tissue changes occur** as a result of the gradually decreased intracellular levels of iron-dependent enzymes caused by prolonged iron depletion.

2. **Symptoms of iron deficiency**

a. **Symptoms and signs pertaining to anemia**

(1) **Nonspecific symptoms** include fatigue, weakness, shortness of breath, and symptoms of congestive heart failure.

(2) **Signs** include pallor, tachycardia, unexplained retinal hemorrhages (in severe and acute-onset anemia), and splenomegaly (in a minority of cases).

b. **Symptoms and signs specific to iron deficiency**

(1) **Atrophic changes in the epithelium** are the most pronounced features of iron deficiency and result from the reduced levels of heme-containing enzymes such as cytochrome c, succinic dehydrogenase, catalase, peroxidase, ribonucleotide reductase, xanthine oxidase, and aconitase. These features fall into three categories:

(a) **Oral lesions,** including **angular cheilosis** (soreness and cracking in the corners of the lips), **atrophy of the tongue papillae with intermittent glossitis,** and **stomatitis** (inflammation and soreness of the tongue and mouth)

(b) **Dysphagia** in middle-aged women caused by postcricoid esophageal webbing (called **Plummer-Vinson syndrome** when it is associated with nail changes)

(c) **Nail lesions** that characteristically begin as a flattening and thinning of the nails and progress to brittle and spoon-shaped nails (**koilonychia**)

(2) **Pica,** the compulsive ingestion of nonnutritive substances, is a symptom specific to iron deficiency that is related to epithelial changes and **may actually contribute to the iron deficiency**.

(a) **In children,** pica often manifests as a craving for and ingestion of clay, dirt, or paint (which often leads to lead intoxication).

(b) **In adults,** pica is expressed as a desire to eat ice (pagophagia), clay, or laundry starch. The latter two substances actually bind dietary iron and prevent its absorption.

C. **Diagnosis. Iron deficiency rarely presents as severe and uncomplicated anemia** with the classic findings of hypochromic, microcytic red cells on blood smear. Rather, **borderline or mild cases of anemia are more often the rule** and are more difficult to diagnose. In addition, several disorders must be excluded in the differential diagnosis.

1. **Laboratory studies**

a. **Peripheral blood findings**

(1) **Red cell indices** will reflect the amount of hemoglobin in the red cells and will vary with the severity and duration of the anemia. In the initial stages of iron deficiency, red cells may display normal indices (see IV B 1 c) with hemoglobin levels of 9–12 g/dl. In general, **an iron-deficient patient with a hemoglobin level below 9 g/dl will display:**

(a) **A low MCV** (55–74 fl)
(b) **A low MCH** (25–30 g/dl)
(c) **An increased RDW** (>16) as determined by an automated blood counting system (see Ch 1 II B 1 c), reflecting the marked variations in the sizes and shapes of the red cells

(2) **Peripheral blood smears** will reveal signs of iron deficiency. Early stages of deficiency will be associated with fairly normal red cell morphology. **In more advanced stages of iron deficiency, the following will be noted.**
(a) **Microcytic, hypochromic red cells**
(b) **Poikilocytes,** which are abnormally shaped erythrocytes such as codocytes, spherostomatocytes, and dacrocytes (see Table 1-1), and **anisocytosis,** which is an excessive variation in the size of erythrocytes in the blood

(3) **Blood counts** will display:
(a) Characteristically, **normal or low reticulocyte counts**
(b) Occasionally, **increased platelet counts** (some cases may exceed 1 million but normalize upon iron replacement)

b. **Serum iron studies**
(1) **The level of serum iron is usually low or normal,** depending on what the patient ate before the measurement was made and the absorption of iron [see III C and IV B 1 b (1)].
(2) **TIBC is usually above 400 μg/dl, and the transferrin saturation is reduced below 15%.**
(3) **The level of serum ferritin is below 12 ng/ml** (normal levels are 40–340 ng/ml in males and 14–150 ng/ml in females). However, the serum ferritin level can be increased by several underlying diseases (gastrointestinal malignancy, lymphoma, and liver cell damage) that can mask the effect of iron deficiency.

c. **Bone marrow studies** are generally not needed to establish a diagnosis of iron deficiency, but the test may be helpful in the differential diagnosis. Characteristic findings include:
(1) **Tissue paper normoblasts,** which have insufficient amounts of cytoplasm and hemoglobin when viewed using Wright's stain
(2) The absence or near absence of both normoblasts and reticuloendothelial iron in macrophages when the sample is subjected to Perls' test

2. **Therapeutic trials.** In addition to laboratory studies, iron deficiency can be diagnosed through a trial of oral iron replacement with careful follow-up to determine if the anemia is improving or responding to therapy. **If the diagnosis of iron deficiency is correct, a characteristic series of changes indicating a positive iron balance will be observed:**
a. **Tissue replacement** with symptomatic improvement of glossitis
b. **Increased hemoglobin level in new red cells** that results in a normal MCV and MCH
c. **Reticulocytosis** that appears within 7 to 10 days
d. **Normal hemoglobin level in mature erythrocytes**
e. **Replacement of iron stores** (i.e., normalization of serum ferritin, which usually takes about 6 months of therapy)

D. **Differential diagnosis. The other causes of hypochromic, microcytic anemia comprise the major differential diagnosis** for iron deficiency, since treatment is quite different in each condition. These conditions can be differentiated from each other by the use of other special tests (see Ch 10 I D 2).

E. **Treatment.** Iron deficiency is not a disease but rather the consequence of the patient's pathologic or physiologic condition. Therefore, **the approach to the patient with iron deficiency is to:**

1. **Determine the cause of iron deficiency or the source of bleeding,** if any.
a. **Analyze stools** for occult blood to determine if there is gastrointestinal tract bleeding; this analysis should be performed three times to avoid missing intermittent blood loss.
b. **Perform a radiologic analysis** of the upper and lower gastrointestinal tract to identify any occult malignancies.
c. **Conduct a urinalysis** for hematuria or hemoglobinuria.
d. **Inspect for pulmonary hemosiderosis** by chest X-ray.
e. **Perform a pelvic examination** in women.

2. **Treat the underlying cause if it is reversible.**

3. **Initiate iron replacement therapy.** Although the patient should be encouraged to maintain a well-balanced diet, proper diet alone is not sufficient for iron replacement in iron deficiency. Iron replacement can take one of two forms:
   a. **Oral iron therapy,** which is preferred for the initial treatment of iron deficiency
      (1) **Preparations**
         (a) **Ferrous sulfate** is the least expensive and best absorbed form of iron therapy, yielding the most elemental iron absorbed per gram administered.
         (b) **Ferrous gluconate and fumarate** have fewer intestinal side effects because they yield less elemental iron absorbed per gram of iron salt in the preparation; they are administered to patients who cannot tolerate ferrous sulfate.
         (c) **Slow-release forms** of iron are generally poorly absorbed.
      (2) **Dosage.** The adult dosage of ferrous sulfate is typically 300 mg/day and is gradually increased to 900 mg/day if tolerated.
      (3) **Adverse effects.** The most common side effects are gastrointestinal irritation and intolerance, including nausea, cramping, and diarrhea. These side effects are related to the amount of elemental iron released from the salt in the intestinal tract and can be minimized by adjusting the dose or changing the preparation administered.
   b. **Parenteral iron therapy**
      (1) **Indications.** Parenteral iron therapy is indicated when the patient:
         (a) Cannot tolerate the side effects of oral therapy
         (b) Suffers from inflammatory bowel disease or peptic ulcer
         (c) Does not comply with prescribed dosages
         (d) Displays documented iron malabsorption
         (e) Suffers from a condition such as hereditary hemorrhagic telangiectasia in which the rapid loss of iron from continuous slow bleeding cannot be compensated by oral iron therapy
      (2) **Preparations**
         (a) **Intramuscular injection of iron dextran (Imferon)** is the preferred route of parenteral iron therapy. However, the patient is at risk for a hypersensitivity reaction (anaphylaxis) to the dextran and for permanent skin discoloration at the injection site. The latter can be avoided by using the Z technique of intramuscular injection: The skin is pulled to one side, the iron dextran is injected, and the skin is allowed to fall back into place, preventing leakage under the skin.
         (b) **Intravenous injection of iron can rapidly replete iron stores,** but its hazards are of sufficient concern that it should be used as little as possible.
         (c) **Transfusion of whole blood or packed red cells is generally not indicated** unless a rapid increase in the hematocrit is critical to the patient because of the risks of hepatitis, acquired immune deficiency syndrome (AIDS), and congestive heart failure resulting from volume overload.

4. **Maintain iron replacement therapy** beyond the point where the anemia is corrected for a period of usually 6 months in order to replenish depleted stores of iron.

5. **Monitor the patient response** to iron replacement therapy. **A failure to respond should suggest the following:**
   a. **An incorrect diagnosis**
   b. **Continued loss of iron,** which is usually due to continued blood loss (e.g., in hereditary hemorrhagic telangiectasia, which can be treated by either local cautery of bleeding sites or estrogen therapy)
   c. The presence of a **chronic infection or inflammation** that is suppressing bone marrow activity
   d. **Lack of patient compliance** with dosage schedule
   e. **Ineffective release of iron** from a sustained-release preparation into the duodenum, where absorption should occur
   f. **Malabsorption of iron**

V. HEMOCHROMATOSIS

A. **Definition. The accumulation of high levels of storage iron** (ferritin and hemosiderin) in macrophages, hepatocytes, pancreatic tissue, and cardiac muscle tissue may cause potentially fatal tissue damage. An arbitrary distinction has been made in the amount of iron that is accumulated.

1. **Hemosiderosis** is the term applied to **a modest increase in iron stores.**
2. **Hemochromatosis** is the term applied to **a substantial increase in iron stores that requires therapeutic intervention.**

B. Etiology. There are two major causes of hemochromatosis.

1. **Chronic transfusion therapy.** Patients with refractory anemias, and other forms of anemia for which there are no specific therapies, will chronically require transfusions of red cells to maintain comfortable hemoglobin levels. These **patients receive 250 mg of iron with each unit of blood** every 2–4 weeks; **they are unable to eliminate iron at an equivalent pace** and will accumulate a tremendous amount of iron over time.
2. **Hereditary hemochromatosis.** Increased levels of iron storage for which no underlying cause can be demonstrated can be attributed to the autosomal recessive inheritance of hemochromatosis. A mutant gene on the short arm of chromosome 6 is expressed as an **increased rate of gastrointestinal absorption of iron** that, in time, results in the accumulation of large amounts of storage iron.

C. Clinical features. Hemochromatosis manifests as tissue damage caused by the accumulation of excessive iron and is classified by organ system.

1. **Cardiac manifestations.** Damage to cardiac muscle is manifested as **abnormal electrical conduction and reduced cardiac muscle strength**. The patient with cardiac damage presents with abnormal cardiac rhythms and signs and symptoms of congestive heart failure that frequently give a clinical picture of generalized cardiomyopathy. This condition is refractory to standard treatment; more than half of the patients with hemochromatosis die of cardiac complications.
2. **Hepatic damage.** The excessive storage of iron may damage liver cells, leading to cirrhosis and liver failure that result in enlargement of the liver and spleen and portal hypertension. Hepatoma is a frequent consequence of this liver damage. In alcoholics with liver cirrhosis, the excessive storage of iron is exacerbated by the consumption of dark red wine, which is rich in iron.
3. **Endocrine manifestations.** Iron accumulation in the pancreatic isles, pituitary gland, and adrenal glands can lead to the development of diabetes mellitus, hypogonadism, and adrenal insufficiency.
4. **Other complications.** Storage iron overload can result in the increased pigmentation of the skin caused by increased levels of dermal melanin, not hemosiderin, giving the patient a bronze-colored skin. Some forms of arthritis that typically affect the joints of the hands are also observed.

D. Diagnosis. Hemochromatosis is diagnosed in a patient with so-called **bronze diabetes displaying the following test results**:

1. **Liver iron stores** of 3 to 4+, on a scale of 0 to 4+ (>5.6 mg/g dry weight), which is the best indicator
2. **Serum iron concentration** above 180 μg/dl and transferrin saturation of 60% or greater
3. **Serum ferritin level** above 1000 ng/ml, which is a useful but less sensitive indicator

E. Treatment. The **removal of excess iron** reverses cardiac and liver abnormalities and substantially prolongs life. Unfortunately, **diabetes is often irreversible, and hepatomas are refractory** to any effective treatment. It is important to investigate asymptomatic family members of patients who present with hereditary hemochromatosis and to treat affected individuals before tissue damage occurs. Hemochromatosis is treated by removing the excess iron through either:

1. **Chelation**
   a. **Mechanism of action.** Chelators are molecules that possess several metal-binding sites that allow the agent to **complex tightly with free iron;** the complex is subsequently excreted from the body.
   b. **Administration. Deferoxamine is the chelating agent of choice;** it is administered continuously by **subcutaneous pump** since only about 0.01% of the total iron stores is available for complexing at any one time. Chelators can be administered on an outpatient basis through the utilization of portable pumps. Chelation therapy is ideal for the treatment of patients who cannot undergo phlebotomy. When iron stores reach normal levels, maintenance therapy that relies on less frequent administration can be initiated.

2. **Phlebotomy** is a very effective means of **removing 250 mg of iron per unit of blood in nonanemic patients.**

VI. ANEMIA OF CHRONIC DISEASE (ACD)
is a common type of anemia that occurs in patients who present with any of several chronic inflammatory and malignant diseases. ACD is often a contributing factor in the chronic anemias of complex origin that are associated with liver or renal insufficiency or that appear after extensive trauma or surgery.

A. Mechanisms of action.
ACD results from several mechanisms.

1. **Relative iron deficiency.** A relative deficiency of iron is created by the action of two proteins.
   a. **Apolactoferrin** is an iron-binding protein that is released into the bloodstream by phagocytes in response to inflammation. Apolactoferrin **short-circuits the metabolic pathway of iron utilization by stripping iron from circulating transferrin and returning it to the mononuclear phagocytes,** which then reconvert the iron to ferritin and hemosiderin. Reticulocytes are thus deprived of valuable iron despite increased storage levels in the marrow.
   b. **Interleukin-1 (IL-1)** is released by monocytes and macrophages at sites of inflammation. IL-1 **causes fever and stimulates the increased retention of iron by macrophages,** thereby limiting the amount of iron available for bacterial growth and, unfortunately, also limiting the amount available for erythropoiesis.
2. **Shortened red cell life span.** A modest shortening of the life span of red cells **from 120 days to 60–90 days** is seen in chronic disease. The red cells in these patients are normal, and normal red cells transfused from healthy donors will have a similarly shortened survival. The mechanism for this shortened life span is unknown.
3. **Relative bone marrow failure.** The average patient with ACD has been shown to have **serum erythropoietin (EPO) levels that are lower than the levels in non-ACD anemic patients**. This lower serum EPO level is thought to contribute to a bone marrow failure that is defined as relative because it is not due to any of the bone marrow failure syndromes (see Ch 3 II) or myelodysplastic syndromes (see Ch 3 IV). However, half of ACD patients have adequate levels of EPO, indicating that other factors may be involved in their marrow failure.

B. Etiology.
Several clinical conditions are associated with ACD, including many chronic infections, connective tissue disorders, and malignant tumors.

1. **Chronic infectious inflammatory diseases** associated with ACD include tuberculosis, pneumonia, bacterial endocarditis, and osteomyelitis.
2. **Chronic noninfectious inflammatory diseases** causing ACD include sarcoidosis, systemic lupus erythematosus (SLE), and rheumatoid arthritis.
3. **Malignancies** involved in the pathogenesis of ACD are carcinoma, lymphoma, and sarcoma.

C. Clinical features.
ACD usually develops slowly over a period of 6 weeks or more. The hematocrit gradually falls to a new level and remains there, establishing a new steady state.

1. **Hematocrit** of **25%–35% is typical;** about 5% of patients have a hematocrit below 20%, which could be an indication that there is another cause for the anemia, such as blood loss.
2. **Most patients have normocytic anemia with normal MCV;** 30% of patients have **microcytic, hypochromic anemia with low MCV** (70–80 fl, which is mild).
3. **RDW is normal,** indicating a uniformity of red cell shape and size.
4. **White cell and platelet counts are normal.**

D. Diagnosis.
Establishment of a diagnosis of ACD is usually based on confirmation of more than one of the following in the absence of a more obvious cause:

1. **Chronic inflammatory disease or malignancy**
2. **Low or normal level of serum iron in association with a decreased TIBC** (TIBC is increased in iron deficiency) **and a transferrin saturation of less than 15%**
3. **A normal or increased level of serum ferritin** (intestinal carcinomas and lymphomas can cause ACD and may secrete ferritin)

4. **Abundant hemosiderin** appearing as coarse granules (>5 μm) in marrow macrophages observed after bone marrow smears are stained with Prussian blue

E. **Treatment.** The anemia in ACD is usually mild, slow to develop, and asymptomatic. The anemia **does not respond to iron therapy** despite the low serum iron; however, it is usually reversed when the underlying disease is ameliorated or eliminated.

VII. HEME SYNTHESIS.

The biosynthesis of heme is a straightforward process that culminates in the addition of iron to porphyrin in the mitochondria of erythrocyte precursors. There are three major steps in this synthesis (see Figure 5-2).

A. **Synthesis of δ-aminolevulinic acid (ALA).** ALA, the five-carbon building block of heme, is produced by the action of the enzyme **ALA synthetase,** which **joins glycine and succinyl coenzyme A (succinyl CoA)** end to end. This synthesis requires **pyridoxal phosphate,** the active form of pyridoxine (vitamin B_6), which is of clinical importance in the therapy for hereditary sideroblastic anemia [see IX B 1 b (1)].

B. **Synthesis of tetrapyrroles.** This synthesis occurs in the cytoplasm in two steps.

1. Two molecules of ALA are condensed to form the monopyrrole **porphobilinogen (PBG)** in a reaction catalyzed by **PBG synthetase.**
2. Four molecules of PBG are condensed to form the tetrapyrrole **uroporphyrinogen III (UROGEN III)** in a single step catalyzed by **PBG deaminase,** which removes a molecule of ammonia from each molecule of PBG during the condensation and cosynthesis.

C. **Synthesis of heme.** Heme is formed from the synthesis of protoporphyrin and addition of iron in three successive steps.

1. CO_2 molecules are cleaved from the acetate side chains of uroporphyrinogen III to produce **coproporphyrinogen III (COPROGEN III).**
2. Two nonadjacent propionate side chains of coproporphyrinogen III are oxidized by the removal of two or more molecules of CO_2, producing **protoporphyrinogen IX (PROTOGEN IX).**
3. The protoporphyrinogen IX ring is oxidized to **protoporphyrin IX (PROTO IX),** and the enzyme **ferrochelatase** catalyzes the insertion of an iron atom into the center of the porphyrin ring, forming heme.

VIII. PORPHYRIA

A. **Definition.** Porphyria is a metabolic condition in which a **deficiency of enzymes specific to the synthesis of heme** causes a decreased heme production. This biosynthetic blockage **results in the accumulation of intermediate porphyrins** (most notably ALA) and their subsequent increased rate of excretion. Heme synthesis is usually controlled by a feedback mechanism by which the end product, heme, inhibits the action of the rate-limiting enzyme (ALA synthetase) of the synthetic reaction. The initial lack of heme causes the unchecked production of porphyrin intermediates until their accumulation eventually pushes heme synthesis back toward normal. However, **the accumulation of porphyrin intermediates is toxic and causes the clinical manifestations of porphyria.**

B. **Classification and description.** The classification of porphyria **depends on the intermediate metabolite that is in excess,** which is itself determined by the restriction point in the porphyrin synthesis pathway created by the enzyme deficiency. There are two types of porphyria: hereditary and acquired (Figure 5-3).

1. **Hereditary porphyrias**
   a. **Definition.** Hereditary porphyria is an autosomal dominant condition: Its symptoms are in evidence in a patient who displays only a 50% reduction in enzyme activity.
   b. **Classification**
      (1) **Acute intermittent porphyria (AIP)** results in the accumulation of both ALA and PBG because of a deficiency of PBG deaminase (see VII B 2).

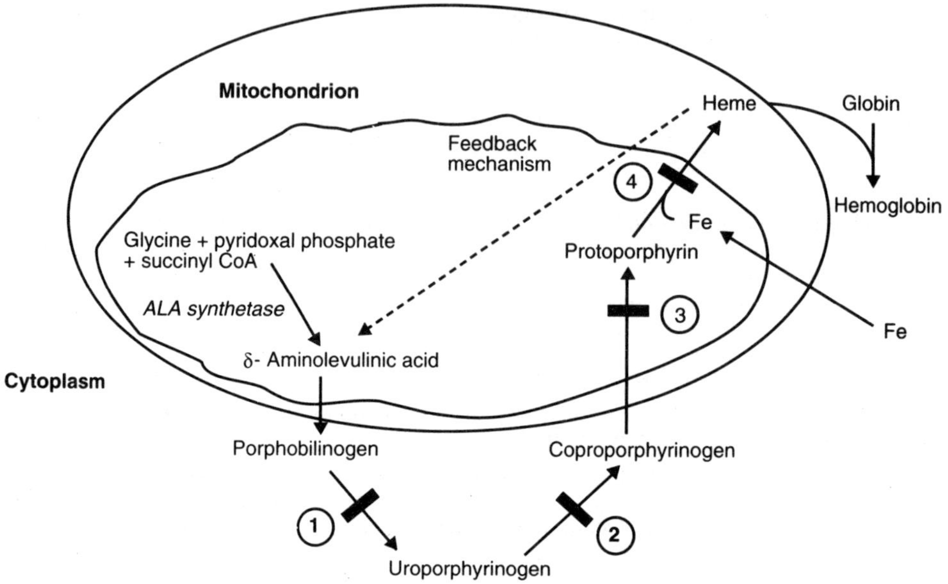

Figure 5-3. Pathophysiology of hereditary porphyria. The *dashed arrow* shows normal heme synthesis; the *numbers* indicate possible sites of blockage in the biosynthetic pathway. Intermediate porphyrins [porphobilinogen (*1*), uroporphyrinogen (*2*), coproporphyrinogen (*3*), protoporphyrinogen (*4*)] accumulate because of the blockage, and decreased heme synthesis compromises the feedback mechanism, further aggravating the condition. The accumulation of intermediates pushes heme synthesis back toward normal, but the resulting toxicity causes the signs and symptoms of porphyria. *ALA synthetase* = δ-aminolevulinic acid synthetase; *Fe* = iron; *succinyl CoA* = succinyl coenzyme A.

(a) **Etiology.** The following **precipitating factors** can trigger an attack of AIP:
  (i) **Menses**
  (ii) **Infection**
  (iii) **Acidosis**
  (iv) **Drugs** that can induce the formation of hepatic drug-metabolizing enzymes such as cytochrome P_{450} **(e.g., barbiturates, birth control pills)**

(b) **Clinical features.** AIP is identified by the **neurotoxicity caused by the accumulation of PBG,** which mimics a neurotransmitter, **causing neurologic abnormalities in different areas of the central and peripheral nervous system**.
  (i) In the **cerebral cortex,** PBG causes **psychosis and convulsions.**
  (ii) In the **brain stem,** PBG causes **disordered thermoregulation and disordered blood pressure control.**
  (iii) In the **autonomic nervous system,** PBG causes **abdominal and pelvic pain.**
  (iv) In the **peripheral nerves,** PBG causes **paralysis and neuropathy.**

(2) **Porphyria cutanea tarda** results in the **accumulation of uroporphyrinogen III** because of the reduced activity of uroporphyrinogen decarboxylase (see VII B 2).
  (a) **Etiology.** The precise cause of porphyria cutanea tarda is not known and often there is no family history of disease; however, liver damage in alcoholics leading to cirrhosis contributes to the severity of the disease.
  (b) **Clinical features.** The accumulation and deposition of porphyrin intermediates in the skin leads to **photosensitivity, the major clinical feature**. The exposed areas of the skin such as the hands and face are affected, and the damage may cause scarring, irregular pigmentation, and hair growth.

(3) **Other porphyrias** have been identified according to other enzyme deficiencies in the heme synthesis pathway; their clinical and laboratory features are listed in Table 5-3.
(a) Hereditary coproporphyria
(b) Variegate porphyria
(c) Erythropoietic protoporphyria
(d) Erythropoietic porphyria

2. **Acquired porphyrias** are the result of intoxication by environmental pollutants, primarily lead and hexachlorobenzene.
a. **Lead intoxication. Lead inhibits the activity of ALA synthetase, heme synthetase,** and other enzymes. Initially, this increases the amounts of ALA and red cell protoporphyrin in the urine and eventually increases the amount of urinary coproporphyrin (see X).
b. **Hexachlorobenzene toxicity. Hexachlorobenzene inhibits uroporphyrinogen decarboxylase;** thus, it mimics porphyria cutanea tarda: Affected individuals will be photosensitive and will pass red urine.

C. **Diagnosis** of any porphyria is made by **demonstrating the appropriate porphyrin precursors in the urine and stools**. Porphyria is usually suggested as a differential diagnosis in patients with recurrent, ill-defined abdominal pain for which no cause could be found in previous workups. Patients with this complaint or with the characteristic skin manifestations and family history should undergo the following laboratory tests to confirm the diagnosis.

1. **Watson-Schwartz screening test.** Porphyrinogen in freshly voided urine will oxidize when exposed to air for a few hours, coloring the urine a deep red.

2. **Urine, stool, and red cell analysis.** The specific porphyria can be identified through the analysis of porphyrin precursors present in the urine and stools. Accumulation in red cells can be detected by fluorescence microscopy.

D. **Treatment**

1. **AIP**
a. **Initiate the following therapies during an attack.**
(1) **Administer heme (hematin) intravenously** to decrease the level of PBG. The heme will inhibit the heme synthesis pathway by stimulating the feedback mechanism.
(2) **Administer phenothiazines.** Phenothiazines appear to antagonize the effects of PBG on the nervous system.
b. **Advise the patient to take the following actions between attacks.**
(1) **Avoid precipitating factors** [see VIII B 1 b (1) (a)] as much as possible.
(2) **Eat a high-carbohydrate diet** to help prevent acidosis.

Table 5-3. The Porphyrias and Their Manifestations

			Clinical Manifestations	
Porphyria	**Enzyme Deficiency**	**Porphyrin Excreted**	**Photosensitivity**	**Neurovisceral Symptoms**
Acute intermittent porphyria	HMB synthase	ALA, PBG	−	+
Porphyria cutanea tarda	URO decarboxylase	URO, COPRO	+	−
Hereditary coproporphyria	COPRO oxidase	ALA, PBG, COPRO	+	+
Variegate porphyria	PROTO oxidase	ALA, PBG, COPRO, PROTO	+	+
Congenital erythropoietic protoporphyria	URO synthase	URO, COPRO	+ + +	−
Erythropoietic protoporphyria	Ferrochelatase	PROTO	+	−

ALA = aminolevulenic acid; COPRO = coproporphyrin; HMB = hydroxymethylbilane; PBG = porphobilinogen; PROTO = protoporphyrinogen; URO = uroporphyrinogen. (Adapted from Desnick RJ, Anderson KE: Heme Biosynthesis and Its Disorders: the Porphyrias and Sideroblastic Anemias. In *Hematology Basic Principles and Practice*. Edited by Hoffman R, Benz EJ Jr, Shattil SJ, et al. New York, Churchill LIvingston, 1991, p 353.)

2. **Porphyria cutanea tarda. Phlebotomy** is used to remove excess iron from the liver. This relieves the inhibition of uroporphyrinogen decarboxylase, permitting the porphyrin precursors to return to their normal levels, and helps reduce the feedback inhibition of heme synthesis.

3. **Other porphyrias.** Patients diagnosed as having other porphyrias and presenting with photosensitivity should be advised to avoid sunlight and should undergo phlebotomy to remove excess iron from the liver.

IX. SIDEROBLASTIC ANEMIAS

A. Definition. The sideroblastic anemias are a diverse group of disorders with various clinical manifestations caused by the blockage of heme synthesis at the early level of ALA participation. All of these anemias can be identified by the following characteristics:

1. **Ringed sideroblasts in the bone marrow,** which are erythroblasts that display rings of Prussian blue-staining granules around their nuclei

2. **Decreased levels of porphyrins without accumulations of pyrroles,** which are characteristic for the porphyrias

3. **Excess stores of iron in the mitochondria**

B. Classification

1. **Hereditary sideroblastic anemia** is a very uncommon, **sex-linked, recessive, inherited disorder** transmitted by females and expressed in males. Rarely has this disorder been autosomally linked.
   a. **Clinical features.** Hereditary sideroblastic anemia **manifests during adolescence** with the following features:
      (1) Mild to moderate anemia and low MCV
      (2) Hepatosplenomegaly
      (3) Signs and symptoms of iron overload or hemochromatosis
   b. **Treatment**
      (1) Clinical trials of high-dosage vitamin B_6 therapy (300 mg/day of pyridoxine or its active form pyridoxal phosphate) have had limited success but are the preferred therapy.
      (2) Therapeutic phlebotomy or iron chelation may be indicated.

2. **Acquired sideroblastic anemia** may be primary, related to the myelodysplastic syndromes, or secondary to exposure to toxic drugs or agents.
   a. **Primary acquired sideroblastic anemia** is primarily a disease of the elderly.
      (1) **Clinical features**
         (a) **Blood** sampling reveals **both normochromic and hypochromic** (to varying degrees) populations of red cells that may be associated with **abnormal platelet and white blood cell counts** and are usually associated with an **increased MCV**.
         (b) **Bone marrow** sampling reveals **increased populations of early myeloid cells or megaloblastoid cells or dysplastic changes; nonrandom chromosomal abnormalities** may be detected.
      (2) **Treatment.** Primary acquired sideroblastic anemias are **usually refractory to treatment;** the following therapies have been tried with little success:
         (a) Folic acid or vitamin B_{12}
         (b) Pyridoxine
         (c) Androgens
         (d) Splenectomy, which may precipitate an acute thrombocytosis (platelet count > 1 million) with increased risk of thromboembolism
         (e) Adrenocorticosteroids
         (f) Supportive therapy with transfusions
      (3) **Prognosis. The patient usually succumbs to complications of cytopenia** such as heart failure, infections, or bleeding **or to complications of transfusion such as iron overload, or the disease transforms into acute leukemia**.
   b. **Secondary acquired sideroblastic anemia** can result from exposure to the following agents:
      (1) Drugs that interfere with pyridoxine, such as **isoniazid**

(2) Drugs that inhibit heme synthesis, such as **azathioprine and chloramphenicol**
(3) Drugs that induce the myelodysplastic syndrome over time, such as **alkylating agents,** in particular, melphalan and the nitrosoureas
(4) Agents directly toxic to the mitochondria, such as **alcohol** (however, the anemia that results from exposure to these agents is transient, reversing rapidly upon withdrawal of the toxin)

X. LEAD POISONING.

Lead inhibits enzymes, including ALA synthetase, that catalyze steps in the synthesis of heme. Lead poisoning can present with symptoms common to both porphyria and sideroblastic anemia.

A. Clinical manifestations

1. **Symptoms common to porphyria** include abdominal pain and motor neuropathy.
2. The **feature shared with sideroblastic anemia** is the formation of ringed sideroblasts in the bone marrow.
3. **Features that distinguish lead poisoning** from other disorders of heme formation include:
   a. **Normal levels of PBG** in the urine
   b. **No photosensitivity** (the protoporphyrins are bound to hemoglobin and do not pass to the skin)
   c. **Prominent neurologic abnormalities and psychoses** (e.g., patients with acute poisoning can present with acute encephalopathy with increased intracranial pressure, papilledema, and coma)
   d. **Renal failure, hypertension, and gout**
   e. **Presence of the so-called lead line** in patients with poor oral hygiene (a bluish black deposit at the gingival margin that is diagnostic for lead and other heavy metal poisoning)

B. Diagnosis.

The possibility of lead poisoning should be considered for any patients at increased risk of exposure: painters working in old buildings, battery factory workers, children living in old homes who may be ingesting flakes of lead-based paint. The following laboratory test results will confirm a diagnosis of lead poisoning:

1. **Microcytic, hypochromic anemia with basophilic stippling** (see Table 1-1)
2. **Sideroblastic bone marrow changes**
3. **Elevated levels of serum iron and red cell porphyrins**
4. **The presence of ALA and coproporphyrin,** but not PBG, in the urine
5. **Elevated levels of lead** in the serum or urine

C. Treatment

1. **Eliminate the source of exposure**
2. **Administer chelating agents** to remove excess levels of lead from the tissues and to promote urinary excretion of lead (see V E 1)

STUDY QUESTIONS

Directions: Each of the numbered items or incomplete statements in this section is followed by answers or by completions of the statement. Select the **one** lettered answer or completion that is **best** in each case.

1. Iron deficiency can develop in all of the following clinical conditions EXCEPT

(A) nontropical sprue
(B) excessive menstrual flow
(C) bacterial endocarditis
(D) occult colonic carcinoma
(E) pulmonary hemosiderosis

2. A 58-year-old woman who complains of easy fatigue and weakness is found to be mildly anemic, presenting with a hemoglobin level of 10 g/dl and ferritin of 16 ng/dl. Of the following courses of management, which one is best suited to this patient?

(A) Encourage the maintenance of a well-balanced diet and monitor the anemia
(B) Prescribe oral ferrous sulfate for 6 months to replace iron stores
(C) Prescribe sustained-release iron capsules to avoid gastrointestinal discomfort and help ensure patient compliance
(D) Order bone marrow studies to identify iron deficiency as the source of the anemia
(E) Order stool analysis to detect the presence of occult blood

3. Normal or increased bone marrow iron stores are found in all of the following forms of hypochromic, microcytic anemia EXCEPT

(A) anemia caused by lead intoxication
(B) sideroblastic anemia
(C) iron deficiency anemia
(D) anemia associated with rheumatoid arthritis

Directions: Each item below contains four suggested answers, of which **one or more** is correct. Choose the answer

A if **1, 2, and 3** are correct
B if **1 and 3** are correct
C if **2 and 4** are correct
D if **4** is correct
E if **1, 2, 3, and 4** are correct

4. Failure of a microcytic anemia to respond to oral iron replacement may be due to

(1) presence of an inflammatory bowel condition
(2) malabsorption of iron
(3) continued blood loss
(4) sustained-release iron preparation

5. Causes of anemia of chronic disease (ACD) include which of the following?

(1) Uncomplicated diabetes mellitus
(2) Tuberculosis
(3) Hypertension
(4) Rheumatoid arthritis

1-C
2-E
3-C
4-E
5-C

6. Prussian blue staining may demonstrate ringed sideroblasts in a bone marrow sample from which of the following patients?

(1) A painter being treated for lead intoxication
(2) A patient on isoniazid (INH) therapy for tuberculosis
(3) An alcoholic who was recently on a binge
(4) A patient with osteomyelitis

7. True statements regarding porphyria include which of the following?

(1) The neurologic manifestations of porphyria are the result of the accumulation of porphobilinogen
(2) Lead intoxication mimics porphyria because of the photosensitization that results from the accumulation of protoporphyrins in the skin
(3) Porphyria should be considered in the differential diagnosis of ill-defined, recurrent abdominal pains when previous workups and laparotomy have had negative findings
(4) All forms of porphyria are inherited

8. True statements regarding sideroblastic anemias include which of the following?

(1) Alkylating agents such as melphalan and nitrosoureas can induce a refractory anemia with ringed sideroblasts (RARS) that is usually preleukemic
(2) Most primary sideroblastic anemias respond to high doses of pyridoxine
(3) The inhibition of heme synthesis by drugs such as azathioprine and chloramphenicol can cause sideroblastic anemia
(4) Most primary acquired sideroblastic anemias occur in the young patient

9. Chronic lead poisoning can be manifested clinically by which of the following? It can

(1) induce acute leukemia
(2) cause bluish-black deposits to form in the gingiva
(3) cause macrocytic, hyperchromic anemia
(4) increase levels of ALA in the urine and cause sideroblastic bone marrow changes

6-A
7-B
8-B
9-C

ANSWERS AND EXPLANATIONS

1. The answer is C *[IV A 1; Table 5-2].*
Iron deficiency does not develop in bacterial endocarditis. Iron stores can be depleted by nontropical sprue, excessive menstrual flow, occult colonic carcinoma, and pulmonary hemosiderosis. Bacterial endocarditis and other chronic diseases that cause anemia are characterized by the increased storage of iron in the bone marrow but poor iron reutilization. Iron stores can be depleted by three mechanisms: inadequate iron intake (as in infants who are fed an unsupplemented diet of milk), iron malabsorption (as in patients with tropical or nontropical sprue), and chronic occult blood loss (as in cases of excessive menstrual bleeding, occult gastrointestinal bleeding in colonic carcinoma, or increased blood loss through the respiratory tract in pulmonary hemosiderosis).

2. The answer is E *[IV E 1 a].*
The best course of action to take in the management of this woman is to order stool analysis to detect the presence of occult blood. Although it is important to replace iron stores in an iron-deficient patient, it is more important to identify and treat the underlying cause of the deficiency. This is especially true for older patients in whom iron deficiency may be the presenting sign of a more serious disorder, most commonly occult gastrointestinal bleeding and malignancy. Therefore, stool analysis to detect the presence of occult blood is the best course of action in the management of this 58-year-old woman. Iron replacement should also be instituted, preferably with oral ferrous sulfate, since it contains 60 mg of elemental iron in each 300 mg tablet, is well absorbed, and is inexpensive. Administration of sustained-release forms of oral iron should not be the first choice for the management since they are not well absorbed. Bone marrow studies may be required at some point in the patient management, but they should not be used as the first step in determining the cause of the iron deficiency. Diet alone cannot supply enough iron to replace deficient stores.

3. The answer is C *[IV A, IX A 3, X B 3].*
Normal or increased bone marrow stores are not found in iron deficiency anemia. The basic defect in hypochromic, microcytic anemia is a quantitative reduction in the synthesis of hemoglobin, which ultimately results in the production of red cells with reduced hemoglobin contents. Disorders of hemoglobin synthesis may involve either the heme component or the globin component. In iron deficiency, there are insufficient marrow iron stores for optimal heme synthesis, which results in hypochromic anemia. In lead poisoning, heme synthesis is impaired by the presence of lead, which inhibits the activity of certain critical enzymes; however, iron stores in the bone marrow are abundant. Sideroblastic anemia refers to a diverse group of disorders that all have impaired heme synthesis; the ultimate result is hypochromic anemia and iron loading. Anemia of chronic diseases such as rheumatoid arthritis is associated with increased iron storage with impaired iron reutilization for heme synthesis.

4. The answer is E (all) *[IV A 3, E 5].*
A patient may not respond to iron therapy for several reasons. The presence of an underlying chronic disease is the most common cause of a patient's failure to respond to iron therapy. Patients who do not absorb iron well may also have a malabsorption syndrome or subtotal gastrectomy, in which an insufficient amount of gastric acid interferes with the conversion of iron from the dietary to soluble form. Oral iron therapy may not be sufficient to replace the iron lost through the continued bleeding that occurs in such conditions as hereditary telangiectasia. Sustained-release iron preparations may be prescribed to avoid the gastrointestinal discomfort often associated with oral iron therapy. However, not enough iron may be available in the duodenum, where absorption should occur.

5. The answer is C (2 and 4) *[VI B 1 a, b].*
Anemia of chronic disease (ACD) can be caused by both tuberculosis and rheumatoid arthritis, which are inflammatory diseases in which there are activated macrophages in the reticuloendothelial system. This activation stimulates the secretion of apolactoferrin, an iron-binding protein found in phagocytic cells, into the circulation. Apolactoferrin promotes both the removal of circulating ferritin and the formation of hemosiderin, the storage form of iron. Iron stored as hemosiderin is less accessible for the synthesis of hemoglobin in erythroid cell precursors. Patients with diabetes mellitus may be highly susceptible to infections, but there is no underlying activation of the phagocytic cells. Hypertension is also not considered an inflammatory disease, and no relationship to ACD has been noted.

6. The answer is A (1, 2, 3) *[IX B 2 b; X B 2].*
Causes of secondary acquired sideroblastic anemias include lead intoxication, which interferes with the synthesis of porphyrin at the level of aminolevulinic acid synthetase (ALA synthetase), isoniazid, which interferes with pyridoxine, and alcohol, which is directly toxic to the erythroblast mitochondria. Osteomyelitis is a chronic disease that can increase the level of hemosiderin in the bone marrow but does not induce the formation of the pathologic ringed sideroblasts.

7. The answer is B (1 and 3) *[VIII B 1 b, 2, C; X A 3 b].*
Acute intermittent porphyria (AIP) results from the accumulation of porphobilinogen (PBG), which behaves as a neurotransmitter, interfering with central nervous system (CNS) and peripheral nervous system functions. Porphyria is usually suggested in the differential diagnosis of recurrent, ill-defined abdominal pain in patients for whom no cause could be found in previous workups. Lead intoxication will increase the levels of protoporphyrins in red cells, but these are bound to hemoglobin and do not pass to the skin. Thus, there is no photosensitization in lead intoxication. AIP and porphyria cutanea tarda are inherited forms of porphyria, but lead toxicity and hexachlorobenzene toxicity are acquired forms.

8. The answer is B (1 and 3) *[IX B 2].*
A secondary cause of acquired sideroblastic anemia are the alkylating agents that are indications of a phase preceding transformation to acute leukemia. Other drugs that inhibit protein and heme synthesis are azathioprine and chloramphenicol; the effects of azathioprine are dose dependent and reversible, in contrast to the idiosyncratic aplastic anemia that results from chloramphenicol administration. The majority of primary sideroblastic anemias are acquired, occur in the elderly, and are unresponsive to pyridoxine.

9. The answer is C (2 and 4) *[X A].*
Lead poisoning mimics porphyria and sideroblastic anemia; patients present with the accumulation of porphyrin and sideroblasts among other symptoms. The induced sideroblastic form is not preleukemic. Patients with poor oral hygiene may present with abnormal bluish black deposits (so-called lead lines) at the gingival margins.

6
Anemias Associated with DNA Synthesis

Emmanuel C. Besa

I. INTRODUCTION. There is a high turnover rate of cells in certain tissues in the body due to normal wear or damage; in particular, hematopoietic tissue and the epithelial lining of the gastrointestinal tract are involved. The rapid turnover of cells sensitizes the tissues to deficiencies of factors involved in DNA synthesis, such as vitamin B_{12} and folate.

II. PHYSIOLOGY OF NUCLEAR MATURATION. Nuclear maturation is **dependent on DNA synthesis**. DNA synthesis can occur by the **de novo pathway (DNA replication)** through deoxyuridine and by the **salvage pathway (excision and repair)** through thymidine (Figure 6-1). Folate and vitamin B_{12} are the two important vitamins involved in the salvage pathway.

A. Structure and function of folate (Figure 6-2). **Folic acid** (pteroylglutamic acid) **is the active form of folate**.

1. **Structure.** Folic acid consists of three parts (see Figure 6-2A):
   a. Pteridine double ring
   b. *p*-Aminobenzoic acid
   c. L-Glutamic acid

2. **Formation.** Folic acid is a monoglutamate that is formed by the reduction of dietary polyglutamic folic acid as it is digested in the small bowel and absorbed by the microvilli (see Figure 6-2B).

3. **Activity.** Only the reduced forms of folic acid are active as coenzymes. Folic acid is reduced in the presence of dihydrofolate reductase through the stepwise addition of four hydrogen atoms at positions 5, 6, 7, and 8 to form **tetrahydrofolate (THF)**.

4. **Dietary requirements and sources.** The average adult requires 100 μg/day of folate. Foods rich in the polyglutamate form of folate are **green vegetables** such as asparagus, broccoli, spinach, lettuce, and green beans. Cooking destroys the non–protein-bound folates in vegetables. The average daily diet contains 400–600 μg of available folate.

5. **Storage.** The total amount of folate acid stored in the liver is small—6–10 mg in the normal person. Consequently, only 2–3 months of dietary deprivation exhausts the body stores of folate and the signs and symptoms of folate deficiency develop.

6. **Absorption and transport.** The proximal jejunum is the primary site of folate absorption, which proceeds as follows.
   a. **Ingested polyglutamic folic acid undergoes enzymatic deconjugation** in the microvilli of the small intestine to the monoglutamate, diglutamate, and triglutamate forms that are then absorbed into the cells.
   b. Within the cells, a substantial amount of **monoglutamate folate is reduced and methylated**.
   c. The resultant **5-methyltetrahydrofolate (5-methyl THF) emerges in the mesenteric circulation** and is the only form of folate found in the circulation. It is loosely bound to albumin. The laboratory value of serum folate normally ranges from 5 to 20 ng/ml.

7. **Function.** Folate functions as a coenzyme in purine and pyrimidine synthesis by acting as a donor of single-carbon units, such as methyl, methylene, and formyl groups. The units are attached to nitrogens in position 5 or 10, or in both positions, of the purine or pyrimidine model.

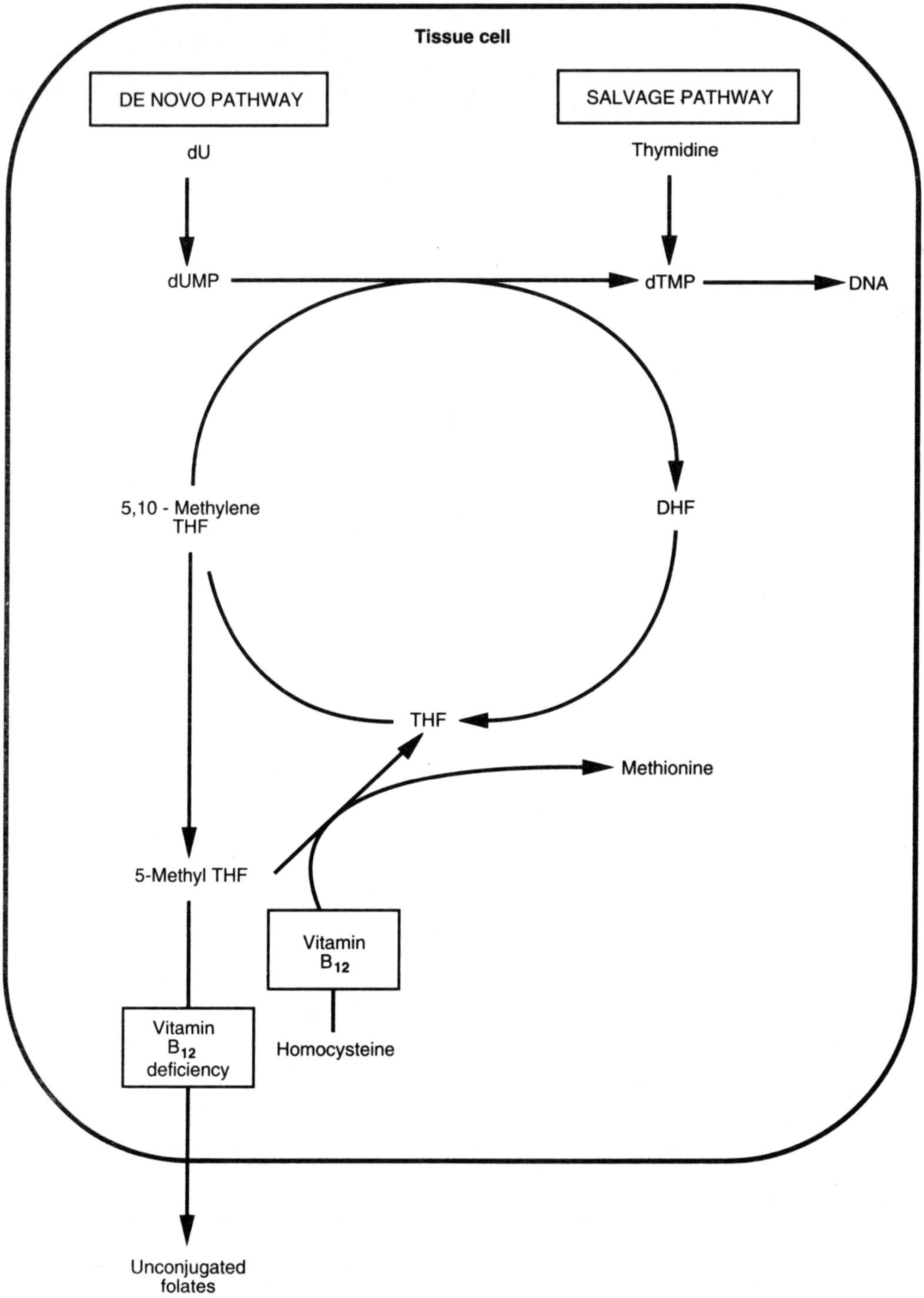

Figure 6-1. The de novo and salvage pathways for DNA synthesis. Folate and deoxythymidine monophosphate (*dTMP*) are important in "salvaging" DNA and helping to replace the uridylate form. During this transfer of a one-carbon fragment from methylene tetrahydrofolate (*THF*) to deoxyuridine monophosphate (*dUMP*), the folate is oxidized from THF to the metabolically inert dihydrofolate (*DHF*), which is reduced to the active form of THF by dihydrofolate reductase. Vitamin B_{12} is important in keeping the active THF form of folate from leaking out of tissue cells by facilitating its conjugation by demethylation. In vitamin B_{12} deficiency, folate is "trapped" in the unconjugated form and leaves the cells without contributing to the DNA synthesis. *dU* = deoxyuridine.

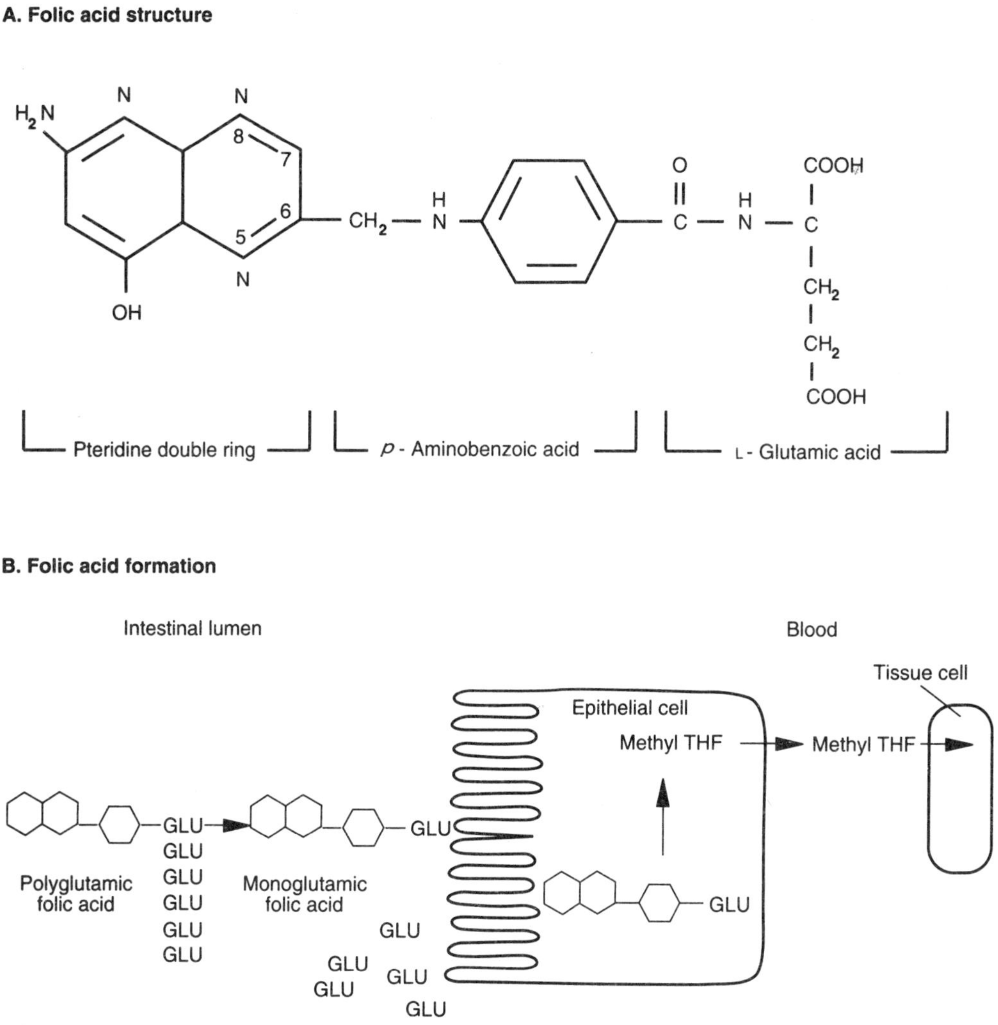

Figure 6-2. (*A*) There are three parts to the folic acid molecule: a pteridine double ring, *p*-aminobenzoic acid, and L-glutamic acid. (*B*) Folate is transformed in the intestinal tract from polyglutamic acid to monoglutamic acid to enable the molecule to enter intestinal epithelial cells for absorption. The folic acid is then converted to methyltetrahydrofolate (methyl *THF*) inside the cell and is transported in its active form via the bloodstream into tissue cells for use in DNA synthesis.

B. Structure and function of vitamin B_{12}

1. **Structure.** The three parts of vitamin B_{12} (cobalamin) are shown in Figure 6-3.
   a. A **porphyrin structure** with a cobalt atom at the center is called the **corrin ring**.
   b. A unique nucleotide base is connected to the corrin ring and is bonded to the cobalt atom through a nitrogen atom.
   c. **A β group,** which determines the form of the molecule, is attached to the cobalt atom from the nucleotide.

2. **Absorption and transport**
   a. **Dietary sources and requirements.** Vitamin B_{12} is found primarily in foods containing **animal protein,** such as meat, fish, eggs, and milk, although ultimately it is derived from microbial synthesis in the gastrointestinal tract.
      (1) The normal daily requirement is 1 μg/day.
      (2) A normal diet provides 5–7 μg/day of vitamin B_{12}; a strict vegetarian diet usually provides none.

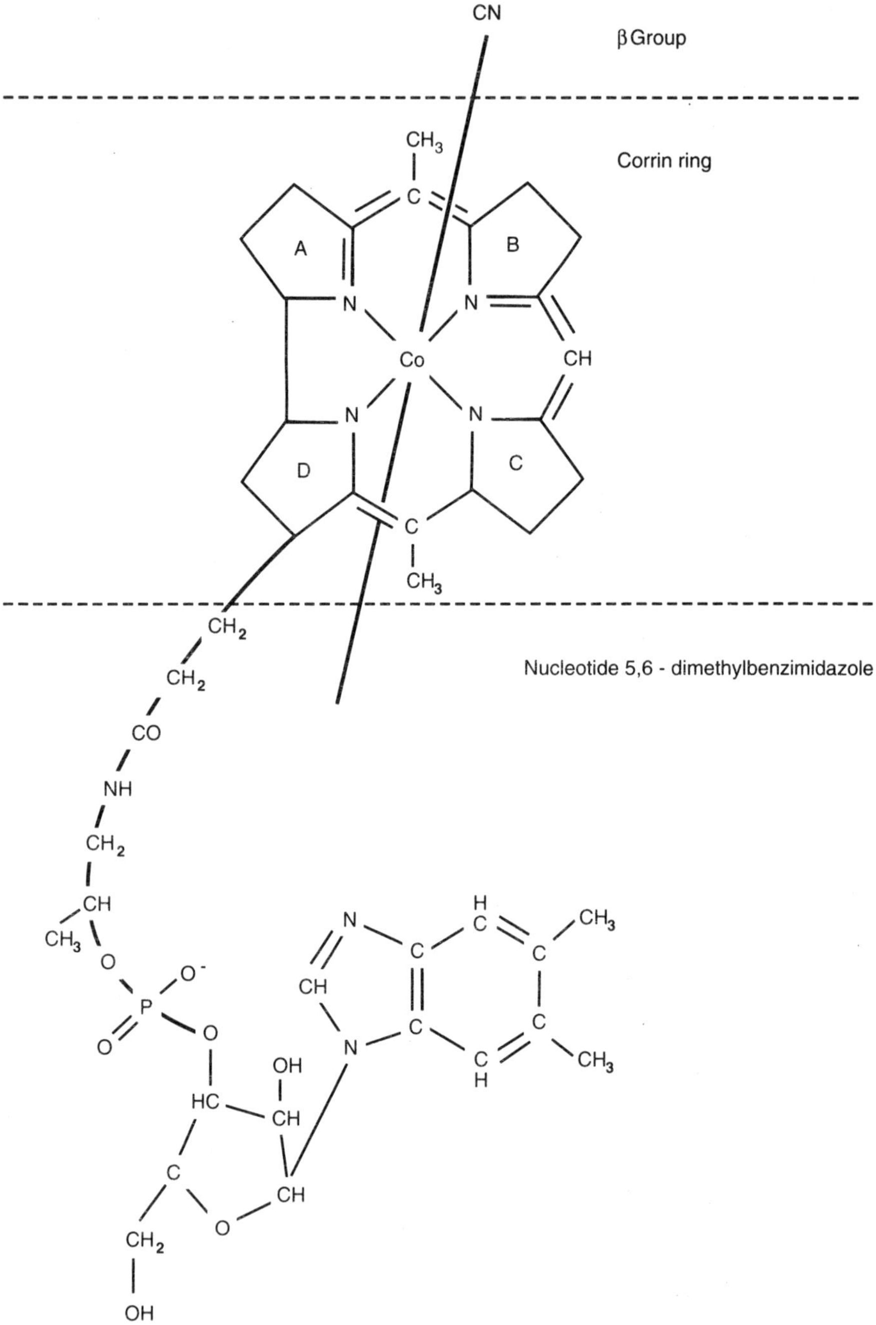

Figure 6-3. Cyanocobalamin structure. Cyanocobalamin is composed of three parts: the β group, the corrin ring, and the nucleotide base. The β group determines the form; that is, cyano- (*CN*), methyl- (*CH_3*), or adenosylcyanocobalamin. *CO* = cobalt.

(3) About 2–5 mg are stored in the liver, the major storage site.
(4) If no vitamin B_{12} is being supplied because of diet or malabsorption, a net loss of 1–3 μg/day will ensue, which will develop into a vitamin B_{12} deficiency in 2 to 12 years.

b. Absorption of vitamin B_{12} (the extrinsic factor) [Figure 6-4] is **dependent on intrinsic factor,** a glycoprotein produced by the parietal cells in the gastric mucosa that binds vitamin B_{12} tightly from foods. Intrinsic factor is crucial to the utilization of vitamin B_{12}; **lack of intrinsic factor will result in megaloblastic anemia and disease. Intrinsic factor functions as follows.**
(1) Intrinsic factor binds with vitamin B_{12} on a mole-for-mole basis and protects it from enzymatic degradation as the complex travels the length of the intestinal tract.
(2) The intrinsic factor–vitamin B_{12} complex attaches to specific receptors on the microvilli of the distal 3–4 ft of the ileum, the major absorptive site, where it is taken up by endocytosis. Intrinsic factor is then removed, but it is not known if this occurs at the cell surface or inside the cell.

c. Transport
(1) Transcobalamin (TC II), which does not contain carbohydrate, is the crucial carrier protein for vitamin B_{12}. A lack of TC II causes megaloblastic anemia and disease.
(a) TC II carries vitamin B_{12} from the intestinal epithelial cells to the target tissues of the liver (for storage) or to the bone marrow (for DNA synthesis).
(b) TC II is produced in the epithelial cells involved in vitamin B_{12} absorption, and it is destroyed by lysosomes in the target cells in the liver and bone marrow.
(c) Serum TC II is measured indirectly from total serum vitamin B_{12} and the vitamin B_{12} binding capacity.
(2) **Rapid electrophoretic mobility (R) binders,** which are other carrier proteins for vitamin B_{12}, are found in plasma and in other body fluids, such as the saliva. Examples of R binders are TC I and TC III, whose functions are not known since complete absence in the plasma and cells does not result in any abnormalities.

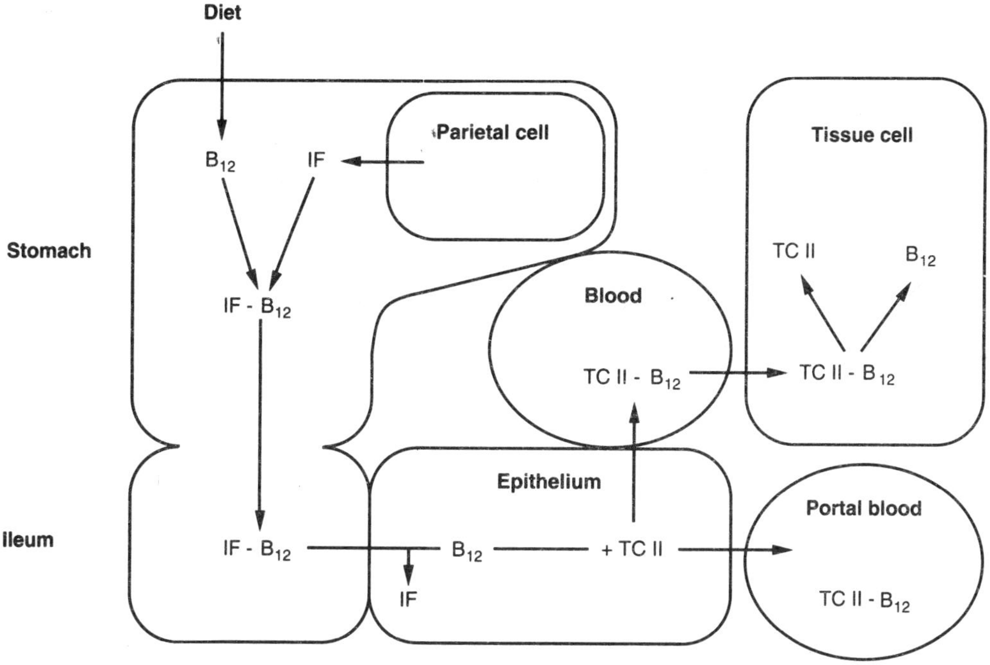

Figure 6-4. Absorption of vitamin B_{12}. Cobalamin (vitamin B_{12}) in the stomach binds to intrinsic factor (*IF*), which protects B_{12} from destruction by enzymes and enables the complex to enter ileal epithelial cells through receptors on the mucosal cells. Vitamin B_{12} binds to a new carrier, transcobalamin II (*TC II*), in the epithelial cell and is released into the bloodstream. The TC II–B_{12} complex then attaches to receptors on the surface of tissue cells, which take up the complex. Vitamin B_{12} is released from the complex so it can be used by the cells in metabolism.

C. Interaction of folate and vitamin B_{12}

1. **Active form of vitamin B_{12}.** Vitamin B_{12} is important in the synthesis of DNA, especially in the form of methylcobalamin. The tissue forms of cobalamins are hydroxycobalamin and cyanocobalamin, which are converted to the coenzyme-active forms of methylcobalamin and adenosylcobalamin.

2. **Folate trap hypothesis.** The function of vitamin B_{12} is believed to be closely related to that of folic acid, since the ability of the cell to use active 5-methyl THF is related to its ability to keep, or "trap," the folate inside the cell. This is achieved by vitamin B_{12} converting the folate from a small monoglutamate to a larger polyglutamate form to prevent its escape into the extracellular space.

3. **Effect of vitamin B_{12} on folate**
   a. **Vitamin B_{12} is required for the demethylation** of folate that has been taken up by the cell, **allowing it then to be conjugated** (i.e., supplied with a polyglutamate tail), a reaction that prevents the folate from leaking out of the cell. When deficient, the 5,10-methylene derivative of THF causes DNA synthesis to decrease because the conversion of deoxyuridylate to thymidylate decreases.
   b. **Vitamin B_{12} deficiency prevents the cells from retaining folate** because demethylation becomes impaired, resulting in defective conjugation, **with the following consequences:**
      (1) Elevated levels of 5-methyl THF
      (2) Decreased levels of intracellular polyglutamate folate caused by increased leakage of solute from the cell

III. MEGALOBLASTIC ANEMIA

A. Introduction

1. Megaloblastic anemia is a descriptive term that refers to the **abnormal changes in blood cell formation** that demonstrate a nuclear and cytoplasmic maturation dissociation in all myeloid and erythroid cell lines, **leading to macrocytic anemia and varying degrees of pancytopenia**.

2. This abnormality affects all cells that have a rapid turnover, such as the gastrointestinal mucosal cells and epidermal cells.

3. Megaloblastic anemia is the **result of abnormal DNA synthesis** because of a single or combined deficiency of folate or vitamin B_{12}.

B. Hematologic changes.
Certain hematologic changes are evident in megaloblastic anemia and are the **result of nuclear maturation that is delayed compared with cytoplasmic development**. These changes manifest as the following.

1. **Bone marrow changes.** A nucleus–cytoplasm dissociation is evident in all cell lines and results in:
   a. **Erythroid cell changes,** such as the appearance of **megaloblasts** (macrocytic erythroblasts), karyorrhexis and fragments such as **Howell-Jolly bodies** (bluish black oval fragments of nuclear material), and **Cabot's rings** (ring forms or figures of eight in red cells)
   b. **Myeloid cell changes,** such as the appearance of **large band forms and hypersegmentation** of polymorphonuclear cells

2. **Ineffective erythropoiesis.** Erythropoiesis becomes ineffective because of an increased rate of intramarrow death of red cells and the premature destruction of defective red cells in the circulation. This may possibly affect granulopoiesis and thrombopoiesis and cause mild pancytopenia. Elevation of lactate dehydrogenase (LDH) and bilirubin levels reflects the high marrow cellular turnover.

3. **Peripheral blood cell changes**
   a. **Red cells** appear as macrocytic ovalocytes. The mean corpuscular volume (MCV) is increased and the reticulocyte count is low. As the anemia worsens, a marked poikilocytosis with red cell fragmentation occurs.
   b. **Leukocytes** display increases in cell size. The number of lobes in mature granulocytes is increased as is the number of polymorphonuclear leukocytes with six or more lobes.

C. Clinical manifestations

1. Gradual and insidious development of the progressive signs and symptoms of **anemia**

2. Pale yellow skin associated with **mild jaundice** as a result of the red cell breakdown in the bone marrow, **purpura** from thrombocytopenia, and, rarely, a reversible, widespread **melanin pigmentation**
3. **Glossitis,** presenting as a beefy, red, sore tongue, and angular stomatitis
4. **Mild malabsorption and weight loss** from the megaloblastic epithelial abnormality in the gastrointestinal tract

D. Etiology. Megaloblastic anemia [especially pernicious anemia (PA)] can result from folate deficiency or vitamin B_{12} deficiency.

1. **Folate deficiency**
   a. **Biochemical mechanism.** Folate deficiency is the result of an **abnormality in the metabolism of deoxyuridine monophosphate (dUMP)** [Figure 6-5].
      (1) Normally, dUMP is converted almost entirely to deoxythymidine monophosphate (dTMP).
      (2) In folate deficiency, the conversion to dTMP is impaired, and dUMP is converted instead to deoxyuridine triphosphate (dUTP). The following cycle is then initiated.
         (a) The intracellular level of dUTP increases, and dUTP replaces dTMP in newly synthesized DNA.
         (b) The dUTP in DNA is detected, and error-correcting mechanisms begin excising dUTP. However, these attempts are futile since the excised dUTP is replaced only with more dUTP.
   b. **Causes of folate deficiency.** There are four causes of folate deficiency (Table 6-1).
      (1) **Nutritional deficiency,** most often as a consequence of alcoholism, is caused primarily by inadequate diet, decreased hepatic folate storage, and malabsorption of folate. Factors that may contribute to a nutritional deficiency of folate include hyperalimentation, insufficient diets such as tea and toast diets in the elderly, and the simple overcooking of vegetables.

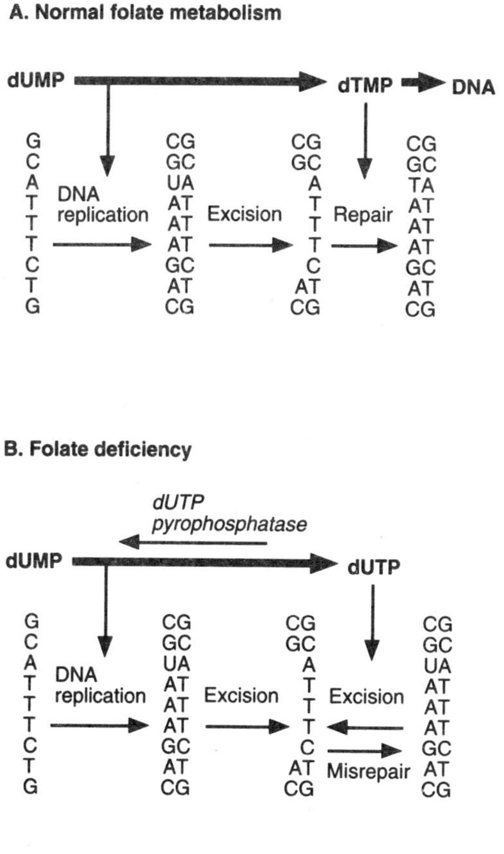

Figure 6-5. The biochemical mechanism of folate deficiency is compared with the normal pathway for DNA synthesis in the presence of folate. (*A*) In normal metabolism, deoxyuridine monophosphate (*dUMP*) is converted almost entirely to deoxythymidine monophosphate (*dTMP*). This is important for repairing and replacing the uracil for the stable thymidine form in DNA. (*B*) In folate deficiency, this conversion is impaired. As a result, deoxyuridine triphosphate (dUTP) increases intracellularly and replaces dTMP in newly synthesized DNA. This initiates a futile cycle in which uracil-containing stretches of DNA are excised by an error-correcting mechanism, only to be replaced by new uracil-containing stretches. The megaloblastic changes are the morphologic expression of this high-slippage mode of DNA replication.

Table 6-1. Causes of Folate Deficiency

Reduced intake of folate
Poor nutrition
Alcoholism
Anorexia nervosa
Hyperalimentation
Poor diet in the elderly
Malabsorption
Alcoholism
Loss of normal mucosa
Celiac and tropical sprue
Crohn's disease
Regional ileitis
Infiltration of submucosa
Intestinal lymphoma
Amyloidosis
Loss of absorbing surface through jejunal resection and shunting
Anticonvulsant drug therapy
Increased folate requirements
Pregnancy
Hemolytic anemias
Exfoliative dermatitis and psoriasis
Impaired folate utilization
Alcoholism
Administration of folate antagonists trimethoprim and methotrexate
Inborn errors of folate metabolism

(2) **Malabsorption of folate** results from:
   (a) **Loss of normal mucosa** (tropical sprue and celiac disease)
   (b) **Infiltration of the submucosa** (amyloidosis and lymphoma)
   (c) **Loss of absorptive surface** in the intestine (surgical resection or shunt)
   (d) **Administration of anticonvulsant drugs,** such as phenytoin, which is believed to result in reduced absorption of folate
(3) **Increased folate requirements** can lead to the exhaustion of folate stores when folate intake does not keep pace. This can occur in conditions such as those listed.
   (a) **Pregnancy** increases the folate requirement anywhere from fivefold to tenfold by the third trimester. The fetus is remarkably efficient in accumulating folate despite a severe deficiency in the mother.
   (b) There are increased folate requirements in **increased hematopoietic states,** such as all types of hemolytic anemias, especially those diseases that require the continuous replacement of blood such as sickle cell anemia, thalassemia syndromes, hereditary spherocytosis, paroxysmal nocturnal hemoglobinuria (PNH), and myeloproliferative disorders.
   (c) **Exfoliative skin disorders,** such as psoriasis, which is aggravated by treatment with methotrexate, have increased folate requirements.
   (d) **Neoplastic diseases,** such as carcinoma or leukemia, increase DNA synthesis. In these diseases there is preferential utilization of folate by tumor cells over host tissues. When these neoplastic diseases involve the intestinal tract, nutritional intake is reduced because of the loss of appetite and malabsorption.
(4) **Impaired cellular utilization of folate**
   (a) **Alcohol** ingested in excessive amounts will inhibit the cellular utilization of folate despite normal dietary intake and normal serum levels.
   (b) **Folate antagonists** are a group of drugs that inhibit dihydrofolate reductase (see II A 3). These drugs are used to treat cancer (methotrexate), bacterial infections (trimethoprim), and parasitic infections (pyrimethamine and pentamidine) and can cause megaloblastic pancytopenia.

c. **Diagnosis** of folate deficiency is dependent on the level of serum folate.
   (1) Normal levels in the serum range from 5 to 15 ng/ml.
   (2) A serum folate level between 3 and 5 ng/ml is inconclusive. Measurements should be

made of the level of folate in the red cells, which is more accurate and reflects the intracellular level and is not affected by the recent intake of folate in the diet.

(3) A red cell folate level below 1 ng/ml (normal > 1.9 ng/ml) is diagnostic.

d. Treatment. Irrespective of etiology, folate deficiency is treated by the **oral replacement of 1 mg/day**.

(1) Replacement therapy should be initiated before any attempts are made to determine the cause of the deficiency.

(2) Alcoholics in particular should be advised to stop drinking and should be offered help to do so since the continued ingestion of alcohol may prevent cellular uptake despite the initiation of replacement therapy.

2. Vitamin B_{12} deficiency

a. Biochemical mechanism. Vitamin B_{12} is present primarily in two coenzyme forms: methylcobalamin and the highly stable cyanocobalamin, whose ligand is a cyanide group and is the form for commercially available therapeutics. **Vitamin B_{12} deficiency results from the disturbance of two enzymatic reactions:**

(1) Methylmalonate–succinate isomerization, which is involved in the conversion of propionate to succinyl coenzyme A (CoA) and in the synthesis of myelin in the central nervous system (CNS)

(2) Methylation of homocysteine to methionine, which is involved in maintaining the active form of folate inside the cell and available for DNA synthesis

b. Causes of vitamin B_{12} deficiency. Vitamin B_{12} deficiency is the result of several causes (Table 6-2) in addition to PA, which is discussed in III D 3.

(1) Nutritional deficiency results from a vegetarian diet, since vitamin B_{12} is found only in food of animal origin.

(2) Gastrectomy syndromes can occur after a partial or total gastrectomy because of the removal of the source of intrinsic factor. Vitamin B_{12} deficiency has been observed in 10% of patients within 5 years of partial gastrectomy.

(3) Intestinal disorders can impair the absorption of the intrinsic factor–vitamin B_{12} complex because of the involvement of the mucosa of the distal ileum in such diseases as regional ileitis, tropical sprue, tuberculosis, and lymphoma of the ileum or resulting from surgical resection of the distal ileum.

(4) Parasitic infestations of organisms such as fish tapeworm (*Diphyllobothrium latum*), which is transmitted by the ingestion of raw fish, can deplete stores of vitamin B_{12} by utilizing the dietary supply as it passes through the small bowel.

Table 6-2. Known Causes of Vitamin B_{12} Deficiency

Depletion by decreased dietary intake
Vegans and vegetarians
Poor absorption
Absence of intrinsic factor
Pernicious anemia (PA)
Gastrectomy
Corrosive chemical damage to stomach epithelium
Infiltration of the stomach (by lymphoma or carcinoma)
Increased bacterial utilization of vitamin B_{12} in areas of overgrowth (blind-loop syndrome)
Gastrointestinal bypass surgery
Small bowel (jejunal) diverticula
Intestinal stasis and obstruction due to strictures
Parasitic infestation
Fish tapeworm (*Diphyllobothrium latum*)
Pathology in absorption sites
Tuberculosis of the ileum
Lymphoma of the small intestines
Tropical sprue
Regional enteritis
Others
Congenital absence of transcobalamin II (TC II) [rare]
Nitrous oxide abuse (inactivates vitamin B_{12} by oxidation of the cobalt atom)

(5) **Bacterial overgrowth** results from the development of **blind-loop syndrome** in the small intestine. The intestine fails to empty completely, allowing the overgrowth of *Escherichia coli* and other gram-negative organisms that utilize the supply of vitamin B_{12} passing through the intestine. Bacterial overgrowth can form in diverticula or as a result of strictures, jejunal surgery, or scleroderma with involvement of the intestinal tract.

3. **Pernicious anemia** is a significant cause of cobalamin deficiency, which contributes to megaloblastic anemia.
   a. **Epidemiology.** PA typically appears in late middle age, although it occasionally appears in late childhood or adolescence. There is a genetic predisposition to PA among northern Europeans, and it has been associated with age-related chronic atrophic gastritis. In the United States, it is found with equal frequency among blacks and whites. The disease tends to occur early in the black population with a preponderance among women.
   b. **Etiology.** PA is believed to be the consequence of long-standing gastritis, which leads to atrophy of all of the secretory cells of the stomach. Some indirect evidence points to an autoimmune mechanism (Figure 6-6).
      (1) **Anti–intrinsic factor antibodies** are found in 75% of patients with PA and are specific for the condition. These polyclonal antibodies (either IgG or IgA) are usually found in the saliva, gastric juice, and serum of patients diagnosed with PA. Two types of anti–intrinsic factor antibodies have been identified.
         (a) **Blocking anti–intrinsic factor antibodies** are clinically significant since they prevent vitamin B_{12}–intrinsic factor binding.
         (b) **Non-blocking anti–intrinsic factor** antibodies are present in patients with PA but do not interfere with the binding and absorption of vitamin B_{12}. The presence of these antibodies is used to support the diagnosis of PA, but their role in the pathogenesis of the disorder is undetermined.
      (2) **Other antibodies** have been identified, specifically those to parietal cells in the gastric fundi that secrete intrinsic factor. However, the specificity of these antibodies for PA is less than that of anti–intrinsic factor antibodies, since they occur in patients with atrophic gastritis (60% positive) and in relatives of PA patients (30% positive), as well as in some normal individuals (<10% positive).
      (3) The **lymphocytic infiltration of the gastric mucosa** suggests a local immunologic process, which can lead to achlorhydria.
   c. **Clinical manifestations.** In addition to megaloblastic anemia, PA displays certain clinical manifestations associated with severe vitamin B_{12} deficiency but distinct from those displayed in folate deficiency.
      (1) **Subacute, combined degeneration of the spinal cord** results in a progressive neuropathy that affects its posterior and lateral columns and the peripheral sensory nerves. This condition presents clinically as neuropathy of the lower limb, causing tingling in the feet, abnormal gait, and loss of proprioception, which causes the patient to fall in the dark.
      (2) **Optic nerve atrophy** occurs occasionally due to cobalamin deficiency.
      (3) **Megaloblastic madness or psychosis,** a severe psychiatric symptom, is an associated abnormality.
      (4) PA is **associated with other autoimmune diseases,** such as Hashimoto's thyroiditis.
   d. **Diagnosis.** The diagnosis of PA is made by demonstrating the following:
      (1) **Macrocytic anemia** with hyperlobulated granulocytes and megaloblastic bone marrow
      (2) **Low serum vitamin B_{12}**
      (3) **Intrinsic factor and parietal cell antibodies** [see III D 3 b (1), (2)]
      (4) **Positive Schilling test.** The Schilling test determines the absorption of radiolabeled vitamin B_{12} (Figure 6-7) and is **the most specific test for establishing a diagnosis of PA,** differentiating the other causes of vitamin B_{12} deficiency (Table 6-3). There are three parts to the Schilling test.
         (a) **Part I.** Vitamin B_{12} absorption is measured by determining the fraction of an oral dose of radioactive vitamin B_{12} excreted in the urine over a period of 24 hours.
            (i) A large parenteral dose of unlabeled vitamin B_{12} is administered in order to saturate the levels of TC I and TC II. Radioactive vitamin B_{12} is then given orally. Because the transcobalamins have already been saturated, any labeled vitamin B_{12} absorbed by the intestines is carried unbound and is excreted in the urine.

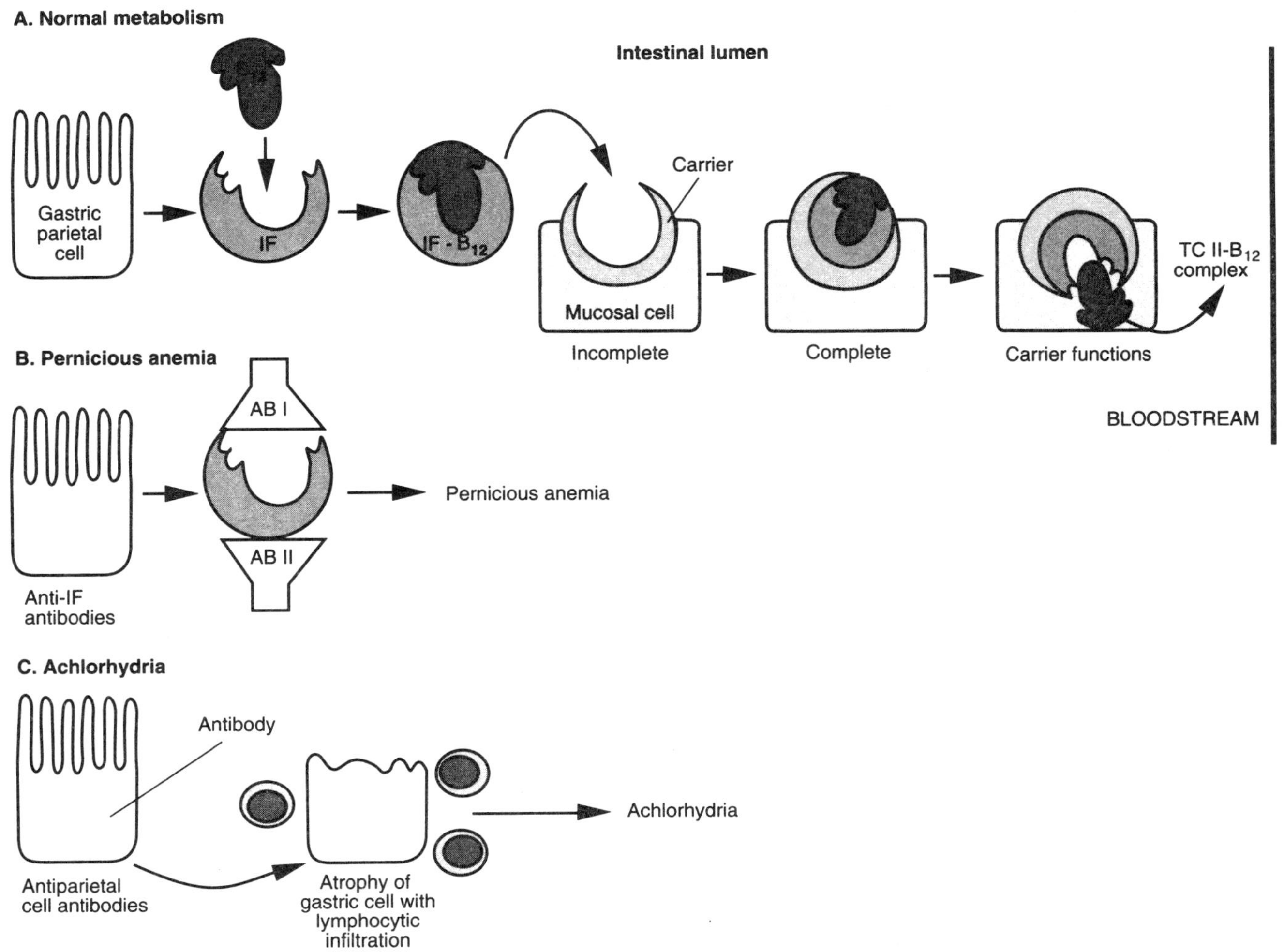

Figure 6-6. Normally, intrinsic factor–vitamin B_{12} complex (*IF-B_{12}*) binds to receptor sites on the mucosal cells of the terminal ileum and is absorbed. In pernicious anemia (PA), anti–intrinsic factor antibodies of the blocking type (*AB I*) prevent B_{12} from complexing with intrinsic factor, and anti–intrinsic factor antibodies of the binding type (*AB II*) prevent the complex from binding with receptors in the ileal mucosa. Antiparietal cell antibodies (found in 90% of PA patients) react with the cytoplasm of these cells, leading to cellular atrophy, lymphocytic infiltration, and eventually to achlorhydria.

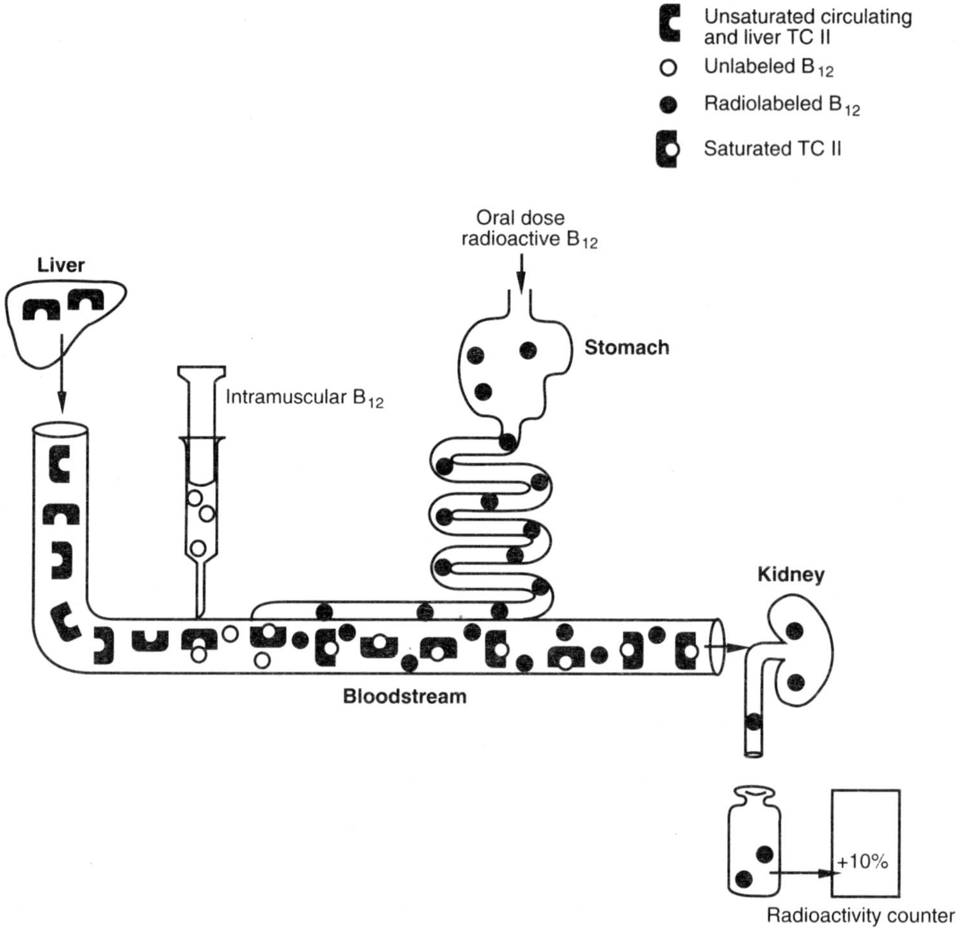

Figure 6-7. In part I of the Schilling test, an oral dose of radioactive vitamin B_{12} is given, followed by an intramuscular injection of unlabeled B_{12}. The latter is given to saturate the circulating binders and liver binders (transcobalamin II; TC II) with unlabeled B_{12}, so the radioactive B_{12} absorbed through the intestine will remain free in the bloodstream and be rapidly excreted in the urine. The urinary radioactive B_{12} is measured as percent radioactivity compared with the total administered by mouth. A positive excretion is expressed as 10% radioactivity in the urine. Part II of the test is performed if part I is abnormal; intrinsic factor is added orally to the radioactive B_{12}. Part III is performed only if part II is abnormal; antibiotics are administered for 1 week to control bacterial overgrowth, and part I is repeated.

(ii) Decreased excretion (in normal renal function) indicates poor absorption but does not distinguish the mechanism of the abnormality. Parts II and III distinguish these causes.

(b) Part II. If less than 9% of the labeled vitamin B_{12} is excreted during the 24-hour urine collection, intrinsic factor is administered orally with a second dose of labeled vitamin and the test is repeated. Cobalamin malabsorption of gastric origin is corrected by this procedure, whereas vitamin B_{12} malabsorption resulting from ileal disease is not.

(c) Part III. Part II may not demonstrate any excretion of labeled vitamin because of ileal disease or competition for the vitamin from overgrown intestinal flora, suggesting the initiation of the optional part III of the Schilling test. Oral antibiotics are administered for 1 week, and part II is then repeated to determine if bacterial overgrowth in the intestine is responsible for the nonabsorption of vitamin B_{12}. In the presence of ileal disease, the results of part III will be negative.

Table 6-3. Differential Diagnosis Based on Schilling Test Results

	Excretion of Labeled Vitamin B_{12}		
Condition	**Part I**	**Part II**	**Part III**
Normal	>8%	. . .	. . .
Vegan diet	>8%	>8%	. . .
Pernicious anemia (PA)	<8%	>8%	. . .
Blind loop syndrome	<8%	No change	>8%
Malabsorption	Usually <8%	No change	No change
Absence of ileum or ileal fistula	<8%	No change	No change

(Reprinted with permission from Mazza J: *Manual of Clinical Hematology,* Boston, Little, Brown, 1988, p 343.)

e. Treatment

(1) **Blood transfusions should be avoided** since circulatory overload may result. However, if transfusion is needed to treat anoxia, 1 or 2 units of packed cells can be administered slowly with the concurrent administration of diuretics or phlebotomy on the other arm.

(2) Treatment specific to severe megaloblastic anemia depends on the patient.

(a) The **average patient** should receive vitamin B_{12} replacement therapy—hydroxycobalamin at an intramuscular dosage of 6000 μg/week for 2–3 weeks initially and 1000 μg every 3 months thereafter.

(b) The **severely anemic patient** who urgently needs therapy but whose vitamin deficiency is not clearly known should be given both folate and vitamin B_{12}. If this patient receives folate for what is actually a vitamin B_{12} deficiency, neurologic abnormalities may precipitate or worsen.

(c) **Elderly patients with heart failure** should receive diuresis and oral potassium supplements for 10 days to prepare for potential hypokalemia. Intramedullary cell destruction and a decreased rate of release of intracellular potassium can occur when the vitamin B_{12} deficiency is corrected, resulting in a decrease in serum potassium.

f. Prognosis. In general, patients will feel better within 24–48 hours of correct vitamin replacement.

(1) The **reticulocyte count will increase** by the second or third day and will peak at 7 days.

(2) The **platelet and white cell counts will increase,** peaking in 7–10 days.

(3) **Peripheral neuropathy may improve gradually** within weeks to several months.

(4) **Spinal cord damage is irreversible.**

STUDY QUESTIONS

Directions: Each of the numbered items or incomplete statements in this section is followed by answers or by completions of the statement. Select the **one** lettered answer or completion that is **best** in each case.

1. All of the following statements are true of patients with pernicious anemia (PA) EXCEPT

(A) about 75% of PA patients exhibit anti–intrinsic factor antibodies in serum
(B) PA is associated with another autoimmune disease called Hashimoto's thyroiditis
(C) older vegetarians develop PA because of disuse of intrinsic factor
(D) about 90% of patients display antibodies to gastric parietal cells
(E) PA is a consequence of long-standing gastritis, which leads to atrophy of the secretory cells of the stomach

2. All of the following findings are present in both folate and vitamin B_{12} deficiencies EXCEPT

(A) macrocytic red cells
(B) peripheral neuropathy
(C) Howell-Jolly bodies and Cabot's rings in the bone marrow
(D) high levels of lactate dehydrogenase (LDH) and indirect bilirubin resulting from ineffective erythropoiesis
(E) hypersegmented neutrophils with six or seven lobes

Directions: Each group of items in this section consists of lettered options followed by a set of numbered items. For each item, select the **one** lettered option that is most closely associated with it. Each lettered option may be selected once, more than once, or not at all.

Questions 3–6

For each patient with megaloblastic anemia, select the associated cause or finding.

(A) Alcoholism
(B) Subacute combined degeneration of the spinal cord
(C) Abnormal results for the three parts of the Schilling test
(D) Bilobate polymorphonuclear cells
(E) Blind loop syndrome

3. A 54-year-old white male with chronic peptic ulcers and a previous gastrectomy presents with anemia, a mean corpuscular volume (MCV) of 110 fl, a red beefy tongue, a normal level of serum folate, a low level of serum vitamin B_{12}, and a normal neurologic examination.

4. A 43-year-old man presents with anemia, a MCV of 101 fl, a platelet count of 70,000/μl, a low level of serum folate, and a normal serum level of vitamin B_{12}.

5. A 72-year-old woman who presented to a neurologist with complaints of falling is found to have anemia, a MCV of 115 fl, a platelet count of 50,000/μl, a white blood cell count (WBC) of 2200/μl, an elevated level of serum folate, and a low serum level of vitamin B_{12} (20 ng/L).

6. A 45-year-old woman who had multiple bowel surgeries for Crohn's disease presents with anemia, a MCV of 110 fl, a WBC of 5700/μl, a platelet count of 150,000/μl, normal serum folate, and a low serum level of vitamin B_{12}.

1-C 4-A
2-B 5-B
3-E 6-C

Questions 7–10

For each set of laboratory test results listed below, select the likely associated condition.

(A) Strict vegetarian diet
(B) Pregnancy
(C) Jejunal resection
(D) Pernicious anemia (PA)
(E) *Diphyllobothrium latum* infestation

7. Low serum level of vitamin B_{12}, normal or high level of serum folate, and an abnormal result for part I and a normal result for part II of the Schilling test

8. Low serum level of vitamin B_{12}, high level of serum folate, and a normal result for part I of the Schilling test

9. Normal serum level of vitamin B_{12}, low level of serum folate, and a normal result for part I of the Schilling test

10. Low serum level of vitamin B_{12}, normal level of serum folate, and abnormal results for parts I, II, and III of the Schilling test

---

7-D
8-A
9-B
10-E

ANSWERS AND EXPLANATIONS

1. The answer is C *[III D 3 b].*
Vegetarians do well with the oral replacement of vitamin B_{12} and develop megaloblastic anemia as a consequence of a lack of animal-derived food in their diet and not because of abnormal intrinsic factor. Rather pernicious anemia (PA) is a consequence of chronic gastritis, which causes atrophy of the stomach secretory cells. Most PA patients display anti–intrinsic factor antibodies in serum, saliva, and gastric juice as well as antibodies to the cytoplasm of gastric parietal cells. This evidence, as well as an association with other immune disorders in these patients such as Hashimoto's thyroiditis (antibodies to thyroid tissues), points to the possibility of an autoimmune mechanism for PA.

2. The answer is B *[III B, D 1, 2].*
Both folate-deficient and vitamin B_{12}-deficient patients exhibit macrocytic red cells, Howell-Jolly bodies and Cabot's rings in the marrow, high levels of lactate dehydrogenase (LDH) and indirect bilirubin resulting from ineffective erythropoiesis, and hypersegmented neutrophils displaying six or seven lobes. However, only vitamin B_{12}-deficient patients develop neurologic abnormalities because vitamin B_{12} is required in myelin metabolism.

3–6. The answers are 3-E *[III C 1, 3, D 2 b, 3 d; Table 6-2],* **4-A** *[III D 1 b (1), (4) (a)],* **5-B** *[II B 2, C; III D 3 c],* **6-C** *[III D 2 b (3), 3 d (4)].*
A patient with megaloblastic anemia and a previous history of gastrectomy should respond positively to part II of the Schilling test. However, the development of blind loop syndrome is common in gastrectomy patients and will cause a negative response to part II. This condition should respond favorably to antibiotic administration and result in a normal part III response.

Folate deficiency in patients from Western countries who present with megaloblastic anemia is most likely due to alcoholism. Alcohol also directly suppresses bone marrow activity and may decrease the platelet counts.

In severe vitamin B_{12} deficiency in pernicious anemia (PA), subacute combined degeneration of the spinal cord and pancytopenia manifest as neurologic symptoms. Poor conjugation of folate allows it to escape from cells into the bloodstream, causing elevated levels of serum folate (the folate trap hypothesis).

Surgical resection of the distal part of the ileum in patients with Crohn's disease is very common. The distal ileum is the site of absorption of vitamin B_{12}. The absorption deficit will not be corrected by the administration of antibiotics in part III of the Schilling test.

7–10. The answers are 7-D *[III D 3 d],* **8-A** *[II A 4, B 2 a (2); III D 2 b (1), 3 d (4) (a)],* **9-B** *[III D 1 b (3) (a), 3 d (4)],* **10-E** *[III D 2 b (4), 3 d (4)].*
The typical findings in a patient with pernicious anemia (PA) are a low serum level of vitamin B_{12}, a normal or elevated level of serum folate, and a failure to absorb orally administered radiolabeled vitamin B_{12} (an abnormal response to part I of the Schilling test) that is corrected with the addition of intrinsic factor (a normal part II response).

Patients who adhere to a strict vegetarian (vegan) diet may display a low serum level of vitamin B_{12}, which is available only in food of animal origin, and a high level of serum folate (vegetables are a rich source of folate, and its concentration is increased by the vitamin B_{12} deficiency). The result for part I of the Schilling test is normal since there is no abnormality associated with the absorption of oral vitamin B_{12}.

Pregnancy can cause folate deficiency by increased utilization of the easily depleted stores. Stores of vitamin B_{12} are much larger and not so easily depleted. The Schilling test would not be indicated in this patient and would show normal results if performed.

Infestation with the fish tapeworm (*Diphyllobothrium latum*) can cause vitamin B_{12} deficiency as the parasite utilizes vitamin B_{12} passing through the intestine. This condition cannot be corrected by the administration of oral antibiotics unless they are prescribed specifically to treat this infestation. Therefore, the result for part III of the Schilling test would be abnormal.

7
Hemolytic Anemia

Emmanuel C. Besa

I. INTRODUCTION

A. Red cell turnover and life span. Approximately 2.5 million red cells are removed from the circulation every second. To replace exhausted red cells, the bone marrow produces 200 billion new red cells (reticulocytes) each day. These cells will survive for about 120 days before they are removed from the circulation by the macrophages of the reticuloendothelial system (RES) in the bone marrow, liver, and spleen. Both cellular and environmental factors affect red cell life span.

1. **Cellular factors.** Red cell metabolism gradually deteriorates because cellular enzymes are not replenished and the cell becomes nonviable and dies.

2. **Environmental factors**
   a. **Physical and chemical stresses.** Circulating red cells are subjected to various chemical and physical stresses that constantly challenge their physical integrity, hastening the aging process, and excluding the aged cells that cannot withstand these stresses. For example, the anucleated red cells have a diameter of 8 μm and have to maintain their biconcave shape while squeezing through the 2–3 μm wide orifices of the splenic cords and capillary arterioles where the exchange of oxygen and carbon dioxide occurs.
   b. **Immunologic challenge.** Recognition of red cell antigens is a means by which old cells are identified and destroyed and healthy cells are injured.

B. Definition of hemolytic anemia. Hemolytic anemia is a decrease in the total number of circulating erythrocytes that is caused by the premature destruction or removal of red cells from the circulation. Since bone marrow erythropoietic hyperplasia and extension may compensate for this decrease severalfold, it may take awhile before the patient displays anemia (compensated hemolytic disease), depending on the rate of destruction or removal of the red cells.

II. BIOCHEMICAL BASIS OF RED CELL SURVIVAL

A. Normal disposal of red cells

1. **The red pulp of the spleen is the site of red cell removal and phagocytosis.** The red cell enters the Billroth cord from a terminal arteriole or capillary, passes through the fine spaces formed by reticular fibers and macrophages, and exits to a splenic sinusoid through pores in the basement membrane. Old or injured red cells are recognized by macrophages via membrane-bound antibodies or complement and are phagocytized.

2. **The components of hemoglobin are liberated by the breakdown of red cells.**
   a. **Iron** is carried by **transferrin** in the plasma to marrow erythroblasts.
   b. **Protoporphyrin** is broken down to **bilirubin**.
      (1) **Bilirubin** then circulates to the **liver,** where it is conjugated with **glucuronide** and excreted into the gut via the bile.
      (2) In the gut, bilirubin is converted to **stercobilinogen,** and this is largely excreted in the feces, where oxidative reactions lead to the formation of **stercobilin**. These compounds are partially reabsorbed, but a small amount is excreted in the urine.
   c. A small fraction of **protoporphyrin** is also converted to **carbon monoxide** and excreted via the lungs.
   d. **Globin chains** are broken down into **amino acids** that are **reutilized for general protein synthesis** in the body. There is little intravascular red cell breakdown of globin.

B. Cellular factors that affect red cell survival. To achieve maximal survival, the red cell must **maintain membrane integrity and its cytoplasmic contents,** protecting itself from the stresses of the circulatory environment.

1. **Red cell membrane** (Figure 7-1A). The red cell membrane can deform to allow the cell to squeeze through vessels that are one-fourth the size of its diameter. After delivering oxygen to tissues, the cell bounces back to its previous shape. The outer surface of the membrane is composed of a **lipid bilayer,** which is attached firmly to a **cytoskeleton.**
   a. **Proteins** traverse the lipid bilayer and **are responsible for the antigenic property** (i.e., blood type) **and shape** of the red cell. The **membrane proteins** penetrating the lipid bilayer are band 3 and glycophorin C.
      (1) **Band 3,** a protein named for its electrophoretic mobility, is the principal intrinsic protein. It forms an anion transport channel through which chloride and bicarbonate can be exchanged rapidly.
      (2) **Glycophorin C** serves as an attachment site for the cytoskeleton.
   b. **Cytoskeleton** (see Figure 7-1B). This tough, interwoven net of proteins underlies the plasma membrane and gives the red cell its shape and ability to withstand the stress of deformation while squeezing through narrow capillaries. Four major **proteins** combine to form the cytoskeleton.
      (1) **Spectrin,** the principal protein of the cytoskeleton, consists of entwined pairs of alpha (α) and beta (β) chains that can associate to form tetramers and higher oligomers. This spectrin network is responsible for the flexibility of the red cell.
      (2) **Ankyrin** (band 2.1) is attached to the cytoplasmic domain of band 3 and anchors the cytoskeleton.
      (3) **Band 4.1** forms a complex with actin and spectrin.
      (4) **Actin** is a principal component of the cytoskeleton to which the tail end of spectrin is attached to form a complex with protein 4.1—allowing spectrin filaments to branch and form a two-dimensional skeleton.
   c. **Lipids provide structure to the cell membrane;** the lipid molecule is composed of a central nonpolar group with polar groups at both ends. Carbohydrates associated with the lipids are found only at the external surface of the membrane.
      (1) **Composition**
         (a) **Phospholipids comprise 60%** of the total lipid component and are arranged in a bilayer with a negatively charged phosphate group toward the external surface of the membrane and the aliphatic fatty acid chains oriented toward the internal surface.
         (b) **Cholesterol comprises 30%** of the lipid component and is found within the hydrophobic core of the phospholipid; it exchanges readily with free plasma cholesterol.
      (2) **Function.** Lipids help to preserve the biconcave shape of the red cell by maintaining a certain amount of surface area. Energy is needed to maintain normal lipid levels in the membrane as it interacts with the plasma. As the red cell reaches senescence and runs out of energy, membrane lipid levels increase, increasing cell volume and marking the cell for removal by the spleen.
         (a) **Increased plasma cholesterol levels** cause the red cell membrane to take up more lipid, resulting in an increased membrane surface area with no change in cell volume. As a result, redundant membrane folds up, particularly in the middle of the cell, giving the narrow center of the cell a target appearance (target cell). If the process continues, more bumps form and the cell assumes a burr-like appearance (burr cell; see Table 1-1).
         (b) **Decreased plasma cholesterol levels** reduce the level of cholesterol in the membrane, resulting in **decreased osmotic resistance.**
         (c) **Serum lipoproteins** also affect the red cell membrane—abnormalities of either the protein or lipid component of the membrane will cause abnormal cell shapes.

2. **Hemoglobin.** Energy is needed to maintain the red cell's high hemoglobin concentration (30 mg/dl) in solution at body temperature. Red cells that are exhausted of their energy supply will not attain the normal 4-month life span. **Mutations** in the hemoglobin molecule itself **can cause hemolysis by altering solubility and cellular stability.** Several enzymes and cofactors help maintain the functional properties of hemoglobin.

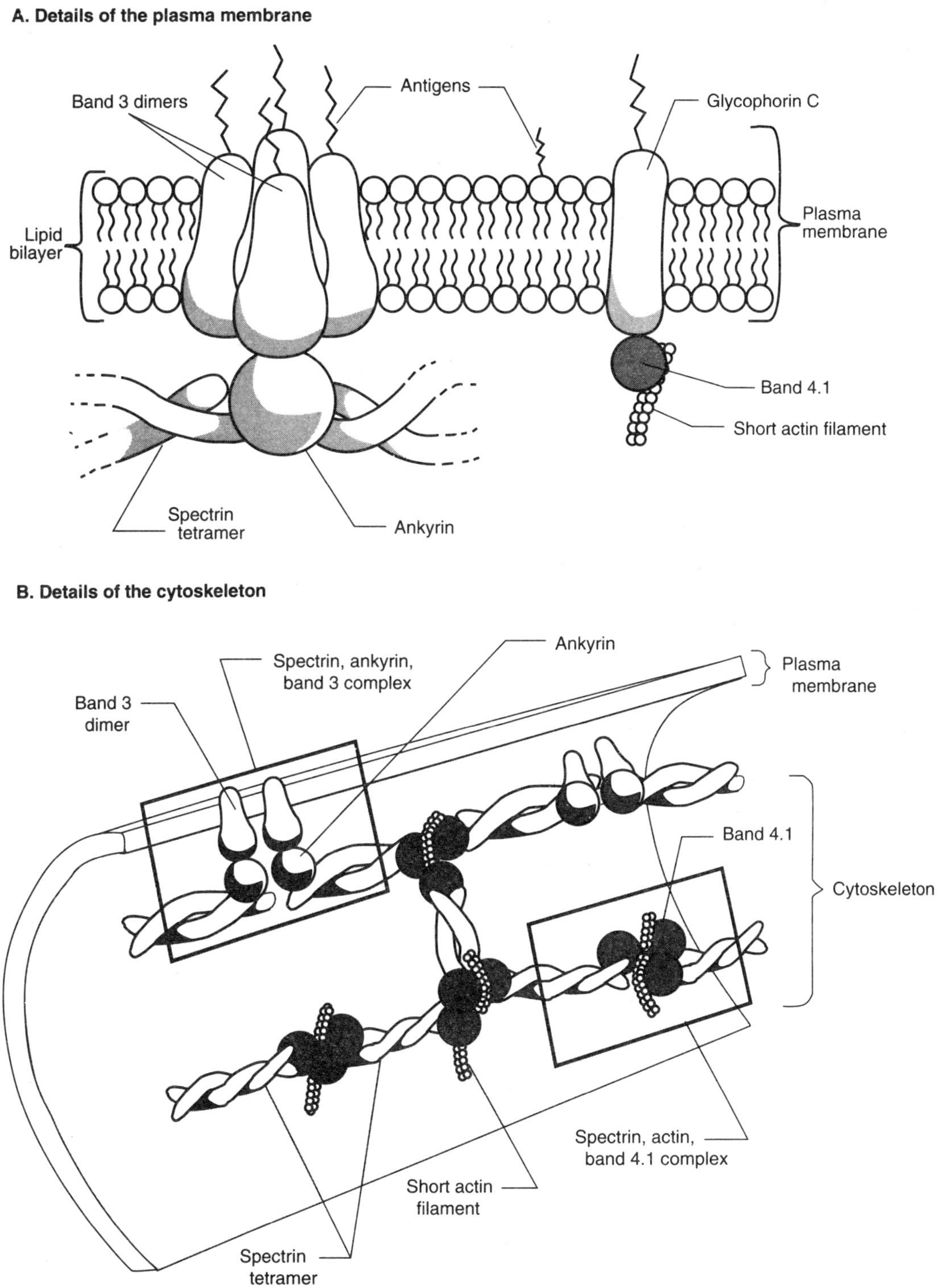

Figure 7-1. The red cell membrane is composed of a plasma membrane and a cytoskeleton. (*A*) The *plasma membrane* is a bipolar lipid layer penetrated by certain membrane proteins (*band 3* and *glycophorin C*). (*B*) The *cytoskeleton,* located beneath the plasma membrane, is composed of four major proteins: *ankyrin, spectrin, band 4.1,* and *actin*. Ankyrin anchors the cytoskeleton to the plasma membrane by coupling with band 3. Spectrin, which is composed of entwined alpha (α) and beta (β) chains, forms complexes with ankyrin and band 3 and with actin and band 4.1.

3. Enzymes

a. **Red cell remodeling enzymes,** active in reticulocytes, remove the organelles (e.g., mitochondria, ribosomes) that remain after maturation is complete. Pyrimidine-5′-nucleotidase facilitates the removal of residual ribonucleotides in reticulocytes.

b. **Red cell housekeeping enzymes** maintain red cell function and integrity by preventing oxidative damage, reducing methemoglobin to hemoglobin, preserving cell membrane structure and function, and salvaging nucleotide enzymes that generate energy and cannot be synthesized from precursors. Many of the housekeeping enzymes function in the Embden-Meyerhof pathway and pentose-phospate shunt (Figure 7-2).

(1) The **Embden-Meyerhof pathway** for glycolysis provides energy for:

(a) **Na^+-K^+ and Ca^{2+} pumps** in the cell membrane, which maintain the normal ionic concentrations within the red cell

(b) **Phosphorylation** of membrane components and **synthesis of glutathione** for protection from oxidative damage

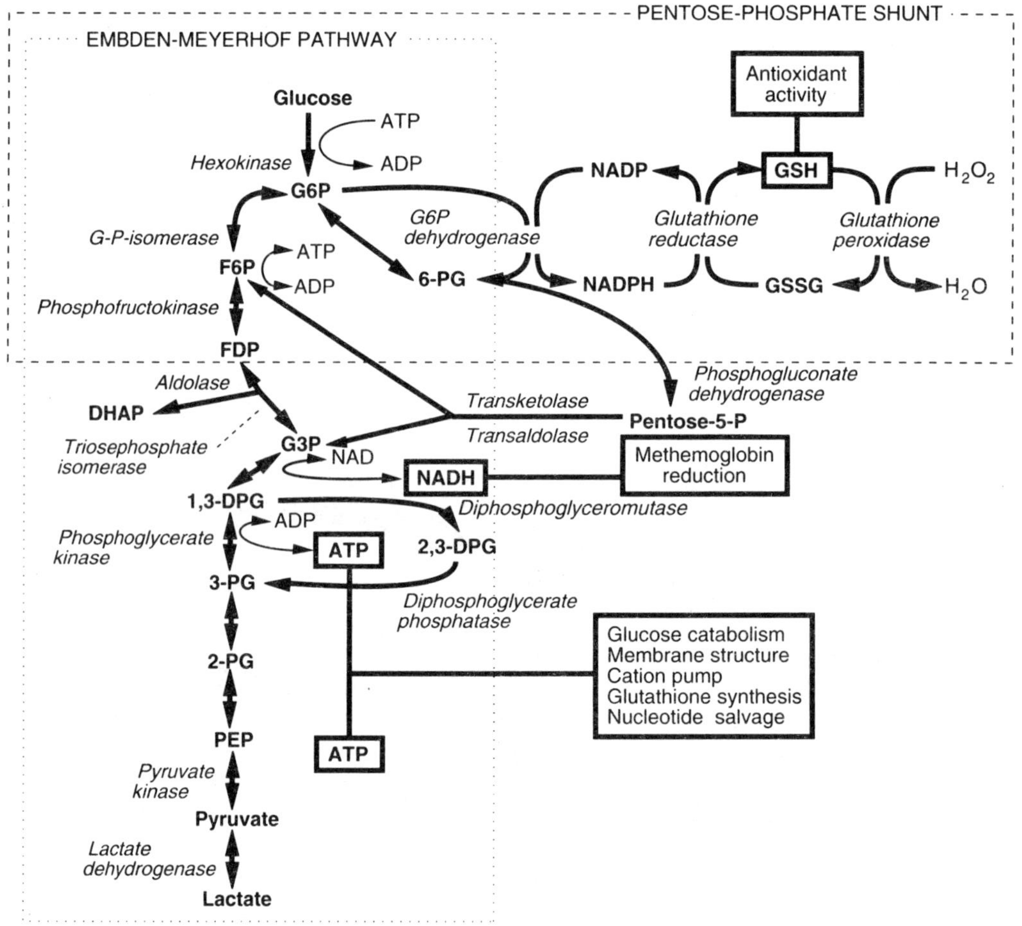

Figure 7-2. Glucose metabolism via the Embden-Meyerhof pathway, anaerobic glycolysis, and pentose-phosphate shunt (hexose-monophosphate shunt) in the human red cell. The roles of specific enzymes in maintaining red cell function and integrity are shown in *boxes*. Inherited enzyme deficiency may involve any enzyme shown with the exception of transketolase and transaldolase. *DHAP* = dihydroxyacetone phosphate; *1,3-DPG* = 1,3-diphosphoglycerate; *2,3-DPG* = 2,3-diphosphoglycerate; *FDP* = fructose-1,6-diphosphate; *F6P* = fructose-6-phosphate; *G-P-isomerase* = glucose-phosphate isomerase; *GSH* = glutathione (reduced form); *GSSG* = glutathione (oxidized form); *G3P* = glucose-3-phosphate; *G6P* = glucose-6-phosphate; *NAD* = nicotinamide-adenine dinucleotide; *NADH* = nicotinamide–adenine dinucleotide (reduced form); *NADP* = nicotinamide-adenine dinucleotide phosphate; *NADPH* = nicotinamide-adenine dinucleotide phosphate (reduced form); *pentose-5-P* = pentose-5-phosphate; *PEP* = phosphoenolpyruvate; *2-PG* = 2-phospho-D-glycerate; *3-PG* = 3-phosphoglycerase; *6-PG* = 6-phosphogluconate.

(c) **Reduction of nicotinamide-adenine-dinucleotide (NAD)** to NADH, which is important in reducing methemoglobin to hemoglobin

(2) The **pentose-phosphate shunt** (hexose-monophosphate shunt) maintains levels of the reduced form of nicotinamide-adenine dinucleotide phosphate (NADPH), which is important in the reduction of oxidized glutathione (GSSG) to **reduced glutathione (GSH)**. GSH is important in:

(a) Destroying the ubiquitous oxidant hydrogen peroxide with glutathione peroxidase

(b) Maintaining sulfhydryl in hemoglobin, in various enzymes, and within the cell membrane

C. Environmental factors that affect red cell survival

1. **Excessive mechanical stress**
   a. Malfunction of a mechanical heart valve can create turbulent flow that can damage red cells.
   b. The fibrin strands that are deposited in the microcirculation in intravascular coagulopathies can damage passing red cells.
2. **Increased temperature.** Above 49° C, membrane destabilization and fragmentation of red cells, as seen in patients with severe burns, may result.
3. **Exposure to toxic chemicals**
   a. Inorganic toxins, such as arsenic and copper
   b. Organic toxins, such as bacterial endotoxins

D. Immunologic factors that affect red cell survival. Red cell antigens have been implicated in immune reactions. The chemical nature of the antigens, their relationship to structural elements of the red cell membrane, their density, and their topographical distribution, as well as the temperature, contribute to an immune reaction. **Aspects of the immunologic mechanism that are important in the survival of red cells are:**

1. **The nature of the antibody,** including its class (IgG or IgM) or subclass (e.g., IgG1, IgG2, IgG3), and other factors that affect the kinetics of the antibody–antigen reaction
   a. Normal human IgG binds with senescent red cells by recognizing age-dependent membrane neoantigens.
   b. This is one mechanism by which macrophages in the spleen identify old erythrocytes for removal and disposal.
2. **The role of the nonimmunoglobulin components of the immune reaction,** most notably the complement system, in mediating red cell injury
3. **The interaction of antibody-injured red cells with RES elements such as macrophages**

III. MEASURING RED CELL SURVIVAL

A. Technique

1. The survival of red cells is determined by using **standard red cell counting techniques** (see Ch 1 II B 2 a).
2. However, the **red cells are first labeled with radioactive chromium (^{51}Cr),** and the drop in radioactivity of the blood samples is measured over time to enumerate the red cell half-life.

B. Normal survival curve (Figure 7-3). The survival curve produced by this method is nonlinear, with a half-life of 25 days. This curve underestimates the actual half-life of 60 days (normal red cell survival is 120 days) due to the different ages of tagged red cells in the sample, leaching of ^{51}Cr from the cells into the blood, and premature red cell death.

C. Clinical applications

1. This is an accurate and reproducible test for identifying premature or increased red cell destruction in **patients with no clear cause of anemia**.
2. Liver and spleen scanning can reveal red cell sequestration and the site of destruction, thus influencing the therapeutic decision to perform splenectomy in **patients with unrelenting hemolytic anemia**.

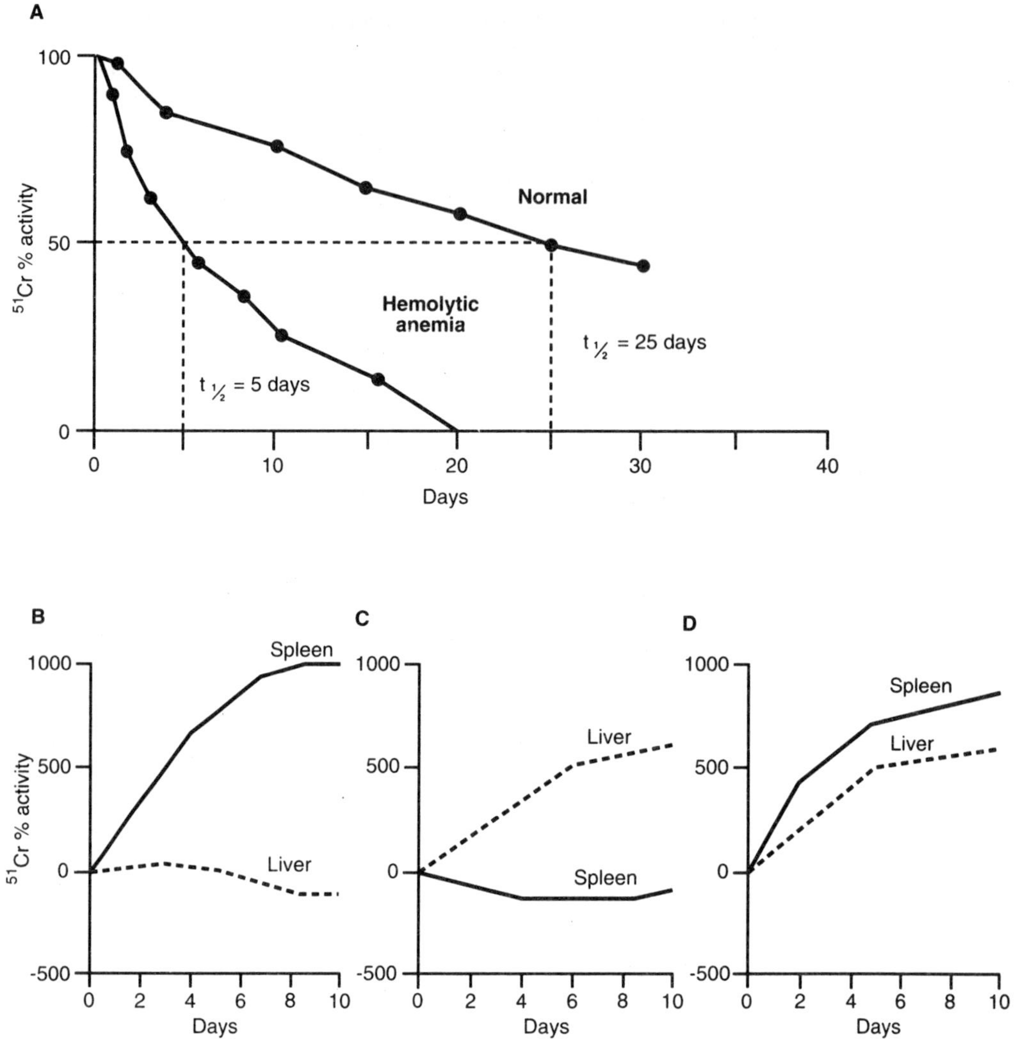

Figure 7-3. (*A*) Normal red cells labeled with radioactive chromium (*^{51}Cr*) have a half-life (*Cr $t_{1/2}$*) of 25 days. Red cells from patients with hemolytic anemia display a reduced survival (Cr $t_{1/2}$ = 5 days). Surface scans conducted during these survival studies show predominantly splenic destruction in hereditary spherocytosis [HS] (*B*), predominantly liver destruction in sickle cell disease (*C*), and a combined pattern in some cases of autoimmune hemolytic anemia (*D*).

IV. HEMOLYSIS. There are many ways to classify hemolytic disease, but the categories tend to overlap. The following are some of the more common means for classifying these disorders.

A. Acute versus chronic hemolysis

1. Acute hemolysis

a. **Anemia** can result from decreased numbers of circulating red cells, with signs of pallor and cardiac dysfunction and symptoms of fatigue, weakness, and shortness of breath.

b. **Red cell hyperplasia and increased numbers of reticulocytes** in the peripheral circulation can result from the increased production of red cells by the bone marrow to compensate for the anemia.

c. **Decreased serum haptoglobin** can result from the increased release of hemoglobin, and breakdown in the liver can overwhelm the normal disposal mechanism, resulting in **jaundice and an increase in indirect bilirubin**.

2. **Chronic hemolysis** and hemoglobin breakdown can lead to the formation of bile gallstones and cholecystitis.

B. Hereditary versus acquired hemolysis (Table 7-1). The patient history helps to determine the type of hemolysis.

1. **Hereditary hemolysis** can be determined by identifying:
   a. Anemia refractory to treatment **early in infancy and childhood**
   b. Any family member with a history of anemia, jaundice, unexplained splenomegaly, splenectomy, or cholecystectomy at an early age

2. **Acquired hemolysis** is suggested by:
   a. The **rapid appearance of signs and symptoms** of hemolysis, such as anemia without blood loss
   b. An **underlying disease process** with a high incidence of immune hemolysis, such as lymphoproliferative disorders, collagen vascular disease, or the use of certain drugs (see V A 3 c)

C. Intracorpuscular versus extracorpuscular hemolysis. Table 7-2 lists a variety of factors inside or outside the red cell that may be involved with destruction of the cell.

D. Intravascular versus extravascular hemolysis (Table 7-3)

1. **Intravascular red cell destruction,** which occurs in the peripheral circulation, is indicated by the following.
   a. **Hemoglobinemia,** manifesting as red plasma and red urine caused by the release of hemoglobin into the plasma, disappears within a few hours after cessation of hemolysis. In hemoglobinuria, the urine will be darkly colored and will test positively for the presence

Table 7-1. Classification of Hemolytic Anemia According to Type of Defect

Hereditary
Membrane defect
HS
Hereditary elliptocytosis
Metabolic defect
G6PD deficiency
PK deficiency
Hemoglobinopathies
Thalassemias
Sickle cell diseases
Other hemoglobinopathies
Acquired
Immunologic defect
Drug-induced hemolysis
Isoimmune and alloimmune hemolysis (neonatal and delayed transfusion reactions)
Mechanical defect
Rapid turbulent flow of blood
Malignant tumors
Malignant hypertension
Tight aortic stenosis
Prosthetic valve leaks
Intravascular coagulopathy (DIC, TTP)
March hemoglobinuria
Infection
Endotoxins of bacterial infections
Parasitic infections
Bartonella bacilliformis
Plasmodium (malaria)
Membrane abnormality (stem cell abnormality)
PNH

DIC = disseminated intravascular coagulation; G6PD = glucose-6-phosphate dehydrogenase; HS = hereditary spherocytosis; PK = pyruvate kinase; PNH = paroxysmal nocturnal hemoglobinuria; TTP = thrombotic thrombocytopenic purpura.

Table 7-2. Classification of Hemolytic Anemia According to Site of Defect

Intracorpuscular factors	Extracorpuscular factors
Red cell membrane abnormalities	Antibodies
HS and related abnormalities	Autoimmune hemolytic anemia
PNH	Transfusion-related hemolytic reactions
Hemoglobinopathies	Drug-related hemolytic reactions
Thalassemias	Mechanical or traumatic factors
Sickle cell disease and related hemoglobinopathies	Prosthetic heart valves
	High-flow red cell damage
Methemoglobinemia	Intravascular coagulopathy
Unstable hemoglobin diseases	Infections
Enzymopathies	Bacterial
G6PD deficiency	Parasitic
Others	Cell membrane lipids
	Liver disease
	Lipid disorders

G6PD = glucose-6-phosphate dehydrogenase; HS = hereditary spherocytosis; PNH = paroxysmal nocturnal hemoglobinuria.

of blood. Hemoglobinuria must be differentiated from myoglobinuria and hematuria, which also test positively for the presence of blood in the urine.

b. **Methemoglobinemia,** manifesting as brown plasma, disappears within 2–3 days after cessation of hemolysis.

c. **Increased serum lactate dehydrogenase (LDH)** is the result of red cells releasing their rich intracellular stores of LDH.

d. **Hemosiderinuria,** the presence of hemosiderin in the blood, appears after the proximal tubule cells take up hemoglobin and convert the iron to hemosiderin; the cells are then shed into the urine.

2. **Extravascular red cell destruction,** which occurs in the RES cells (macrophages) of the liver and spleen, presents as splenomegaly and hepatomegaly due to increased removal and disposal of red cells by these organs. This can be considered an exaggeration of the normal mechanisms of red cell disposal.

V. HEMOLYTIC DISORDERS.

There are five categories of hemolytic disorders: immune hemolysis, oxidant hemolysis, red cell membrane disorder, traumatic hemolysis, and intravascular hemolysis resulting from infection.

Table 7-3. Classification of Hemolytic Anemia According to Site of Hemolysis

Intravascular hemolysis	Extravascular hemolysis
Traumatic hemolysis (Waring blender syndrome)	Autoimmune hemolytic anemia
G6PD deficiency	Red cell membrane defects
Type A form	HS
Mediterranean form	Others
Immune hemolysis	Spur cell anemia
Hemolytic transfusion reactions (ABO incompatibility)	Liver disease
	Abetalipoproteinemia (very rare)
Donath-Landsteiner antibody	Red cell metabolism defect
PNH	PK deficiency
Infections	Severe hypophosphatemia
Clostridium perfringens toxin	Pyrimidine-5′-nucleotidase deficiency
Bartonella bacilliformis (Oroya fever)	Unstable hemoglobin diseases
Plasmodium (malaria)	

G6PD = glucose-6-phosphate dehydrogenase; HS = hereditary spherocytosis; PK = pyruvate kinase; PNH = paroxysmal nocturnal hemoglobinuria.

A. Immune hemolysis

1. **Definition.** Immune hemolytic diseases are blood disorders in which the red cell life span is shortened because **abnormalities in the components of the immune system are specifically directed against the patient's own erythrocytes.**

2. **Coombs' test** (also called direct antiglobulin test, or DAT) is used to demonstrate immune hemolysis.
   a. The **direct Coombs' test** detects antibodies on red cells.
      (1) The patient's red cells are washed with normal saline at body temperature to remove plasma with antibodies from the red cell surface. Then, antihuman rabbit IgG or anti-complement component C3 is added to the suspension.
      (2) If the patient's red cells have autoantibodies of IgG or activated C3, they will bind the rabbit antibodies, forming bridges to adjacent cells. Agglutination indicates a positive test result.
      (3) Autoantibodies of IgM may be missed if antihuman IgG is used alone. Instead, IgM may be detected as positive for anti-C3, since IgM activates complement to produce hemolysis.
   b. The **indirect Coombs' test** detects circulating antibodies in the serum.
      (1) The patient's serum is mixed with normal red cells that are then washed and reacted with antihuman rabbit IgG or anti-C3.
      (2) If the cells then agglutinate, the test is positive.

3. **Major clinical types of immune hemolysis**
   a. **Autoimmune hemolytic anemia** presents with different clinical pictures that correlate reasonably well with the properties of the specific autoantibodies and those of the red cell antigens. The autoantibodies can be activated by either heat or cold.
      (1) **Warm-reactive autoimmune hemolysis.** Warm-reactive autoantibodies usually are IgG, which react maximally at 37° C. These are the most commonly occurring antibodies in autoimmune hemolytic anemia. Warm-reactive antibodies may cause hemolysis with or without fixing complement, and they usually are specific for the Rh antigen.
         (a) **Causes.** Warm-type hemolysis may be **idiopathic or secondary to:**
            (i) **The administration of drugs** such as methyldopa
            (ii) **Underlying connective tissue diseases** such as systemic lupus erythematosus or refractory anemia
            (iii) **Lymphoproliferative disorders** such as chronic lymphocytic leukemia (CLL) or Hodgkin's and non-Hodgkin's lymphomas
         (b) **Clinical manifestations.** The rapid development of anemia causes tiredness and fatigue; elderly patients with underlying atherosclerosis may experience chest pain. Splenomegaly and jaundice usually are noted but may be absent in the early acute phase. Abdominal pain and fever may also occur.
         (c) **Diagnosis** of warm-type hemolysis relies on a positive direct Coombs' test combined with absence of haptoglobin and presence of spherocytosis, reticulocytosis, increased serum LDH, and indirect bilirubinemia. The indirect Coombs' test is positive in about 75% of cases.
         (d) **Treatment**
            (i) **Removal of the underlying cause** (e.g., ceasing methyldopa administration).
            (ii) **Administration of high doses of corticosteroids,** such as 1 mg/kg of prednisone, with a subsequent slow tapering of the dose if the patient is responsive to therapy. It may be necessary to maintain some patients on chronic low-dose therapy.
            (iii) **Removal of the spleen** in patients who display steroid failure or who are refractory to other treatments. Patients who have been treated with IgG or IgG with complement respond the best to splenectomy, patients who have been treated with IgA are less responsive, and patients who have been treated with IgM are unresponsive to splenectomy.
      (2) **Cold-reactive autoimmune hemolysis.** Cold-reactive autoantibodies usually are IgM, although occasionally IgG may be implicated. The reactivity to cold resides in the antigen, not the antibody; low temperature makes the antigen more prominent on the membrane, and, so, more accessible for antibody interaction. Warm temperature has the opposite effect, hiding the antigen below the lipid component of the membrane and preventing antibody-antigen binding.

(a) **Causes** of cold-type hemolysis may be idiopathic or secondary to infection (e.g., mycoplasmal pneumonia, infectious mononucleosis) or lymphoma.

(b) **Pathogenesis and clinical effects**

(i) As the circulation brings blood from the warm body cavities to the body surface, blood temperature drops to near room temperature. This activates the autoantibodies to cause agglutination, impairing the circulation and producing symptoms of cyanosis, pallor, and ischemic pain (Raynaud's phenomenon) in extremities.

(ii) IgM binds only temporarily with antigen, but during this time it fixes complement. IgM then disengages from the red cell and is free to attach to another cell.

(iii) The fixed complement remains and activates C5 though C9, causing membrane holes and hemolysis. C3-sensitized red cells are removed from the circulation by Kuppfer cells in the liver (i.e., reticuloendothelial cells rich in C3 receptors). This explains why cold-reactive autoantibody hemolysis does not respond to splenectomy.

(c) **Diagnosis.** Cold-type hemolysis is diagnosed by:

(i) **A positive direct Coombs' test** that reveals only complement (C3) on the red cells

(ii) **IgM antibodies present in high titer,** which **react best at 4° C** with "thermal amplitude" (i.e., there is a range from 4° C to 32° C in which activity can be demonstrated) and **show specificity to I antigen and anti-i** (anti-i is seen in infectious mononucleosis but often does not cause hemolysis since most adult red cells are poorly reactive to anti-i)

(iii) **Autoantibodies** IgM and IgG, which are **usually monoclonal** in cases of lymphoma and **may be polyclonal** in cases of infection

(d) **Treatment** is directed at the cause of the hemolysis.

(i) **Infections** typically are transient and self-limited, but patients should be given supportive care, including transfusions when needed, and advised to avoid exposure to cold temperatures.

(ii) **Lymphomas** require specific treatment according to their histology and involvement of other organs.

(iii) **Idiopathic hemolysis,** which is most common, generally is unresponsive to corticosteroids or splenectomy. Refractory cases may respond to alkylating agents.

(e) **Paroxysmal cold hemoglobinuria** is an unusual form of cold-associated hemolysis caused by the **Donath-Landsteiner antibody**.

(i) **Pathogenesis.** The Donath-Landsteiner antibody is a unique antibody that binds to red cells in cold temperatures and causes complement-mediated hemolysis in warm temperatures. The antibody is an IgG that activates complement specific for blood group antigen P—a very common antigen that exists not only on red cells but also on lymphocytes and fibroblasts.

(ii) **Clinical manifestations.** Paroxysmal cold hemoglobinuria may occur in association with syphilis or following chickenpox, measles, or other viral infections. The condition is an acute, fulminating, intravascular hemolysis that produces aching pain in the back, legs, or abdomen; hemoglobinuria; and vasospastic or anaphylactic reactions.

b. **Transfusion-related hemolysis** (ABO incompatibility). For a complete discussion of this immune hemolysis, the reader is referred to Chapter 17.

c. **Drug-related immune hemolysis** can occur by three mechanisms.

(1) The **hapten mechanism** applies to drugs that can firmly bind proteins on the red cell surface; penicillin is such a drug. High doses of penicillin (as required for the treatment of subacute bacterial endocarditis) can cause formation of antibody against penicillin or its active metabolites, which may or may not result in hemolysis.

(a) IgG antibodies cause hemolysis of varying severity, which subsides after discontinuation of the drug.

(b) IgM antibodies commonly occur with penicillin treatment but do not cause hemolysis.

(2) The **"innocent bystander" mechanism** applies to drugs that form immune complexes with antibody (usually IgM), which then attach to the red cell membrane and target

the cell for immune destruction, presumably by fixing complement. Such drugs include sulfonamides, chlorpropamide, phenacetin, and para-aminobenzoic acid.

(3) The **autoantibody mechanism** applies to drugs that can induce the formation of antibodies (usually IgG) to a patient's own red cells, thus producing true autoimmune hemolytic anemia. Prolonged administration of α-methyldopa (usually over 5 years) can induce a positive direct Coombs' test in about 10%–20% of patients and true hemolytic anemia in a few patients. Hemolysis improves after the drug is discontinued, but the Coombs' test remains positive.

(a) The autoantibody usually is specific for Rh antigen and may be associated with other autoantibodies (e.g., antinuclear antibodies, rheumatoid factor).

(b) The mechanism is postulated to be a prolonged effect on immunoregulatory T cells.

B. Oxidant hemolysis (enzymopathy) results from a **deficiency of enzymes critical to the operation of the pentose-phosphate shunt and Embden-Meyerhof pathway** (see Figure 7-2) in erythrocytes and reticulocytes. The deficiency is caused by an **inherited disorder that creates mutant unstable forms of the enzymes** of the metabolic pathways, resulting in increased breakdown and decreased activity of the enzyme. The most common enzymatic deficiencies contributing to oxidant hemolysis are glucose-6-phosphate dehydrogenase (G6PD) deficiency and pyruvate kinase (PK) deficiency.

1. **G6PD deficiency,** the more common of the two enzyme deficiencies, is an X-linked disorder and the **most frequent clinically apparent cause for hemolysis**. G6PD is important in the pentose-phosphate shunt (see Figure 7-2) for the generation of both nicotinamide-adenine dinucleotide phosphate (NADP) and its reduced form (NADPH) as well as glutathione, which is required for reduction or protection of sulfhydryl groups in critical regions that are subjected to oxidative denaturation.

a. **Enzyme variants**

(1) **Normal forms.** Two forms of G6PD have normal activity. The **B form** is found in whites and most blacks; the **A form** (or **A+ form**) is found only in blacks, many of whom are AB heterozygotes.

(2) **Deficiency forms.** The many other forms of G6PD all are associated with deficiency. The enzyme may exist at normal intracellular levels but have decreased activity, or it may be unstable and prone to increased breakdown in red cells. These mutant enzymes confer a natural resistance to malaria and are thought to be an adaptive mechanism for people living in endemic areas. Two important mutant forms of G6PD are the **A− isoenzyme** and the **Mediterranean isoenzyme** [see V B 1 b (2)].

b. **Pathophysiology.** In the daily wear and tear of red cells, hemoglobin is constantly being oxidized to methemoglobin, but a special protective mechanism that uses the Embden-Meyerhof pathway [see II B 3 b (1)] reduces it back to hemoglobin. This is important because methemoglobin dissociates into heme and globin and then precipitates as an insoluble mass (**Heinz body**). Red cells that form Heinz bodies are nondeformable and have difficulty passing through the spleen. Splenic removal of Heinz bodies damages the red cell membrane, forming spherocytes and causing hemolysis.

(1) **Precipitating factors.** Hemolysis may be precipitated in G6PD deficiency by a variety of factors, including oxidant drugs, ingestion of fava beans (broad beans containing pyrimidine derivatives with potent oxidant properties), infection, and other stressful conditions (Table 7-4).

(2) **Clinically relevant G6PD mutations**

(a) The **A− isoenzyme,** seen only in blacks, is similar to the A+ form but has an additional amino acid substitution and decreased activity or increased catabolism. Red cells are released with adequate amounts of G6PD whose activity decays too rapidly, so that by 1 month the cells have no more G6PD and undergo mild hemolysis when exposed to oxidants. Reticulocytes (young red cells) survive since they have not yet lost their G6PD. Hemolysis usually is self-limited, since reticulocytosis with increased G6PD activity occurs, compensating for low enzyme levels.

(b) The **Mediterranean isoenzyme,** seen only in whites from Mediterranean countries such as Greece and Italy, is extremely unstable and has markedly decreased activity, producing severe hemolysis in the presence of oxidants. Nearly all cells (including reticulocytes) lack enzyme activity due to the instability of the isoenzyme.

Table 7-4. Precipitating Factors of Hemolysis in Enzymopathies

Oxidant drugs	Other factors
Antimalarials	Fava beans and pollen
Chloroquine	Infections
Primaquine	Respiratory viruses
Quinine and quinidine	Hepatitis
Antipyretics	Infectious mononucleosis
Aspirin	Bacterial pneumonia
Phenacetin	Septicemia
Sulfonamides and related compounds	Diabetic ketoacidosis
Nitrofurantoin	Uremia
Phenylhydrazine	
Acetanilid	

c. **Clinical manifestations**

(1) **General features.** Patients with G6PD deficiency display signs and symptoms of intravascular hemolysis (hemoglobinemia, hemosiderinuria) and extravascular hemolysis (enlarged spleen). The deficiency usually is episodic and occasionally is chronic, which can give rise to gallstones.

(2) **Patients with the common A− form of G6PD deficiency** generally have mild hemolysis only when stressed (e.g., by oxidant drugs); the hemolysis usually is self-limited, since reticulocytes have high levels of the enzyme, thus compensating for the decreased activity.

(3) **Patients with the rare Mediterranean form of G6PD deficiency** have severe hemolysis when exposed to oxidants or when stressed by surgery or infections. The hemolysis persists as long as the stress or oxidant persists.

d. **Diagnosis**

(1) **Red cell enzyme levels** measured by electrophoresis show very low activity in severe disease and low to normal activity in mild disease, depending on when the test is performed. Since young red cells display normal levels of enzymes, measurements should not be taken at the time of hemolysis and reticulocytosis.

(2) **Heinz bodies** can be demonstrated in red cells with special staining only during the early phase of G6PD deficiency hemolysis, since these cells are rapidly removed from the circulation by the spleen. The finding of Heinz bodies should trigger a search for an oxidant (e.g., a drug or food) or an infection in the patient.

e. **Treatment.** Primary therapy is to **avoid oxidative agents**—the ingestion of fava beans can be catastrophic in the severe form of the disease.

2. **PK deficiency** is one of several enzymopathies responsible for the group of conditions known as **congenital nonspherocytic hemolytic anemias**. PK deficiency, the most common of these rare conditions, is an autosomal recessive defect characterized by an unstable enzyme and decreased generation of ATP in red cells. Impairment of glycolysis also results in increased 2,3-DPG, causing a shift of the oxygen-hemoglobin dissociation curve favoring oxygen release.

a. **Clinical manifestations.** PK deficiency causes a chronic hemolytic syndrome of variable severity. Severe deficiency may be clinically apparent in the neonatal stage, whereas mild deficiency may be asymptomatic. The manifestations are similar to those of other chronic hemolytic disorders from enzyme deficiency, including reticulocytosis, marrow hyperplasia, splenomegaly, jaundice, and gallstones.

b. **Diagnosis.** PK deficiency is best diagnosed by measuring the PK level in red cells. An abnormal osmotic fragility test that is not corrected by incubation of the patient's red cells with glucose also suggests PK deficiency.

c. **Treatment** of PK deficiency varies with the severity of the anemia and consists of supplemental folates and transfusion (when needed) to control the chronic hemolysis. Splenectomy may decrease the need for transfusion in some cases. Management of aplastic crisis with supportive treatment is recommended.

C. **Red cell membrane disorders**

1. **Hereditary spherocytosis (HS)** is the most common of the inherited red cell membrane defects, affecting 1 in 5000 individuals. This disorder is characterized by red cells that appear cup-shaped on electron microscopy and spherical on peripheral blood smear.

a. Pathophysiology

(1) The abnormal red cell shape is caused by a **defective cytoskeleton**. This defect involves a partial deficiency of spectrin, unstable ankyrin (decreasing the incorporation of spectrin into the membrane skeleton), and a defective β spectrin (leading to decreased binding to band 4.1 protein and actin). The spherical shape has two effects on red cells.

(a) They become trapped in the splenic cords.

(b) They have a shortened life span due to rapid depletion of energy (changing shape uses energy).

(2) The abnormal membrane also demonstrates an **increased permeability of sodium,** causing the cell to lose as much as 10 times the normal levels. To compensate for this loss, the red cell uses up an enormous amount of energy (ATP) to retrieve sodium into the intracellular space, thus consuming more glucose than normal red cells.

b. Clinical manifestations. The typical HS patient is relatively asymptomatic, with a well-compensated hemolysis and a palpable spleen. The rare patient with severe HS may present early in childhood with life-threatening hemolysis. HS has the usual features of chronic hemolysis (i.e., symptoms of anemia and splenomegaly and complications of gallstones or aplastic crisis). Family members usually have mild forms of the disorder or are carriers; diagnosis in these individuals usually is made late in life.

c. Diagnosis is suggested by a family history of HS and characteristic findings on blood smear (i.e., spherocytes). Two studies are used to confirm the diagnosis.

(1) Osmotic fragility test (Figure 7-4). Incubation of red cells in hypotonic solution causes the cell to expand as intracellular fluid volume increases. The normal cell, with its flexible and distensible membrane, can withstand a higher volume increase compared to the spherocyte from an HS patient. A positive osmotic fragility test shows hemolysis of the patient's red cells at a saline concentration near isotonic conditions, compared to simple swelling in normal cells.

(2) Autohemolysis test. HS cells consume glucose at higher rates than normal cells. In the autohemolysis test, red cells are incubated in buffer or serum for 48 hours, after which hemolysis is determined by measuring the release of hemoglobin. **Normal autohemolysis is about 1%, while HS cells will display hemoglobin release rates of 3% or more.** The increased autohemolysis of HS cells can be completely prevented by including glucose in the incubation medium, implying that the cells lyse because they use up their glucose and consequently cannot maintain their integrity.

d. Treatment. Asymptomatic patients with compensated hemolysis should receive supportive treatment with folate supplements. Aplastic crisis may require a short period of blood

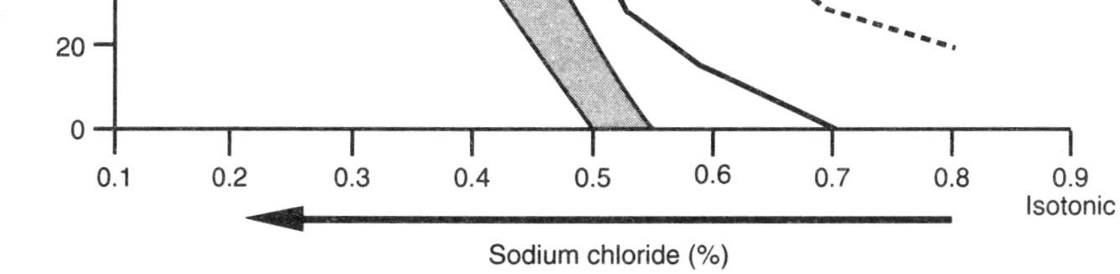

Figure 7-4. In the osmotic fragility test, the lysis of red cells from normal patients is compared with that of red cells from patients with hereditary spherocytosis (HS). HS red cells (*solid curve*) are more sensitive to reductions in the concentration of sodium chloride than are normal cells (*shaded area*), although there are some osmotically resistant HS cells (reticulocytes). HS red cells that have been incubated in sterile, hypotonic saline for 24 hours are more susceptible to reductions in the sodium chloride concentration (*dashed line*) than are fresh HS red cells.

transfusion support. Splenectomy is curative in most cases of HS but is warranted only in certain circumstances. Guidelines for performing splenectomy include:

(1) It should be performed only when necessary (e.g., patients who require blood transfusions).

(2) It should be avoided in children younger than 10 years of age because of associated risks (e.g., fatal pneumonia, sepsis).

(3) It may be performed with cholecystectomy to decrease the amount of hemolysis and the risk for developing more gallstones.

2. Disorders related to HS. Other abnormalities of red cell morphology caused by structural defects are rare. Relatively benign conditions include **hereditary elliptocytosis and stomatocytosis. Hereditary pyropoikilocytosis** is a severe hemolytic condition related to HS.

3. Spur cell anemia. A characteristic cell called the **acanthocyte, or spur cell, develops when the red cell surface area increases without a concurrent increase in the cell volume**. If there is a modest increase in surface area, the cell appears in a blood smear as a **target cell**. Additional increase in surface area results in the formation of spurs, which are long spikes that project in all directions. The spleen will amputate the spikes, causing the spur cell to lose some membrane and acquire an irregular, asymmetric shape.

a. Pathophysiology. Acanthocytes eventually lose membrane and elasticity, leading to a mild type of anemia due to destruction by the spleen.

b. Causes

(1) Severe liver disease is the most common cause of spur cell anemia. The presence of hemolysis and spur cells in a patient with liver disease is an ominous sign suggesting the patient is in end-stage disease.

(a) In severe liver disease (e.g., advanced cirrhosis), esterification of cholesterol is impaired, causing an increase in free (nonesterified) cholesterol in plasma.

(b) When the free cholesterol from the plasma equilibrates with the red cell membrane, there is a marked increase in the normal ratio of free cholesterol to phospholipids. This causes the cell to develop the characteristic spicules and to lose membrane fluidity.

(c) The spleen traps the abnormally shaped red cells and removes them from the circulation, causing a decrease in red cell survival and development of anemia.

(2) Hereditary abetalipoproteinemia. Patients with congenital absence of apolipoprotein β demonstrate prominent acanthocytes in peripheral blood smears but do not present with hemolysis or anemia. Accumulation of sphingomyelin has been implicated, since the red cells have normal cholesterol levels.

4. Paroxysmal nocturnal hemoglobinuria (PNH)

a. Pathophysiology. PNH is an acquired stem cell disorder resulting in three distinct populations of stem cells. Normal stem cells (**PNH I cells**) are identified by a normal sensitivity to the alternative complement system. Abnormal stem cells (**PNH II and PNH III cells**) have varying degrees of surface membrane abnormalities, which affect all blood cell lines including red cells, platelets, and granulocytes.

(1) PNH II and PNH III cells show increased sensitivity to destruction by the alternative complement system because of increased cell surface activation of C3/C5 convertase, which leads to the deposition of C3b and C5b–C9 on the membrane and resultant hemolysis.

(2) Complement activation in PNH bypasses the requirement for antibody-dependent fixation of C1, C2, and C4. The PNH cells are significantly more efficient in completing the sequential addition of C3 and C5–C9 than are normal cells, whether mediated by the bypass mechanism or by antibody.

(3) The **cell membrane defect** has been characterized by a deletion and a depletion.

(a) There is a **deletion** of complement regulatory molecules in blood cells affected by PNH. Decay-accelerating factor, the membrane protein that normally regulates C3bBb, is not present in PNH II and PNH III cells. Decay-accelerating factor normally prevents activation of complement on cell surfaces by accelerating the dissociation of the C3-cleaving enzyme Bb from its membrane-bound cofactor, C3. Addition of decay-accelerating factor will correct the defect only in PNH II cells and not in PNH III cells; thus, this mechanism only partially explains the PNH defect.

(b) There is a **depletion** of acetylcholinesterase, neutrophil alkaline phosphatase, granulocyte Fc receptors, and lymphocyte function antigen. This depletion is the result of a defect in membrane lipid phosphatidylinositol, which attaches the glucoproteins by glycosidic linkages.

b. **Clinical manifestations**

(1) **PNH typically presents with anemia and dark urine on awakening,** indicating the nocturnal exacerbation of hemolysis, presumably through a lowering of blood pH by alveolar hypoventilation during sleep. However, hemolysis can occur at any time. **Iron deficiency is also present** as a result of hemosiderinuria and hemoglobinuria.

(2) **Thrombosis in both the venous and arterial vessels** manifests as the Budd-Chiari syndrome (portal vein thrombosis in the liver) due to spontaneous platelet aggregation caused by activation and release of adenosine diphosphate (ADP) from platelets sensitive to complement. Platelet membrane abnormalities increase the adhesive properties of these cells, favoring intravascular coagulation.

(3) **Bone marrow aplasia and pancytopenia** can result from complement-mediated injury to the hematopoietic stem cell and can induce leukemic transformation in rare cases. These phenomena illustrate the mechanism of the disease's relationship to aplastic anemia.

c. **Diagnosis** of PNH depends on the in vitro demonstration of lysis through the following tests.

(1) **Ham test.** This is a specific test for PNH in which the patient's red cells are incubated with fresh acidified serum. This promotes the activation of complement; **PNH cells are sensitive to complement and will undergo hemolysis while normal cells will not**. The test's sensitivity is compromised because some normal fresh serum may give a negative reaction.

(2) **Sugar water test.** The patient's red cells are incubated in an isotonic sucrose solution. As in the Ham test, complement is activated, **causing the hemolysis of PNH cells while normal cells are not affected**. This test is more sensitive, but less specific, than the Ham test.

d. **Treatment** for PNH depends on the severity of the anemia and hemolysis and the attendant complications.

(1) **Supportive therapy** used in other bone marrow failure syndromes is indicated.

(2) **Iron therapy** for iron deficiency can trigger reticulocytosis and can exacerbate the hemolysis by increasing the number of abnormal cells. Thus, therapy should stop if the hemolysis increases.

(3) **Androgen therapy** has been used with some benefit.

(4) **Antiplatelet therapy** may prevent thrombosis; however, bleeding complications related to pancytopenia or portal hypertension limit its use.

(5) **Bone marrow transplantation** can be considered for severely affected patients who meet the criteria for this therapy.

D. **Traumatic hemolysis (Waring blender syndrome).** The following conditions can result in hemolysis due to physical trauma to red cells.

1. **Rapid blood flow through turbulent regions of the circulation** causes physical damage by shear force on red cells, producing tears and overcoming the distensible property of the cell membrane.

a. **Malignant tumors.** Turbulent blood flow can develop in the neovascularization of malignant tumors that results in highly tortuous and irregular blood vessels. **Kasabach-Merritt syndrome** is an anemia that results from the damage done to red cells as they flow through the deformed blood vessels of a giant hemangioma.

b. **Malignant hypertension** is associated with severe vasoconstriction, increasing blood flow in tight spaces. This increases the risk that red cells will come in contact with vessel walls.

c. **Tight aortic stenosis.** The combination of very rapid blood flow through a very narrow aortic valve and into the large space beyond creates turbulence that can damage red cells.

d. **Prosthetic valve leak.** The back flow through a leaky prosthetic valve that is caused by cardiac contraction can damage red cells when they are drawn quickly through the narrow opening of the rigid valve walls.

2. **Blood flow through regions of intravascular coagulation** causes red cells to be caught in fibrin strands. Once caught, portions of the membrane are sliced off, resulting in red cell fragments

and the formation of schistocytes (helmet cells). Conditions associated with intravascular coagulation include disseminated intravascular coagulation (DIC) and thrombotic thrombocytopenic purpura (TTP).

3. **Repeated trauma to superficial capillaries** of the hands and feet can damage red cells as they flow under the skin surface, causing the cells to break up and form fragments of varying sizes and shapes. Damage of this nature usually is not enough to cause anemia by itself but may aggravate mild anemia from other causes. This so-called **march hemoglobinuria** can be seen in athletes, in soldiers after a long march, in bongo drummers, and in martial artists.

E. **Intravascular hemolysis** is a prominent feature of a few bacterial and parasitic infections, such as:

1. ***Clostridium perfringens* infection,** in which the bacilli **secrete a toxin that can cause hemolysis** by breaking down phospholipids in the erythrocyte membrane
2. ***Bartonella bacilliformis* infection,** which is a rare infection occurring in South America that causes **Oroya fever**
3. ***Plasmodium* infestation,** which is the most prevalent parasitic infestation and the cause of thousands of deaths every year from **malaria**
4. **Human immunodeficiency virus (HIV) infection,** which is seen in patients with acquired immune deficiency syndrome (AIDS) and is associated with autoimmunodeficiency diseases such as **autoimmune hemolytic anemia and idiopathic thrombocytopenic purpura (ITP)**

STUDY QUESTIONS

Directions: Each of the numbered items or incomplete statements in this section is followed by answers or by completions of the statement. Select the **one** lettered answer or completion that is **best** in each case.

1. The ingestion of fava beans can cause severe hemolytic anemia in patients who have which one of the following enzymopathies?

(A) Glucose-6-phosphate dehydrogenase (G6PD) deficiency (type A)
(B) Pyruvate kinase (PK) deficiency
(C) G6PD deficiency (Mediterranean form)
(D) Glutathione synthetase deficiency
(E) γ-Glutamylcysteine synthetase deficiency

2. Hemolysis in disseminated intravascular coagulation (DIC) is due to which one of the following mechanisms?

(A) Removal by the spleen of target cells that were formed when the red cell membrane expanded in response to an excess level of lipids
(B) Pitting of red cells by the spleen to remove Heinz bodies that were formed by the unstable denaturation of hemoglobin
(C) Formation of spherocytes in response to the activation of IgG complement in red cell membrane antigens
(D) Loss of membrane elasticity and formation of spherocytes as a result of a cytoskeletal defect
(E) Formation of helmet cells and cell fragments as red cells flow through small vessels in which the fibrin strands of a clot clothesline the red cells

3. The patient with intravascular hemolysis can present with all of the following clinical and laboratory findings EXCEPT

(A) low levels of serum haptoglobin
(B) increased indirect bilirubin
(C) splenomegaly
(D) hemoglobinuria and hemosiderinuria
(E) increased serum lactic dehydrogenase (LDH)

4. The patient with warm-type antibody autoimmune hemolytic anemia can present with all of the following symptoms and laboratory findings EXCEPT

(A) non-Hodgkin's lymphoma
(B) positive Coombs' test
(C) splenomegaly
(D) spherocytosis
(E) Raynaud's phenomenon

5. The patient with a glucose-6-phosphate dehydrogenase (G6PD) deficiency should be instructed to avoid all of the following EXCEPT

(A) cephalothin
(B) quinidine
(C) chloroquine
(D) fava beans
(E) sulfonamides

6. When recommending therapy to a patient with hereditary spherocytosis (HS), all of the following guidelines should be considered EXCEPT

(A) folates should be given and aplastic crisis should be managed by supportive transfusion therapy
(B) splenectomy should be avoided if possible in children younger than 10 years because of the risk of fulminant sepsis
(C) in patients with gallstones, the spleen should be removed with the gallbladder to avoid further stone formation by continued hemolysis
(D) adult patients should be splenectomized regardless of the degree of anemia since the procedure is usually curative

7. The patient with acute hemolysis may present with all of the following findings EXCEPT

(A) gallstones
(B) erythroid hyperplasia in the bone marrow
(C) increased mean corpuscular volume (MCV) with polychromatophilia
(D) increased serum indirect bilirubin
(E) dark urine that is positive for blood

1-C	4-E	7-A
2-E	5-A	
3-C	6-D	

8. Hemolytic anemia can be associated with all of the following infections EXCEPT

(A) human immunodeficiency virus (HIV)
(B) *Plasmodium*
(C) syphilis
(D) herpes simplex
(E) mycoplasmal pneumonia

Directions: Each group of items in this section consists of lettered options followed by a set of numbered items. For each item, select the **one** lettered option that is most closely associated with it. Each lettered option may be selected once, more than once, or not at all.

Questions 9–12

For each of the hematologic disorders presented below, select the diagnostic test by which it can be identified.

(A) Coombs' test
(B) Ham test
(C) Osmotic fragility test
(D) Heinz bodies test
(E) Donath-Landsteiner antibody test

9. Paroxysmal nocturnal hemoglobinuria (PNH)

10. Autoimmune hemolytic anemia with warm-type antibody

11. Glucose-6-phosphate dehydrogenase (G6PD) deficiency, Mediterranean type

12. Hereditary spherocytosis (HS)

Questions 13–16

For each of the hemolytic disorders presented below, select the mechanism that causes it.

(A) Mechanical or physical trauma (Waring blender syndrome)
(B) Membrane cytoskeletal abnormality
(C) Decay-accelerating factor deficiency
(D) Lipid membrane abnormality
(E) Autoantibodies and complement activation ,

13. Spur cell anemia

14. Paroxysmal nocturnal hemoglobinuria (PNH)

15. Kasabach-Merritt syndrome

16. Methyldopa-associated autoimmune hemolytic anemia

8-D	11-D	14-C
9-B	12-C	15-A
10-A	13-D	16-E

ANSWERS AND EXPLANATIONS

1. The answer is C *[V B 1 c (3)].*
Reticulocytes have higher levels of glucose-6-phosphate dehydrogenase (G6PD), pyruvate kinase (PK), glutathione synthetase, γ-glutamylcysteine synthetase, and other enzymes than do older cells. Once the older cells have been destroyed and replaced with the younger erythrocytes in metabolic enzymopathy, the hemolysis subsides. However, in the Mediterranean form of G6PD deficiency, this enzyme is so unstable that even reticulocytes are susceptible to oxidative damage. They will also hemolyze as long as the oxidative agents are present, and fava beans are a source of pyrimidine derivatives, which have potent oxidative properties.

2. The answer is E *[V D 2].*
The presence of helmet cells and red cell fragments is characteristic of disseminated intravascular coagulation (DIC) caused by intravascular coagulation and the deposition of fibrin in the capillaries. The damage done to passing red cells causes the hemolysis. The expansion of the red cell membrane in response to increased levels of lipids is the mechanism of spur cell anemia. Denatured hemoglobin and Heinz bodies are seen in glucose-6-phosphate dehydrogenase (G6PD) deficiency patients who are exposed to oxidative agents. In autoimmune hemolytic anemia, spherocytes are created when parts of the red cell membrane are removed by macrophages with Fc receptors responding to the presence of IgG. Cytoskeletal abnormality is the mechanism of hereditary spherocytosis (HS).

3. The answer is C *[IV D 1].*
Patients with intravascular hemolysis do not present with an enlarged spleen. Extravascular hemolysis results when the normal destruction of red cells is accelerated primarily through the increased activity of tissue macrophages located in the spleen, thus resulting in splenomegaly. Intravascular hemolysis alters the blood chemistry. Red cells are rich in lactic dehydrogenase (LDH), and their breakdown releases this enzyme to the circulation along with their hemoglobin. The hepatic breakdown products of this hemoglobin overwhelm the normal disposal mechanisms. Haptoglobin is rapidly depleted, and the patient displays hemoglobinuria, hemosiderinuria, and an increase in indirect bilirubin.

4. The answer is E *[V A 3 a (1) (a)–(c), (2) (a)–(c)].*
The patient with warm-reactive autoantibody hemolytic anemia will not present with Raynaud's phenomenon, which results from the agglutination of red cells in the distal vasculature at low ambient temperatures by cold-responsive autoantibodies. The presence of warm-responsive autoantibodies results in splenomegaly (mostly in extravascular hemolysis), a positive Coombs' test, and the presence of spherocytes in the smear. These symptoms can be idiopathic or secondary to lymphoma.

5. The answer is A *[V B 1 b (1); Table 7-4].*
Patients with glucose-6-phosphate dehydrogenase (G6PD) deficiency should avoid all oxidative agents; cephalothin is not an oxidative agent. Quinidine, chloroquine, fava beans, and sulfonamides are all oxidative agents and have been implicated in causing hemolysis in G6PD-deficient patients. Travelers who are contemplating prophylactic antimalarial treatment (quinidine) should be tested for G6PD deficiency.

6. The answer is D *[V C 1 d].*
The patient with hereditary spherocytosis (HS) should not be splenectomized unless warranted by the degree of anemia. The patient with HS can be asymptomatic for a long period of time with good support such as folate replacement therapy without developing anemia. Long-term or chronic hemolysis may result in severe anemia that requires blood transfusion or splenectomy. However, splenectomy is usually delayed if possible until the patient is at least 10 years of age to allow the immune system to mature and to avoid the risk of fulminant infection secondary to splenectomy.

7. The answer is A *[IV A 1].*
The patient with acute hemolysis will not present with bile gallstones or cholecystitis, signs that distinguish chronic hemolysis. The signs and symptoms of acute hemolysis are a compensatory erythroid hyperplasia in the bone marrow, increased reticulocyte counts that may show as increased mean corpuscular volume (MCV) and polychromatophilia, increased breakdown of heme to bilirubin and other indirect forms as a result of the overwhelming of liver function, and hemoglobinuria, which is seen as dark red or brown urine that tests positive for blood.

8. The answer is D *[V E].*
Infection with herpes simplex virus does not cause hemolysis and is not related to a hemolytic process. Human immunodeficiency virus (HIV) infection is associated with autoimmune hemolytic anemia. Malaria (*Plasmodium* infestation) causes intravascular hemolysis by invading red cells. The presence of Donath-Landsteiner antibody and the subsequent paroxysmal cold hemoglobinuria is associated with syphilis. The presence of cold-type antibody is also associated with mycoplasmal pneumonia.

9–12. The answers are: 9-B *[V C 4 c (1)],* **10-A** *[V A 3 a (1) (c)],* **11-D** *[V B 1 b (2), d (2)],* **12-C** *[V C 1 c (1)].*
In the Ham test, the presence of paroxysmal nocturnal hemoglobinuria (PNH) is determined by incubating the patient's red cells in acidified normal serum. A positive result indicates the presence of sensitive, abnormal PNH II and PNH III cells; their hemolysis is the result of the activation of complement. Since some normal serum is inactive in this test and may give a false-negative result, the sugar water test is performed to check if the negative Ham test result is a true- or false-negative.

Although the indirect Coombs' test may give positive results in two-thirds of patients with autoimmune hemolytic anemia, the direct Coombs' test will demonstrate the presence of autoantibodies, complement, or both on the red cell surface. The indirect Coombs' test demonstrates antibodies in the serum, and they are specific to antigens in the donor red cells, causing a delayed hemolytic transfusion reaction.

The formation of Heinz bodies (unstable hemoglobin precipitates) can be seen on crystal violet stain in glucose-6-phosphate dehydrogenase (G6PD) deficiency during episodes of hemolysis. Although the test is nonspecific, diagnosis is made by transiently assaying enzyme levels in red cells during the stable phase.

The test for hereditary spherocytosis (HS) is the osmotic fragility test, in which the patient's red cells are exposed to a series of sodium chloride solutions that vary from isotonic concentration (0.9%) to much lower concentrations. HS is demonstrated when hemolysis occurs at concentrations of 0.6% to 0.8%; normal cells do not demonstrate hemolysis until concentrations of 0.4% to 0.5% are reached. HS red cells are already in the form of spherocytes and do not have much leeway for expansion in response to the low sodium concentration of their test environment. Normal cells are able to withstand much lower sodium concentrations.

13–16. The answers are: 13-D *[V C 3],* **14-C** *[V C 4 a (1) (a)],* **15-A** *[V D 1 a],* **16-E** *[V A 3 c (3)].*
Spur cell anemia is commonly seen in conjunction with liver disease that is associated with hypercholesterolemia. Because of the high levels of serum lipids, the level of lipids in the erythrocyte membrane increases; the membrane surface area thus increases, causing the formation of target cells and acanthocytes. These abnormally shaped cells are removed from the circulation by the spleen, precipitating the anemia.

Paroxysmal nocturnal hemoglobinuria red cells (PNH II red cells) are sensitive to the alternative pathway of complement that is normally inactivated by decay-accelerating factor (DAF); DAF is deficient in these cells.

The Kasabach-Merritt syndrome is a hemolytic anemia found in giant hemangiomas and other malignant tumors. It is due to the physical damage of red cells as they pass through the abnormal, tortuous, irregular blood vessels created as a result of the neovascularization within the malignant tumors.

Methyldopa-associated autoimmune hemolytic anemia is similar to idiopathic autoimmune hemolytic anemia and is a true autoimmune process that is probably due to the prolonged effects of the drug on the T cells, causing an imbalance between helper and suppressor T cells.

8
Globin Synthesis and the Thalassemia Syndromes

Emmanuel C. Besa

I. DEFINITION. The thalassemia syndromes are syndromes that result from **inherited abnormalities in globin synthesis** that lead to decreases in the production of hemoglobin. Hemoglobin synthesis is dependent on a balanced production of heme and globin chains; a decrease of one component will lead to a decrease in hemoglobin and hypochromic, microcytic anemia. The structure of hemoglobin and genetic defects affecting the structure or rate of synthesis of globin chains (hemoglobinopathies) are considered in greater detail in Chapter 9.

II. GLOBIN SYNTHESIS

A. Composition of hemoglobin

1. **Globin chains.** Hemoglobin is composed of pairs of two types of globin chains:
   a. Alpha (α) chains
   b. Non-α chains

2. **Fetal hemoglobin (Hb F)**
   a. Early in embryonic development, two α-like chains [the theta (θ) and zeta (ζ) chains] are produced and combine with a beta (β)-like chain [the epsilon (ε) chain] to form hemoglobin (Gower I, Gower II, and Portland hemoglobins). The β chain is the component that predominates in adult hemoglobin.
   b. Later in the first trimester, α chains combine with other β-like chains [gamma (γ) chains] to form **Hb F**.

3. **Adult hemoglobin**
   a. **Hemoglobin A (Hb A) is the major component of adult hemoglobin** and is composed of pairs of α chains and β chains. The β chains are synthesized early in the individual's development but do not predominate until the third month after birth.
   b. **Hemoglobin A_2 (Hb A_2) is the minor component of hemoglobin** (accounting for 2.5%) and is composed of pairs of α chains and delta (δ) chains, which closely resemble β chains.

B. Genetic control of globin-chain synthesis (Figure 8-1).
There are at least six loci on chromosomes 11 and 16 that direct globin synthesis. The α and β chains of the adult are normally produced in equal amounts, but the genes that control their syntheses are far apart on different chromosomes; those for the α family of globins (α, θ, and ζ) are on chromosome 16, and those for the β family (β, γ, δ, and ε) are on chromosome 11.

1. **Globin gene.** The genes on chromosomes 11 and 16 responsible for globin-chain synthesis have a complex structure. Nucleotides in the genes create the template for globin synthesis. These nucleotides, although arranged in a very precise sequence, are not adjacent. Coding regions of DNA (**exons**) are interrupted by sections of DNA that are not used in coding (**introns**).

2. **Globin synthesis** (Figure 8-2)
   a. **Transcription.** The instructions for the synthesis of globin must first be transcribed from DNA to nuclear RNA. This nuclear RNA includes both exons and introns.
   b. **RNA splicing.** The transcribed RNA is then modified: The introns are excised and the remaining exons are fused, forming messenger RNA (mRNA). A 7-methyl G cap is then added to the 5′ end of the mRNA chain, and a poly-A chain is attached to the 3′ end of the mRNA.

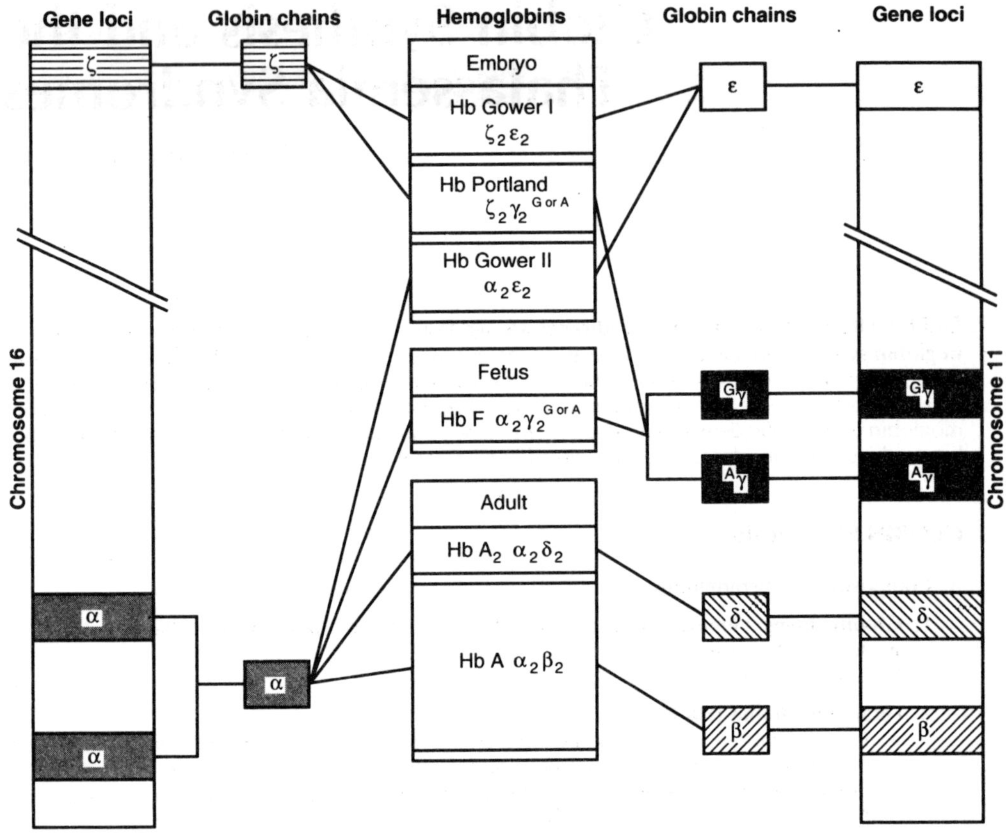

Figure 8-1. The synthesis of globin is under the control of genes on chromosome 16 (for the α family of globins) and chromosome 11 (for the β family of globins). The coding segments of DNA (exons) are separated by noncoding segments of DNA (introns). (Adapted from Schrier SL: Hematology. In *Scientific American: Medicine.* New York, Scientific American, 1991, Section 5, subsection IV, p 22.)

c. **Translation.** The mRNA then moves to the cytoplasm, attaches to ribosomes, and acts as a template, accepting amino acids from transfer RNA (tRNA) in the sequence predetermined by its structure so that they can combine to form the necessary globin chain.

III. PATHOPHYSIOLOGY OF THE THALASSEMIAS.
The thalassemias are caused by mutations in the chromosome regions that contain the globin genes. These genetic defects and their associated thalassemias are shown in Table 8-1.

A. α Thalassemia. Gene deletions are responsible for the decrease in or absence of α chains in most α thalassemias. In some forms of α thalassemia, such as hemoglobin H (Hb H) disease, the α gene is detected. The defect in this situation is presumed to occur without a deletion.

B. β Thalassemia. In contrast to α thalassemia, β thalassemia is **usually due to an mRNA abnormality;** this mutation reduces or eliminates the production of β-globin chains. In general, β thalassemias are the result of point mutations in or near the globin genes, causing, for example, defective splicing (in which splices do not occur or occur at the wrong sites), nonsense lesions (in which chains terminate prematurely), and frameshift. Gene deletions may cause β thalassemias but are more common in α thalassemia.

1. **Gene defects**
   a. **Classification.** The β thalassemia defects fall into three general classes.
      (1) **Substitution** is the **replacement of one base with another** without an alteration in the total length of the DNA molecule.

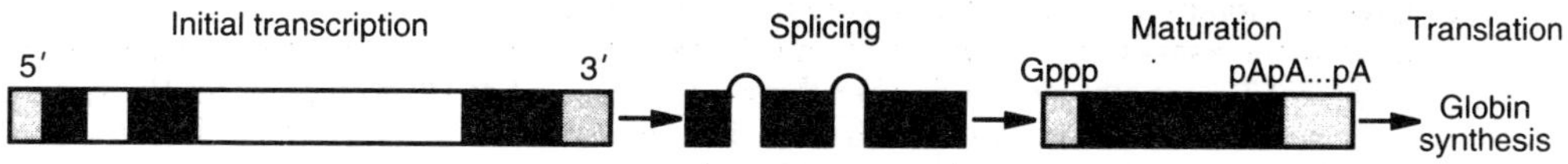

Figure 8-2. Globin synthesis begins with transcription of messenger RNA (mRNA), which starts at the cap (*5′*) and proceeds to the termination site (*3′*). This initial copy includes the exons (*shaded areas*), introns (*unshaded areas*), and flanking sequences (*stippled areas*). The mRNA then undergoes post-transcriptional modifications: (1) Introns are spliced out so that exons can be fused, (2) a 7-methyl G cap is attached to the 5′ end of mRNA, and (3) a poly-A chain is added to the 3′ end of mRNA. The completed mRNA then moves to the cytoplasm, where it participates in the construction of globin chains.

(2) **Deletion** is the **elimination of an entire stretch of DNA** from the molecule, as occurs, for example, in hemoglobin Lepore (Hb Lepore).

(3) **Frameshift** is the **insertion or deletion of a single nucleotide, resulting in the lengthening or shortening of the DNA molecule** by one base pair. Frameshift can occur during transcription to mRNA. The shift changes the reading frame for protein synthesis, resulting in a completely normal protein upstream of the mutation, while downstream of the mutation the protein is totally scrambled.

b. **Expression.** Mutations in the exon may have one of three effects:

(1) **Decreased RNA production due to gene deletions**

(2) **Production of mRNA that codes for an abnormal globin** (e.g., a chain with amino acid substitutions or a chain that is too short or too long because of abnormal termination)

(3) **Minor alterations in RNA that produce a normal globin chain**

2. **Terminal group defects.** A decrease in mRNA production can occur due to delay in the transcription process caused by mutations in the untranslated terminal groups.

IV. CLINICAL MANIFESTATIONS OF THALASSEMIA

A. **β Thalassemias.** The decreased production of β chains results in an **excess of α chains that precipitate** and subsequently are removed by the spleen, **causing hemolysis.**

1. **Pathogenesis of the anemia of β thalassemia.** Decreased β-chain production has two major consequences.

a. **Total hemoglobin synthesis is reduced, leading to microcytic anemia.** In compensation for the reduced levels of Hb A, the concentrations of Hb A_2 and Hb F increase, for example, since they contain other β-like chains.

b. **Free α chains accumulate in the red cells.**

(1) The imbalance between α- and β-chain synthesis causes α chains to accumulate and precipitate (i.e., Heinz bodies are formed) inside the cells. This leads to **hemolysis,** the destruction of these red cells in the bone marrow in β thalassemia major.

(2) The extent to which β-chain synthesis is suppressed determines the degree of anemia seen in β thalassemia—mild anemia in β thalassemia minor to the severe anemia in β thalassemia major that is caused by the **ineffective erythropoiesis.**

(3) Overall red cell production is also greatly increased as a consequence of α-chain accumulation due to **extramedullary hematopoiesis and increased erythropoiesis in the bone marrow.**

Table 8-1. Genetic Defects in the Various Forms of Thalassemias

Type of Thalassemia	Genetic Defect	Region Affected
α Thalassemia	Deletion	Entire α gene
	Short deletion	Intron of α gene
$β^+$ Thalassemia	Substitution	Intron of β gene
$β^0$ Thalassemia	Deletion	Part of β gene
	Substitution	Exon of β gene (new termination signal)
δβ Thalassemia	Deletion	Entire β gene and part of δ gene
Hereditary persistence of fetal hemoglobin (HPFH)	Deletion	Entire β and δ genes

2. Classification of β thalassemias (Figure 8-3; Table 8-2)

a. β Thalassemia major ($\beta^0\beta^0$) is the **most severe** β thalassemia and usually becomes apparent 3–6 months after birth when the switch from Hb F to Hb A takes place. The symbol β^0 indicates that there is a total absence of β-chain production; a γ, δ, or ε chain replaces it in one or both positions, indicated by whether one or two symbols are given. The following signs may be evident.

(1) **Hepatosplenomegaly** may be present due to excessive red cell destruction, extramedullary hematopoiesis, and iron overload. An enlarged spleen increases red cell destruction, pooling, and the need for transfusion. Gallstones are also common.

(2) **Expansion of the bones** may occur because intense marrow hyperplasia leads to prominence of the malar eminences, frontal bossing, and maxillary hypertrophy (chipmunk facies). There may be thinning of the cortex of many bones, with a tendency to fracture, and a hair-on-end appearance of the skull on x-ray.

(3) **Severe anemia with growth retardation and delayed sexual development** may occur.

(4) **Damage to the heart, pancreas, endocrine organs, and liver** similar to that seen in hemochromatosis (see Ch 5) may result from an iron overload caused by repeated transfusions.

b. β Thalassemia intermedia ($\beta^0\beta^0$ or $\beta^+\beta^+$) presents with abnormalities similar to those of thalassemia major. However, the patient suffers only a **moderate degree of anemia** and has only an intermittent or no requirement for transfusion. These patients have chronic disease up to adult life. The symbol β^+ indicates that there is a partial deficiency of β-chain production.

c. Hb Lepore disease is an unusual type of thalassemia that occurs when fusion variations of α and β chains produce an abnormal hemoglobin. The abnormality results when a defect occurs in the recombiation of the α and β chains during meiosis.

d. β Thalassemia trait ($\beta\beta^0$ or $\beta\beta^+$) is a relatively **mild disease** with few or no symptoms; the diagnosis is made only upon conducting a family study.

e. β Thalassemia minor (δβ thalassemia) can be detected only by genetic studies.

f. Hereditary persistence of fetal hemoglobin (HPFH) is clinically different from, although related to, β thalassemia in that β- and δ-chain production are decreased. Production of the adjacent γ chain is enhanced, however, and, therefore, the synthesis of globin chains is more in balance than in β thalassemia. **Anemia is mild or absent** since there is no accumulation of α chains in the red cells. HPFH is characterized by the production of fetal hemoglobin into adulthood.

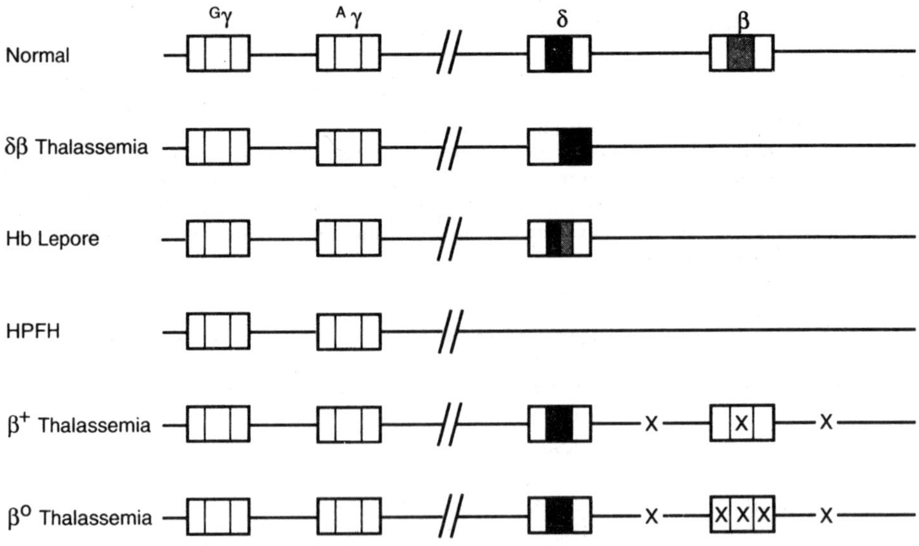

Figure 8-3. Schematic representation of the genetic defects in chromosome 11 observed in the different β thalassemias. *HPFH* = hereditary persistence of fetal hemoglobin; *X* = postulated site of nucleotide change. (Reprinted from Rifkind RA: *Fundamental Hematology,* 3rd edition. Chicago, Mosby-Year Book, 1986, p 90.)

Table 8-2. Clinical Forms of Thalassemias

Thalassemia major
Transfusion-dependent β^0 thalassemia
Homozygous β^+ thalassemia (some types)
Thalassemia intermedia
Hemoglobin Lepore syndromes
Homozygous $\delta\beta$ thalassemia and hereditary persistence of fetal hemoglobin (HPFH)
Combinations of α and β thalassemias
Hemoglobin H disease
Thalassemia minor
β^0 Thalassemia trait
$\delta\beta$ Thalassemia trait
HPFH
β^+ Thalassemia trait
α^1 (α^0) Thalassemia trait
α^2 (α^+) Thalassemia trait

3. **Diagnosis of β thalassemia** is made by the association of the following laboratory findings with a positive family history.
   a. **Nonspecific findings**
      (1) Blood smear reveals microcytic red cells with poikilocytosis and fragmented dacrocytes. The mean corpuscular volume (MCV) is low (around 65 fl).
      (2) Heinz bodies are evident by supravital staining with crystal violet.
   b. **Specific findings.** The definitive diagnosis of β thalassemia is based on the following findings on hemoglobin electrophoresis:
      (1) Findings true of β thalassemia
         (a) Increased proportion of Hb A_2 (to >3.5%; normal is 2%–3%)
         (b) Increased proportion of Hb F in HPFH (to 70%–100%; normal is 1%–3%)
      (2) Differentiating features among β thalassemias
         (a) Decreased proportion of Hb A in β thalassemia trait
         (b) Very little Hb A in β thalassemia major
         (c) Absence of Hb A_2 in β thalassemia minor, HPFH, and Hb Lepore

B. α Thalassemias. In α thalassemia, a decreased synthesis of α chains, leading to the **precipitation of Hb H** (an abnormal hemoglobin composed of four β chains) **or Bart's hemoglobin** (an abnormal hemoglobin composed of four γ chains), results from genetic defects that prevent the formation of some or all of the necessary α globin.

1. **Classification of α thalassemias** (Figure 8-4)
   a. **Hydrops fetalis is the most severe form** of α thalassemia: All four α genes are deleted, resulting in a severely anemic, edematous, stillborn infant. The Bart's hemoglobin causes morbidity and mortality in the infant because of its very high oxygen affinity.
   b. **Hb H disease,** which is clinically similar to β thalassemia major, is the result of the deletion of three α genes. Because of its instability, Hb H precipitates and results in extravascular hemolysis.
   c. **α Thalassemia trait** is the result of the deletion of two α genes. The condition occurs in the offspring of two carrier parents or of an Hb H parent and a normal parent and is clinically similar to β thalassemia minor.
   d. **α Thalassemia carrier** is the result of the deletion of one α gene; these individuals are asymptomatic.

2. **Diagnosis of α thalassemia** is made by the association of the following laboratory findings with a positive family history.
   a. **Nonspecific findings**
      (1) Blood smear reveals microcytic, hypochromic red cells, target cells, and anisopoikilocytosis. The MCV is low.
      (2) Heinz bodies are evident.
   b. **Specific findings.** The definitive diagnosis of α thalassemia is based on the identification of Hb H by hemoglobin electrophoresis.

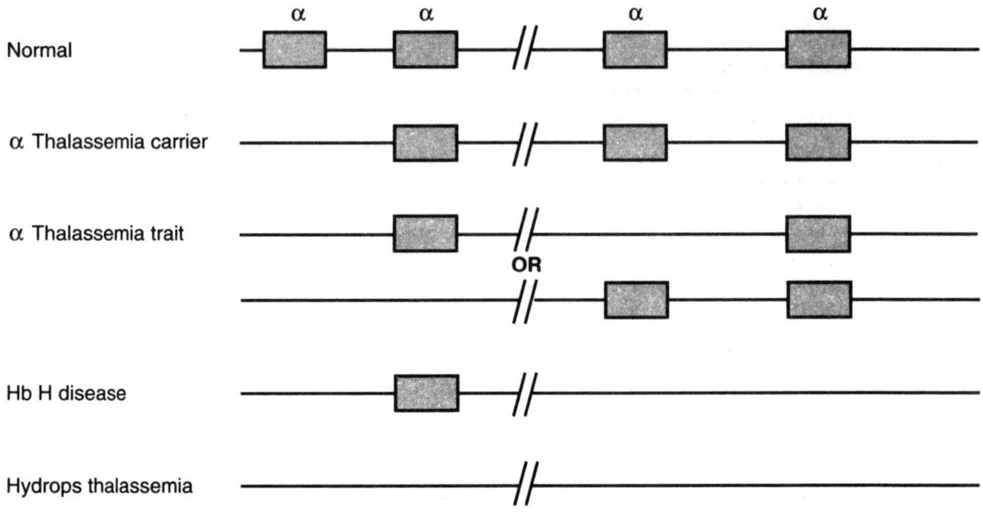

Figure 8-4. Schematic representation of the genetic defects in chromosome 16 observed in the different α thalassemias.

V. TREATMENT OF α AND β THALASSEMIA.

The severity of the anemia dictates treatment, which consists of the following measures.

A. Regular red cell transfusions are needed to maintain hemoglobin levels above 11 g/dl. Separating the larger red cells (neocytes) by density centrifugation and transfusing the neocytes has increased the red cell survival and decreased the frequency of transfusion and iron overload in these patients. Usually, 2 or 3 units are administered every 4–6 weeks. The use of white cell filters lowers the rate of transfusion reactions.

B. Folic acid supplementation should be given to prevent aplastic crisis.

C. Iron chelation is indicated for transfusion-induced iron accumulation. Deferoxamine is administered either with each unit of transfused blood (2 g) or by slow subcutaneous daily infusions by pump (1–4 g over 8–12 hours).

D. Splenectomy is indicated if an enlarging spleen is contributing to increased transfusion requirements.

E. Bone marrow transplantation, although still experimental, is a highly promising form of therapy in severe cases of thalassemia, especially if performed prior to development of hepatomegaly and portal fibrosis.

VI. PRENATAL DIAGNOSIS OF THALASSEMIA.

A prenatal diagnosis may guide parents and physicians in deciding whether to complete a pregnancy. If both parents are known carriers, fetal diagnosis can be conducted either by using a fetoscope to sample fetal venous blood for the determination of the α/β-chain synthesis ratio or by amniocentesis or trophoblast (chorionic villus) biopsy to obtain DNA for hybridization with relevant DNA probes. The use of restriction mapping of the globin genes and cloned DNA probes of human globin gene sequences now allow for the detection of thalassemia from just a few cells. Thus, the parents and physician can make an informed decision through the use of safe procedures that do not expose the mother or fetus to unnecessary risk.

STUDY QUESTIONS

Directions: Each of the numbered items or incomplete statements in this section is followed by answers or by completions of the statement. Select the **one** lettered answer or completion that is **best** in each case.

1. Which of the following findings is specific for a diagnosis of α thalassemia in a patient who is symptomatic and anemic?

(A) Low mean corpuscular volume (MCV)
(B) Target cells and anisopoikilocytosis on blood smear
(C) Hemoglobin H (Hb H) by hemoglobin electrophoresis
(D) Heinz bodies

2. Both members of a couple are carriers of the thalassemia gene. The best method for determining whether their unborn child will be severely affected by thalassemia is

(A) a detailed family tree
(B) statistical calculation of risk
(C) chromosome analysis of the parents
(D) amniocentesis and DNA hybridization

3. Which of the following therapeutic modalities is NOT yet accepted in the United States as standard treatment for thalassemia?

(A) Folic acid supplementation
(B) Bone marrow transplantation
(C) Iron chelation with deferoxamine
(D) Splenectomy

Directions: Each item below contains four suggested answers, of which **one or more** is correct. Choose the answer

A if **1, 2, and 3** are correct
B if **1 and 3** are correct
C if **2 and 4** are correct
D if **4** is correct
E if **1, 2, 3, and 4** are correct

4. Advances in molecular biology have identified the genetics of hemoglobin production and helped clarify the pathophysiology of the thalassemias. True statements concerning the genetics of hemoglobin production include which of the following?

(1) The genes that code for the hemoglobin chains have been found on different chromosomes
(2) The genes that code for hemoglobin are not contiguous on the same chromosome
(3) α and β Thalassemias can be diagnosed prenatally by examining amniotic fluid
(4) β Thalassemia, in contrast to α thalassemia, is usually due to a messenger RNA (mRNA) abnormality rather than a gene deletion

5. Statements true of either α or β thalassemia include which of the following?

(1) An amino acid substitution is the typical form of genetic mutation
(2) Thalassemia trait may manifest as an unexplained microcytic, hypochromic blood picture with mild or no anemia
(3) Patients who are homozygous for thalassemia do not survive childhood
(4) Blood transfusion supplemented by splenectomy, iron chelation therapy, and neocyte transfusions is the mainstay of therapy in thalassemia major

---

1-C
2-D
3-B
4-E
5-C

ANSWERS AND EXPLANATIONS

1. The answer is C *[IV B 2 b].*
The definitive diagnosis of α thalassemia requires identification of hemoglobin H (Hb H) by hemoglobin electrophoresis. Findings that suggest thalassemia include a hypochromic, microcytic anemia [i.e., low mean corpuscular volume (MCV)], Heinz bodies, and a positive family history. Hemoglobin electrophoresis is needed to establish the type of thalassemia (i.e., α or β). Other nonspecific findings in α thalassemia include target cells and anisopoikilocytosis on blood smear.

2. The answer is D *[VI].*
Prenatal diagnosis of thalassemia can be achieved with reasonable safety by fetal blood sampling (using a fetoscope) to measure the α/β-chain synthesis ratio or by amniocentesis or chorionic villus biopsy to obtain DNA for hybridization with relevant DNA probes. These techniques allow the couple, with the guidance of their physician, to consider whether or not this pregnancy should be carried to term in the event that their child will be severely affected.

3. The answer is B *[V E].*
Bone marrow transplantation is still an experimental form of thalassemia treatment in the United States. Standard therapy for severe thalassemia consists of folic acid supplementation (to prevent aplastic crisis), red cell transfusion (for anemia), iron chelation (for transfusion-related iron accumulation), and splenectomy (if splenomegaly is the cause of increased transfusion requirements).

4. The answer is E (all) *[II B; III B; VI].*
Advances of molecular biology have helped to uncover the mechanisms of the genetic control of hemoglobin formation. The genes that code for the hemoglobin chains have been identified. The genes for the α family of globins (α, θ, and ζ) are found on chromosome 16, and those for the β family of globins (β, γ, δ, and ϵ) are found on chromosome 11.

It has become possible to map the genes by breaking up the genome into fragments of sharply defined lengths using restriction endonucleases and then determining which fragments contain the globin genes in a process called restriction mapping. Identification of the fragments containing the globin genes is accomplished by using a radioactively labeled cloned DNA probe (which is made from bacteria in which a small piece of globin gene containing human DNA has been artificially introduced) that binds specifically to globin sequences.

Physicians can now predict with certain accuracy the health of a fetus by establishing fetal globin maps that were inherited from each parent. Safe and effective prenatal diagnosis of α and β thalassemias is now possible by measuring the globin-chain synthetic rates in cord blood. α Thalassemia can also be diagnosed prenatally by examining amniotic fluid cells by restriction mapping; however, β thalassemia is rarely diagnosed by the latter method because, unlike α thalassemia, which results from gene deletions, β thalassemias almost always result from limited mutations that cannot be detected by restriction mapping.

5. The answer is C (2, 4) *[IV A, B; V].*
Most α thalassemias, together with $\delta\beta$ thalassemia and hereditary persistence of fetal hemoglobin (HPFH), are due to gene deletions of major size. On the other hand, most β and β^+ thalassemias seem to be genetic defects that are more localized as substitutions and small deletions. Unlike patients who are homozygous for α thalassemias, which cause hydrops fetalis, patients who are homozygous for β thalassemias can survive childhood, and their life spans can be extended with chronic transfusions and chelation therapy. Patients with α and β thalassemia traits are usually asymptomatic and may not be anemic except for an unexplained microcytosis of their red cells, which would be difficult to diagnose. Efforts to decrease the frequency of blood transfusions in thalassemia patients involve transfusing neocytes or splenectomy to improve red cell survival. Iron chelation therapy is being used to prevent the adverse effects of iron overload, which result from multiple transfusions.

9
Hemoglobin and Hemoglobinopathies

Emmanuel C. Besa

I. HEMOGLOBIN

A. Structure. The structure of hemoglobin is shown in Figure 9-1; the molecule has two components:

1. **Heme moiety,** which contains one ferrous iron atom (Fe^{2+}) carried in a porphyrin ring (the structure and synthesis of porphyrin are described in Chapter 5 II A, C; Figure 5-1)

2. **Globin tetramer,** which is bound to the heme moiety and is composed of two alpha- (α-) globin chains and two non–α-globin chains (the structure and synthesis of the globin chains are described in Chapter 8 II)

B. Differentiation. The **type of hemoglobin is determined by the globin chains that comprise it**. The types of globin chains available for hemoglobin synthesis depend on the developmental stage of the individual.

1. **Embryonic hemoglobin.** Red cell synthesis begins in the yolk sac of 19-day-old embryos, continues in the liver by 6 weeks, and begins in the bone marrow by 4–5 months gestation. The main embryonic hemoglobins present in the first 3–6 months in utero are:
   a. **Gower I ($\zeta_2\epsilon_2$),** which is composed of two α-like globin chains called zeta (ζ) chains and two epsilon (ϵ) chains, a type of globin closely related to the prominent non-α globin in adults called the beta (β) globin
   b. **Gower II ($\alpha_2\epsilon_2$),** which is composed of two α-globin chains and two ϵ-globin chains
   c. **Portland ($\zeta_2\gamma_2$),** which is composed of two ζ-globin chains and two chains of gamma (γ) globin, another β-like globin that is a successor to the ϵ globin

2. **Fetal hemoglobin ($\alpha_2\gamma_2$).** Fetal hemoglobin **(Hb F)** is composed of two α-globin chains and two γ-globin chains and **represents 90%–95% of the in utero hemoglobin** from 8–35 weeks gestation until the switch from fetal to adult hemoglobin occurs.

3. **Adult hemoglobin ($\alpha_2\beta_2$)** is composed of two α- and two β-globin chains, is **designated Hb A, and accounts for 96%–98%** of all adult hemoglobin. Adult hemoglobin **($\alpha_2\delta_2$)** composed of two α-globin chains and two chains of delta (δ) globin, another β-like globin, is **designated Hb A_2 and represents 1.5%–3%** of all adult hemoglobin. Small amounts of **Hb F (0.5%–1%)** also remain in the adult.

C. Function. Hemoglobin is the main solute in the erythrocyte, and its properties affect the red cell's adaptability in size, shape, flexibility, flow, and function.

1. **Oxygen transport.** Hemoglobin takes up oxygen from the pulmonary circulation and delivers it to the tissues.
   a. **Hemoglobin–oxygen (Hb–O_2) affinity.** The affinity of hemoglobin for oxygen at various intracellular and extracellular oxygen tensions (partial pressures) is represented by the sigmoid-shaped oxygen dissociation curve (Figure 9-2).
   b. **Factors that affect Hb–O_2 affinity.** Hypoxia itself creates metabolic conditions that force the delivery of more oxygen to the tissues.
      (1) **Bohr effect.** Tissue hypoxia can cause an acidotic microenvironment. According to the Bohr effect, **as pH is lowered, more oxygen is released from hemoglobin**. Thus, the acidic conditions of tissue with a low oxygen content (40 mm Hg) permit a more efficient delivery of oxygen where it is needed (a right shift of the oxygen dissociation

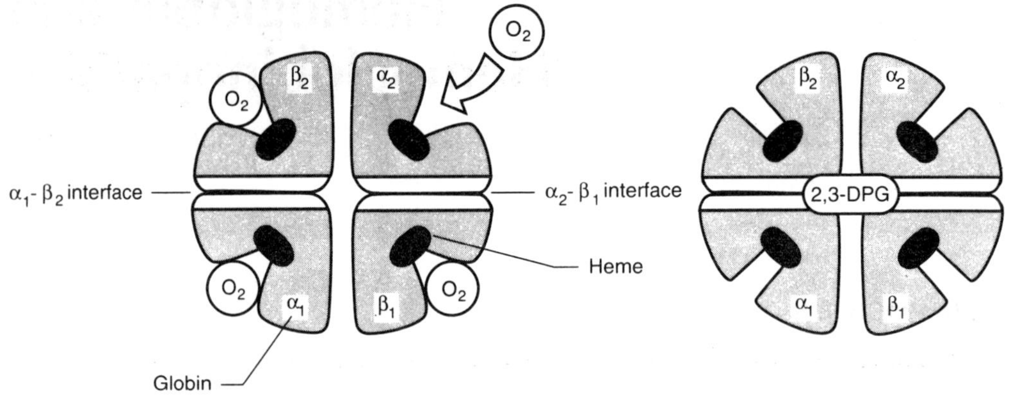

Figure 9-1. Hemoglobin is a tetramer composed of two α-globin chains (α_1 and α_2) and two β-globin chains (β_1 and β_2) linked to four heme molecules, each of which carries iron in a porphyrin ring. The α_1–β_2 and α_2–β_1 interfaces are the areas where the hemoglobin molecule deforms to create the heme crevice that accommodates the oxygen molecule. 2,3-Diphosphoglycerate (*2,3-DPG*) binds in the center of the hemoglobin after the red cell has given up its oxygen and decreases the affinity for oxygen. (Adapted from Hoffbrand AV, Pettit JE: *Essential Haematology,* 2nd edition. Oxford, Blackwell Scientific Publications, 1984, p 10.)

curve), while oxygen can still saturate hemoglobin in the pulmonary alveolar capillaries at their normal tissue oxygen tension level of 100 mm Hg.

(2) **2,3-Diphosphoglycerate (2,3-DPG).** Certain organic intermediates of the glycolytic pathway (i.e., the Rapaport-Leubering cycle of the Embden-Meyerhof pathway) influence the Hb–O_2 dissociation affinity of normal adult hemoglobin (Hb A). The 2, 3-DPG molecule **binds the β chain of Hb A at the N terminal,** which results in a decrease in the oxygen affinity by 3.8 mm Hg for every mM of 2,3-DPG bound. Hb F is unable to bind 2,3-DPG and, therefore, has a higher affinity for oxygen compared to Hb A.

c. **Spatial rearrangement of hemoglobin.** To take up and deliver oxygen, the hemoglobin molecule undergoes considerable spatial rearrangement that gives it its unique oxygen-binding properties. The initial attachment of deoxygenated hemoglobin to an oxygen molecule requires a relatively large increase in oxygen tension because of the very low affinity for oxygen of deoxygenated hemoglobin. After the initial binding, a spacial change in the tetrameric molecule occurs, enhancing the ability of hemoglobin to bind more oxygen molecules.

(1) The **initial effect** is presumably a change in the distal histidine radical linked to the ferrous iron that causes a sliding motion in the α–β contact area, **distorting the molecular shape** and reducing the size of the central cavity.

(2) The **other heme pockets then become more available** as a heme crevice is formed that can accept two more molecules of oxygen with only a slight increase in oxygen tension.

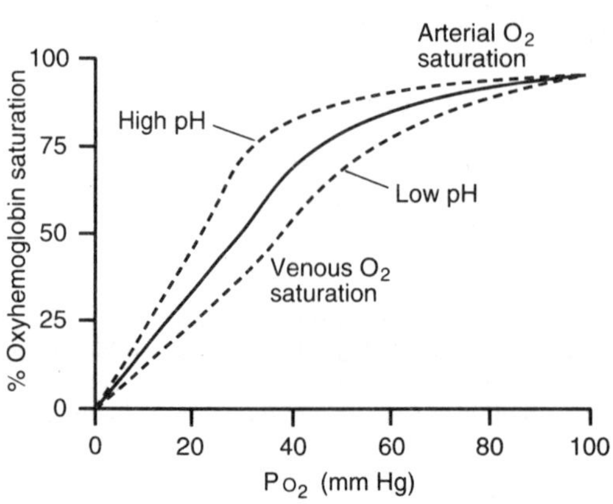

Figure 9-2. The oxygen dissociation curve of hemoglobin (Hb–O_2 dissociation curve) [*solid line*] represents the affinity of hemoglobin for oxygen at various intracellular and extracellular oxygen tensions (Po_2) from venous to arterial saturation. The sigmoid shape of the curve is critical for hemoglobin function, allowing hemoglobin to saturate with oxygen in the lung and to unload oxygen at the relatively high Po_2 at the tissue level. The position of the curve may be shifted by several factors, including the pH and temperature of blood and the concentration of certain organic phosphates. According to the Bohr effect, carbon dioxide is given off at the pulmonary capillaries, raising blood pH and causing a beneficial increase in affinity for oxygen (leftward shift); this allows easier loading of oxygen in red cells. Conversely, as oxygenated red cells enter tissue capillaries that are rich in carbon dioxide, blood pH decreases and causes a decreased affinity for oxygen (rightward shift); this allows better delivery of oxygen to oxygen-deprived cells.

2. **Carbon dioxide transport.** Once hemoglobin unloads oxygen at the tissues, it takes up carbon dioxide for disposal.
   a. As the hemoglobin molecule unloads oxygen, the globin chains shift and the β chains are pulled apart, which permits entry of 2,3-DPG and carbon dioxide, lowers the affinity for oxygen, and causes the sigmoid shape of the Hb–O_2 dissociation curve.
   b. The curve shifts to the right with high concentrations of carbon dioxide, 2,3-DPG, and hydrogen and in the presence of certain hemoglobins such as sickle hemoglobin [Hb S; see II E 1 a (1)].

II. HEMOGLOBINOPATHIES

A. Introduction

1. **Definition.** Hemoglobinopathies are inherited disorders in which **mutations** in or near the globin genes **alter the structure** (amino acid sequence) **or the rate of synthesis of a particular globin chain.** Most pathologic genetic variants result from a single amino acid substitution in one of the normal globin chains (Table 9-1).
2. **Nomenclature.** The hemoglobin tetramers formed by the variant globin plus the normal globin are designated or named by a letter or after the city in which the discovery was first made; a more informative system is to name them according to the actual amino acid substitution.
3. **Classification.** The hemoglobinopathies can be classified according to the effects of the genetic mutations:
   a. Solubility abnormalities
   b. Oxygen transport malfunction
   c. Oxidation–reduction abnormalities
   d. Abnormal monomeric states

B. Solubility abnormalities.
An abnormal solubility of hemoglobin can be the result of a mutation affecting globin chain synthesis or of the formation of precipitates or intracellular inclusion bodies.

1. **Globin chain synthesis.** The **thalassemia syndromes** are inherited disorders arising from globin gene mutations that either reduce or totally abolish the synthesis of one or more globin chains.

Table 9-1. Hemoglobin Mutations and the Resulting Physical Characteristics

Hemoglobin	Mutation	Characteristic
S	$\beta^{6\ glu \rightarrow val}$	Reduced solubility
C	$\beta^{6\ glu \rightarrow lys}$	Reduced solubility
C Harlem	$\beta^{6\ glu \rightarrow val}$ and $\beta^{73\ asp \rightarrow asn}$	Reduced solubility
Chesapeake	$\alpha^{92\ arg \rightarrow leu}$	Abnormal O_2 transport, increased O_2 affinity
Rainier	$\beta^{145\ tyr \rightarrow cys}$	Abnormal O_2 transport, increased O_2 affinity
Hiroshima	$\beta^{146\ his \rightarrow asp}$	Abnormal O_2 transport, increased O_2 affinity
Tacoma	$\beta^{30\ arg \rightarrow ser}$	Abnormal O_2 transport, increased O_2 affinity Unstable molecules, β-chain mutants
Zurich	$\beta^{63\ his \rightarrow arg}$	Abnormal O_2 transport, increased O_2 affinity Unstable molecules, β-chain mutants
Gun Hill	deletion; $\beta^{93-97\ leu}$	Abnormal O_2 transport, increased O_2 affinity Unstable molecules, β-chain mutants
Kansas	$\beta^{102\ asn \rightarrow thr}$	Decreased O_2 affinity
Hammersmith	$\beta^{42\ phe \rightarrow ser}$	Decreased O_2 affinity Unstable molecules, β-chain mutants
Seattle	$\beta^{76\ ala \rightarrow glu}$	Decreased O_2 affinity
Torino	$\alpha^{43\ phe \rightarrow val}$	Decreased O_2 affinity Unstable molecules, α-chain mutants
M Boston	$\alpha^{58\ his \rightarrow tyr}$	Methemoglobins
M Saskatoon	$\beta^{63\ his \rightarrow tyr}$	Methemoglobins
M Hyde Park	$\beta^{92\ his \rightarrow tyr}$	Methemoglobins
Seattle	$\beta^{70\ ala \rightarrow asp}$	Unstable molecules, β-chain mutants
Geneva	$\beta^{28\ leu \rightarrow pro}$	Unstable molecules, β-chain mutants

These imbalances in globin chain synthesis lead to the formation of unstable hemoglobin or to decreased amounts of hemoglobin, leading to microcytic, hypochromic anemia (see Ch 8 IV A 1 a). The thalassemias are named according to the globin chain involved.

2. **Formation of precipitates or intracellular inclusion bodies.** Genetic mutations may cause the formation of unstable hemoglobin (e.g., hemoglobin Geneva) with a reduced solubility that is due to the instability of the hemoglobin quaternary structure that results in spontaneous or drug-induced denaturation.
   a. **Inheritance.** These defects are usually inherited in an **autosomal dominant** fashion. Most of these mutations affect the β-globin chain (80%); the rest affect the α chains.
   b. **Clinical manifestations.** The unstable hemoglobins precipitate and are removed by the spleen, resulting in **hemolysis**. These mutations are **present at childhood** and are associated with jaundice, gallstones, and splenomegaly. They are often episodic and precipitated by infection and the administration of oxidant drugs.
   c. **Diagnosis. Hemoglobin electrophoresis is not helpful** in testing unstable hemoglobin because of electrically neutral amino acid substitution in these mutants. However, the following tests are useful.
      (1) **Peripheral blood smears** show hypochromia, poikilocytosis, anisocytosis, and reticulocytosis with other signs of hemolysis. These precipitated hemoglobins are demonstrated by supravital staining with methyl violet (1%) as Heinz bodies.
      (2) The **isopropanol stability test** demonstrates excessive precipitation of the abnormal hemoglobin at 37° C in a 17% solution of isopropanol compared with normal control hemoglobin.
      (3) The **heat stability test** precipitates unstable hemoglobin on exposure to a temperature of 50° C in an appropriate buffer, as indicated by the appearance of turbidity in the solution.
   d. **Treatment.** The hemolysis that results from the unstable hemoglobin is treated similarly to that resulting from other causes: folate replacement, splenectomy, and transfusion when necessary as well as the avoidance of oxidant drugs (Table 9-2).

C. **Oxygen transport malfunction.** The normal delivery of oxygen to the tissues is dependent on the reversible binding of oxygen at physiologic capillary–venous oxygen tensions. **Changes in Hb–O_2 affinity** does not cause hemolysis but may alter red cell mass because of stimulation or inhibition of the normal erythropoietic control systems. **Abnormal hemoglobin variants** affecting the heme pocket or the α–β contact area can cause a shift to the right and are listed in Table 9-1. These hemoglobin variants can result in an affinity for oxygen that is either higher or lower than normal.

1. **High-affinity hemoglobin. Abnormal hemoglobin** in which there is an amino acid substitution in the heme pocket or in the α–β contact area can shift the Hb–O_2 dissociation curve to the left, the resultant increased affinity **causing tissue hypoxia and compensatory polycythemia** (see Ch 10 II).
   a. **Inheritance.** High-affinity hemoglobin is an **autosomal dominant** inherited trait.
   b. **Clinical manifestations. Patients are asymptomatic, with true erythrocytic polycythemia.** The absence of splenomegaly indicates a nonmyeloproliferative disorder. However, hemolysis and an enlarged spleen may be evident when the hemoglobin mutation is unstable (a rare condition).
   c. **Diagnosis** is made by the low oxygen half-saturation pressure of hemoglobin (P_{50}) and abnormal Hb–O_2 dissociation curve.

2. **Low-affinity hemoglobin.** Hemoglobin with a reduced affinity for oxygen can shift the Hb–O_2 dissociation curve to the right, ensuring that the **tissues are adequately oxygenated.**
   a. **Inheritance.** Low-affinity hemoglobin is an **autosomal dominant** inherited trait in most patients.

Table 9-2. Drugs that Induce Hemolysis in Patients with Unstable Hemoglobins

Antimalarials	Sulfonamides	Others
Pamaquine	Sulfacetamide	Acetanilide
Primaquine	Sulfamethoxazole	Nalidixic acid
Quinacrine	Sulfanilamide	Nitrofurantoin
	Sulfapyridine	Toluidine blue

b. Clinical manifestations. Patients display signs of **cyanosis and low hemoglobin concentration** (pseudoanemia). A mild hemolytic anemia is seen in some cases.
c. Diagnosis is made by performing an Hb–O_2 dissociation study.

D. Oxidation–reduction abnormalities. The normal Hb–O_2 dissociation curve requires that the iron be available in the ferrous, or reduced, (Fe^{2+}) state. Hemoglobin that contains ferric, or oxidized, iron (Fe^{3+}) **[methemoglobin]** appears brownish blue and **binds oxygen tightly, not allowing for normal tissue exchange** at normal oxygen tension. The condition wherein red cells containing methemoglobin are found in the circulation is called **methemoglobinemia**.

1. **Classification.** Methemoglobinemia can be either congenital or acquired.
   a. **Congenital methemoglobinemia can result from two causes.**
      (1) The formation of **hemoglobin M (Hb M)** is due to an α- or β-globin chain mutation in the vicinity of iron in the molecule. An amino acid substitution stabilizes the heme iron in the oxidized (ferric) state instead of in the normal ferrous form. **Heterozygotes may have approximately 25% Hb M in their red cells,** which is enough to cause clinical symptoms.
      (2) **Methemoglobin reductase deficiency results from a deficiency of NADH–cytochrome b_5 reductase** (where NADH represents the reduced form of nicotinamide–adenine dinucleotide) and is **inherited as an autosomal recessive trait;** only homozygous patients can manifest the disease.
         (a) Spontaneous Hb M production is slow, but the cell's ability to reduce the endogenous production is much slower.
         (b) **Levels of 10%–40% Hb M are typical,** indicating that other reducing systems that are dependent on reduced nicotinamide–adenine dinucleotide phosphate (NADPH) are used when the red cell system fails.
   b. **Acquired methemoglobinemia.** Red cells exposed to strong oxidizing agents will produce Hb M, causing clinical symptoms. The most common oxidizing agents to which patients are exposed are:
      (1) Well water contaminated with **nitrates** and **inorganic nitrite (NO_2)**
      (2) **Drugs** such as acetanilid, phenacetin, acetaminophen, sulfonamides, and nitroprusside
      (3) **Local anesthetics** such as benzocaine and lidocaine

2. **Clinical manifestations**
   a. **Patients with congenital Hb M display:**
      (1) Cyanosis from infancy onward
      (2) A brown tinge to the blood that is often a telltale sign that leads to the diagnosis
      (3) Normal arterial oxygen saturation
      (4) Good health apart from symptoms of Hb M
   b. **Patients with acquired Hb M may experience dangerous levels of tissue hypoxia.** When the proportion of Hb M red cells to normal red cells reaches a very high level, oxygen transport becomes seriously reduced because Hb M fixes oxygen too tightly and cannot release it to the tissues. **An Hb M level of 60% represents a medical emergency.**

3. **Diagnosis**
   a. Presence of Hb M is established through spectrophotometry or electrophoresis.
   b. The cause is determined through:
      (1) History of early childhood cyanosis or positive family history of acquired Hb M
      (2) History of exposure to oxidizing agents
      (3) Measurement of methemoglobin reductase to confirm congenital Hb M

4. **Treatment** depends on both the cause of the abnormality and the patient's condition.
   a. Symptomatic patients with known congenital Hb M can be treated by administration of ascorbate or the reducing agent methylene blue.
   b. Treatment limited to the removal of the oxidizing agent in emergency cases of acquired Hb M is not sufficient. Administration of methylene blue is appropriate.
   c. Patients with life-threatening Hb M levels should be given an exchange blood transfusion.

E. Abnormal monomeric states: sickle cell anemia and related hemoglobinopathies. Normally, hemoglobin is present at very high concentrations inside the red cell. Certain hemoglobin mutations, such as sickle cell anemia, can polymerize hemoglobin inside the cell because of amino acid substitutions at the surface of the molecule that produce abnormal interactions between adjacent hemoglobin tetramers.

1. **Physiology of the sickle cell**
   a. **Formation of the sickle cell**
      (1) **Amino acid substitution**. Hb S is a mutant hemoglobin A (Hb A) with an abnormal β chain that contains a valine instead of a glutamate at position 6.
         (a) **Polymerization** is enhanced by the amino acid substitution because the tetrameric hemoglobin molecules are brought together by the removal of the oxygen molecule.
         (b) The bundles of 14-strand fibers that are produced deform the disc-like shape of the cell to a holly-leaf shape, then to an elongated rod or crescent shape. At this point, the cells become rigid and stiff.
         (c) Sickle cells, which cannot traverse the small capillary lumen because of their shape and rigidity, are ingested by the macrophages of the reticuloendothelial system (RES).
         (d) **Reoxygenation of reversibly sickled cells** causes the charge on the molecule to be buried and the polymers to dissolve. The hemoglobin regains its solubility, and the cell regains its normal shape.
         (e) Red cells become irreversibly sickled when repeated interaction between the Hb S and the membrane alters the membrane–skeletal relationship. The membrane loses its flexibility and becomes fragile, regardless of oxygenation, with repeated sickling and unsickling.
      (2) **Stages of polymerization.** Formation of Hb S occurs in the following stages (Figure 9-3).
         (a) **Nucleation** is an early rate-limiting stage in which molecules aggregate to form small 14- to 20-molecule clusters that act as nuclei. The red cells exhibit small surface clumps and are called **granular cells** at this stage.
         (b) **Polymerization** is signaled by a significant increase in viscosity that causes the cell membrane to lose its flexibility. Short 14-strand rods form inside the cell, which then assumes a **holly-leaf shape**.
         (c) **Alignment** of the 14-strand fibers deforms red cells further into stiff sickle-shaped cells.
   b. **Pathophysiologic effects of sickled cells.** Red cells carrying Hb S constantly switch from normal shape on the arterial side to sickled shape on the venous side. Eventually, some cells become irreversibly deformed, resulting in:
      (1) **Extravascular hemolysis.** Conscientious function of the spleen to remove damaged or deformed cells targets the cells that cannot traverse the narrow openings of the splenic sinusoids. The cells are trapped and removed by macrophages.
         (a) The deformed cells compromise the blood supply of the spleen causing repeated small infarctions and eventual **loss of splenic function**.
         (b) Replacement of cells carrying Hb S with the same abnormal cells causes **anemia** because of continuous early destruction of the cells by the spleen and, later, by the RES.
      (2) **Compromise of microcirculation.** As red cells carrying Hb S become sickled and lose their ability to traverse narrow passages, they create a blockage that obstructs blood flow into the tissue.
         (a) The local **anoxia** that results from the blockage increases oxygen extraction from the trapped red cells and further aggravates the **deoxygenation** and polymerization of abnormal hemoglobin.
         (b) The compensatory action of the adjacent vessels releases more oxygen from the cells. This increases sickling and causes exacerbation of the situation.
         (c) Tissue damage from lack of oxygen is the cause of the acute and chronic pain characteristic of sickle cell crises.

2. **Inheritance of Hb S.** Hb S is present as a single gene in 1 of every 10 blacks in North America. This is important clinically since **1 of every 4 children born of parents with the trait will have sickle cell anemia** as an autosomal recessive disease and **1 out of 2 will inherit the trait (i.e., will be carriers)** via autosomal dominant inheritance. These variations in the inheritance of Hb S with other hemoglobinopathies can cause a wide variation of clinical manifestations ranging from a relatively asymptomatic patient to one with symptoms indistinguishable from sickle cell disease (Figure 9-4).

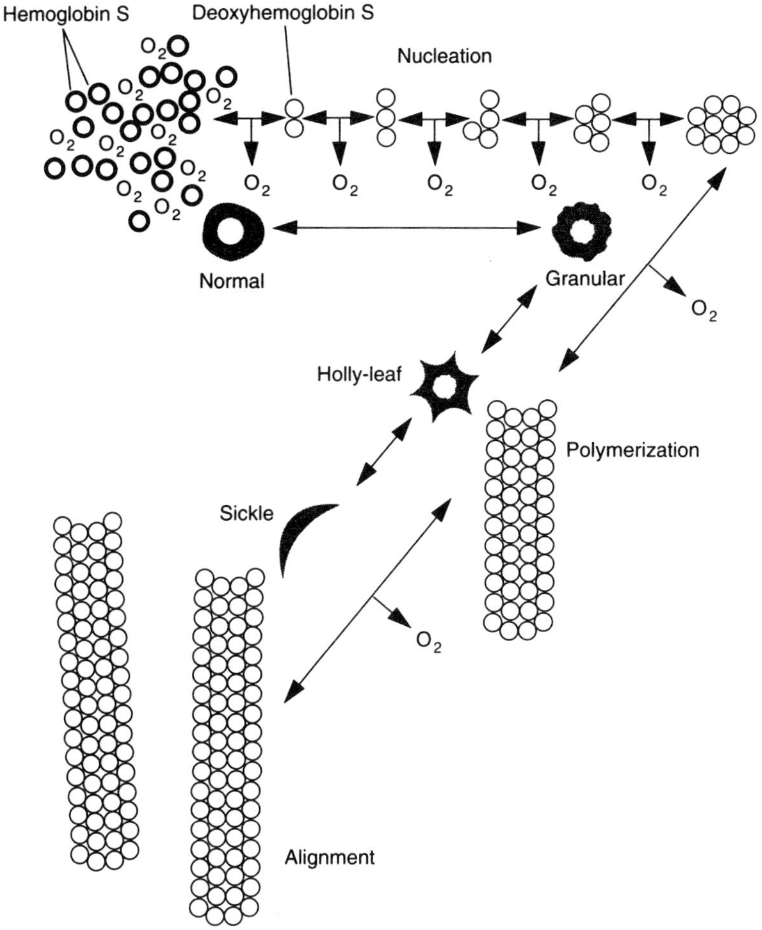

Figure 9-3. Hemoglobin S (Hb S) is in solution with oxygen, and the three stages in the polymerization of deoxyhemoglobin S and red cell shape changes occur as more oxygen is unloaded into the tissues. Nucleation (granular formation of red cells) is the lag period before polymerization; the interval varies from a few milliseconds to more than 1 hour, depending on local conditions such as pH, Po_2, and the intracellular concentration of Hb S. The red cell suddenly increases in viscosity during the polymerization phase (holly-leaf–shape change), loses its flexibility, and finally assumes the sickle form as the 14-strand fibers align into bundles, at a fixed rate of a few seconds. (Adapted from Hofrichter J, Ross PD, Eaton WA: Supersaturation in the sickle cell hemoglobin solutions. *Proc Natl Acad Sci USA* 73(9):3035, 1976.)

a. **Hemoglobin C (Hb C) and hemoglobin SC (Hb SC).** Homozygous Hb C ($\beta^{6\ glu \rightarrow lys}$) will tend to form hemoglobin crystals. Heterozygous Hb C (Hb AC) occurs in 6% of black Americans. The combination of SC in patients results in two abnormal β-globin chains.
   (1) **Clinical manifestations are similar to those of sickle cell anemia,** but these patients have less hemolysis and higher hematocrit levels, fewer painful crises, fewer infections, and generally less vaso-occlusive disease. Patients with Hb SC disease may have persistent splenomegaly.
   (2) **Diagnosis. Hemoglobin electrophoresis** can identify abnormal hemoglobin patterns. Hb C migrates to the position of Hb A_2 in the routinely used gel electrophoresis and can also be identified by column electrophoresis. Another diagnostic finding is the **presence of target cells (Hb C)** with the sickle cells.
   (3) **Treatment** is the same as for sickle cell anemia (see II E 3 d).

b. **Sickle thal disease (Hb S–β thalassemia).** The combination of Hb S and β thalassemia is indistinguishable from sickle cell anemia and results from the inheritance of β^S from one parent and β thalassemia from the other.

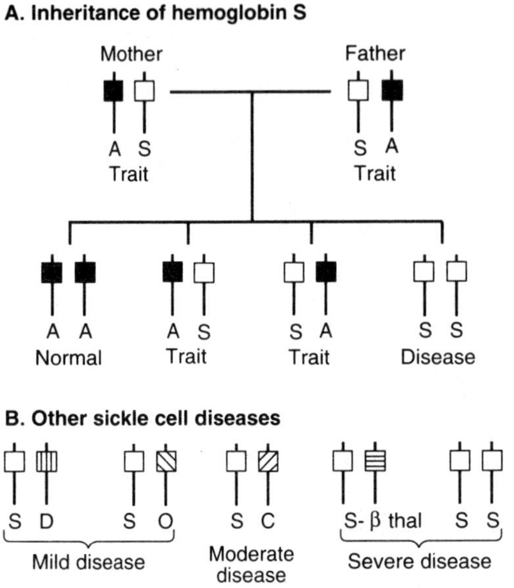

Figure 9-4. (*A*) The inheritance of hemoglobin S (Hb S) [*S*] from parents with sickle cell trait causes disease only in homozygous offspring. (*B*) Other sickle cell diseases are β-globin gene heterozygous, in which one of the genes is Hb S and the other is a gene with a mutation different from Hb S. Consequently, except in sickle thal disease, the red cells contain another hemoglobin that interferes with the polymerization of deoxyhemoglobin S and results in a mild or moderate form of the disease. *A* = hemoglobin A; *D* = hemoglobin D; *O* = hemoglobin O; *C* = hemoglobin C; *β thal* = β thalassemia.

(1) **Clinical manifestations.** Patients with β^0 thalassemia are severely affected since they cannot make any β globin; patients with β^+ thalassemia have normal β globin in 5%–15% of their hemoglobin.

(2) **Diagnosis** is made by the presence of microcytosis or splenomegaly in patients with mild to moderately severe sickle cell syndrome. Examination of the parents' blood will reveal microcytosis and an elevated Hb A_2 in one of the parents.

c. **Hemoglobin SD (Hb SD), hemoglobin SO (Hb SO), and Hb S–α thalassemia** are generally mild syndromes of academic interest since the interaction between the mutant globins results in less polymerization. Hemoglobin D (Hb D) Punjab ($\beta^{121\ glu \rightarrow gln}$) and hemoglobin O (Hb O) Arab ($\beta^{121\ glu \rightarrow lys}$) cause little disease by themselves (mild hemolysis in homozygous patients) but result in sickle cell disease when present with Hb S. In blacks, **Hb S–α thalassemia** is very common and **tends to lessen the severity of sickle cell disease** by reducing the hemoglobin concentration in the erythrocytes. This is characteristically seen in individuals with microcytosis without elevated levels of Hb A_2.

d. **Sickle cell trait (Hb AS)** is mild and **the most common syndrome,** occurring in 8% of North American blacks, but it is not considered a disease. The clinical importance of Hb AS is that it is a carrier state of a lifelong, incurable disease. It also **confers a protective advantage against malaria infection.**

(1) **Clinical manifestations. Hyposthenuria** (the excretion of dilute urine), **papillary necrosis, and hematuria** can occur in Hb AS since hyperosmolar and hypoxic regions in the renal medulla can induce sickling.

(a) Although most patients lead normal healthy lives, sudden deaths have been reported in young athletes who have sickle cell trait and are participating in rigorous physical activities, such as football or military training.

(b) Some of these individuals occasionally experience abdominal pain due to **splenic infarcts** while travelling in unpressurized airplanes.

(2) **Diagnosis.** Levels of Hb S in patients with sickle cell trait are generally lower than 40% because the normal β chains bind faster to the α chains than do the sickle β chains.

3. **Sickle cell anemia (Hb SS). Individuals who have inherited the two β-sickle globin genes (who are, therefore, homozygous)** have sickle cell anemia, and more than 90% of their total hemoglobin is Hb S.

a. **Clinical manifestations** are due to two primary causes.

(1) **Complications from a moderate to severe anemia** associated with **chronic hemolysis** result from a shortened red cell life span of 17 days in Hb SS and 28 days in Hb SC and include the following.

(a) **Slowed growth and development** can occur in children.

(b) In cases of severe anemia, cardiac overload results from compensation for low hemoglobin levels. Cardiac muscles are weakened by small infarcts and scar tissue formation, and **congestive heart failure** occurs eventually.
(c) **Bilirubin stones** from chronic hemolysis can cause hepatic biliary obstruction and **cholecystitis**.
(d) **Aplastic crisis** lasting from 5–10 days can occur following a parvovirus infection that inhibits erythroid cells in the bone marrow. The consequence of this acute and self-limited episode of erythroid aplasia is a rapid fall in hematocrit and reticulocytes to life-threatening levels that require transfusions.

(2) **Consequences of vaso-occlusion** of the microcirculation plugged by sickle cells include the following.
(a) **Sickle cell crisis** (or painful and infarctive crisis), which is the **most common manifestation of Hb SS,** leads to tissue hypoxia and microinfarction. This is commonly manifested as pain in the bones, chest, abdomen, and extremities precipitated by infections, fever, pregnancy, cold, dehydration, psychic stress, and surgery.
(b) **Splenic crisis**
(i) **Splenic sequestration syndrome** occurs when excessive sickling of cells in the spleen of a child with Hb SS causes a massive accumulation of blood in and rapid enlargement of the spleen. Since shock and hypotension can result, an exchange blood transfusion is required when this syndrome is recognized.
(ii) **Autosplenectomy and functional asplenia** occur in early childhood (1–2 years of age) due to repeated infarctions and lead to fibrosis by adulthood. Rarely, an enlarged spleen can be palpated in the adult because sickling in the splenic vein leads to engorgement, but this cannot be visualized on nuclear scanning since the RES is not functional.
(c) **Infections** and acute sepsis from encapsulated organisms, which are increased in these asplenic individuals, are an indication that the **patient is moderately immunocompromised**.
(i) These patients have an impaired antibody response, impaired complement activation (especially of the alternate pathway), and abnormal leukocyte chemotaxis and opsonization.
(ii) Common infections in sickle cell anemia are *Haemophilus influenzae,* pneumococcus, *Salmonella* or *Staphylococcus* (osteomyelitis), and *Mycoplasma pneumoniae.*
(iii) The susceptibility to viral and fungal infections is not increased, but these infections frequently precipitate a painful crisis.
(d) **Central nervous system (CNS) and ophthalmic effects**, which include **cerebrovascular accidents** in up to 8% of patients with Hb SS and 2% in Hb SC, are recurrent in 65% of patients. **Proliferative retinopathy** occurs in the periphery of the retina where repeated occlusion and hemorrhage lead to neovascularization, retinal detachment, and blindness.
(e) **Acute chest syndrome,** which is characterized by chest pain, dyspnea, cough, fever, and a pulmonary infiltration, can be caused by pulmonary infarction or bacterial infection. The syndrome may lead to **chronic pulmonary hypertension** and **cor pulmonale**.
(f) **Gastrointestinal complications.** A diffuse abdominal pain is symptomatic of sickle cell crisis. Upper right quadrant pain must, however, be differentiated from cholecystitis, hepatitis, or obstruction from gallbladder stones and be treated specifically.
(g) **Genitourinary symptoms include painless hematuria,** which is a rare problem that can result from infarction of the renal medulla, and **papillary necrosis**.
(i) Because increased osmolality induces sickling, the medulla of the kidney, where the osmotic gradient in the loop occurs, may become infarcted with high osmolality and poor oxygenation. This results in **hyposthenuria**.
(ii) Other effects, such as priapism, which can occur by sickling in the cavernous sinus of the penis of an individual with sickle cell anemia, and hypogonadism and underdevelopment of the genitalia are also seen.
(h) **Skeletal complications.** Multiple small infarctions in bones and joints, which are characteristic of Hb SS, lead to spontaneous fractures because of abnormalities in bone growth and strength.
(i) The **hand–foot syndrome** most commonly affects young children with sickle

cell anemia. The children experience infarction of the phalanges near the growth plate. This manifests as **leukocytosis,** or as painful and swollen red fingers or toes accompanied by fever. Consequences of hand–foot syndrome observed in adults are marked shortening of the right middle finger and second toes because of infarcts affecting the growth of the epiphysis. The bones and joints are often affected by sickle cell disease.

(ii) Acute arthritis may be due to synovial infarctions or, occasionally, true rheumatoid arthritis.

(iii) Aseptic necrosis of the femoral head can result in spontaneous fracture of the hip.

(iv) Osteomyelitis from secondary infections or from encapsulated organisms such as salmonellae or pneumococci are common.

(i) Skin changes, such as chronic nonhealing ankle ulcers, are common in sickle cell disease. They respond poorly to treatment and are difficult to heal even with skin grafting because of static blood flow and secondary infections.

b. Diagnosis. Homozygous Hb SS is easily diagnosed with the clinical picture of repeated painful crisis, hemolysis, infections, and the presence of sickled red cells in the blood smears. The tests for determining the presence of Hb SS are as follows.

(1) Peripheral blood smear will show sickled cells as well as target cells (Hb SC), Howell-Jolly bodies, nucleated red cells, red cell fragments, thrombocytosis, and occasionally leukocytosis. **Irreversibly sickled cells display an oak leaf shape** and membrane damage.

(2) Hemoglobin electrophoresis is performed under alkaline conditions or with agar or starch gel.

(a) The electrophoretic patterns of normal and abnormal hemoglobins depend on the amount of negative charges that they carry. The net charge varies due to the gain of negative charges in amino acid substitutions as shown in the following equation: Hb A > Hb S ($\beta^{S:\ glu \rightarrow val}$) > Hb C ($\beta^{C:\ glu \rightarrow lys}$), in which the negative charge increases and electrophoretic mobility decreases.

(b) Several abnormal hemoglobins may overlap in their electrophoretic patterns.

(i) Hb S and D overlap as does Hb C with E. The confusion can be allayed with alterations of the pH and manipulation of the electrophoretic conditions.

(ii) For a patient with a mild clinical disease and splenomegaly, electrophoretic patterns that resemble Hb SS should be differentiated from Hb SD.

(iii) Clinical findings may offer the only clue to differentiation between Hb SC and Hb SO Arab for diagnostic purposes.

(3) Screening tests

(a) The **sickling test** is an in vitro method of deoxygenating hemoglobin of red cells to induce sickling. It is performed by adding metabisulfite to a cell suspension on a slide and covering it with a cover slip. Formation of sickle-shaped red cells in the saline suspension indicates a positive result.

(b) The **solubility test** is a modification of the sickling test. It is performed by lysing the red cells to release hemoglobin and adding sodium metabisulfite to a solution of the hemoglobin and distilled water. Formation of a dark precipitate indicates a positive result for Hb S in the patient's red cells.

(4) Antenatal diagnosis is important when both parents have sickle trait and wish to determine if the fetus is homozygous for Hb S. As with thalassemia, sickle cell disease can sometimes be diagnosed prenatally by measuring the βs/βa synthetic ratio in the fetal blood or by demonstrating, through the use of restriction endonuclease, the presence of the sickle mutation in the fetal β-globin gene, whose recognition sequence is altered by the S mutation. The clinical course of homozygous Hb S is highly variable; some patients are relatively symptom-free throughout long and relatively healthy lives.

c. The **clinical course of Hb SS varies widely** from patient to patient for a number of reasons.

(1) The **fetal hemoglobin content** of the red cells of a patient with Hb S may influence the severity of the disease. Because of the high oxygen affinity of Hb F, the sickling of Hb S may be offset, also Hb F does not contain any β-globin chains. Elevated Hb F levels (i.e., to 20%) are responsible for the mild clinical course in Hb S patients.

(2) The **total hemoglobin concentration** affects nucleation, which is impeded at low hemoglobin levels.

(3) The **total number of irreversibly sickled cells** are used occasionally as a measure for disease severity, but the method is not reproducible.

(4) As a rule, most patients exhibit an unpredictable clinical course that cannot be identified by any laboratory parameter.

d. Treatment of sickle cell syndromes is **confined to supportive therapy** since there are no specific approaches to prevent the sickling of red cells or to reduce the effects of sickled cells on the hemodynamics.

(1) Painful vaso-occlusive (infarctive) crises. Once the tissues are infarcted by vaso-occlusion, the damage is irreversible and the objective of therapy is mainly pain relief, prevention of further vaso-occlusion, and preservation of neighboring tissue. These objectives are guidelines for the following measures.

(a) Hydration. Maintain adequate hydration orally and by intravenous fluids (100–200 ml/hr) to maintain a vigorous urine flow and closely monitor the cardiovascular response. Therapy must be individualized.

(b) Precipitating factors such as infections or inflammatory states such as arthritis, cholecystitis, pneumonia, and osteomyelitis should be looked for by the appropriate use of cultures and radiologic and scanning studies. Often, infections of the teeth and gums are missed. A dental examination and x-ray will often reveal an asymptomatic abscess. Specific antibiotics should be started if such an infection is documented.

(c) Oxygen therapy has a poorly defined role; oxygen is still administered by nasal prongs at 3–4 L/min for **acute chest syndromes** but contributes very little in peripheral tissue infarctions.

(d) Analgesics. The administration of analgesics is **important for the pain of infarction,** which persists during healing even after sickling has stopped. Analgesics should be given on a regular basis (never on an "as needed" basis) during the early days of the crisis, with a preference for smaller doses at more frequent intervals rather than larger doses over longer intervals, which produces swings of euphoria and pain. Inadequate dosing leads to inadequate control and prolongation of the hospital stay, promoting drug-seeking behavior that in turn results in further withholding of drugs by nurses and physicians. House officers should realize that there are no reliable tests to confirm or rule out vaso-occlusive crisis; thus, the decision to prescribe analgesics remains largely based on familiarity with the patient, clinical judgment, and intensive searches for other causes of pain.

(e) Exchange transfusion is used **only in certain unusual circumstances** such as acute splenic sequestration (children 2–5 years of age), CNS events (recurrent strokes), retinal lesions, priapism, hematuria, pulmonary crises, dactylitis and aseptic necrosis; leg and ankle ulcers, and aplastic crisis—all of which are refractory to conservative measures. Transfusions in general should be done with care since **multiple transfusions increase the risk for isoimmunization and delayed hemolytic transfusion hemolysis,** which is often difficult to differentiate from painful crises. This is often associated with diffuse intravascular coagulation (DIC) and acute respiratory distress syndrome.

(2) Maintenance therapy and prevention are equally important in the management of sickle cell syndrome patients to avoid frequent and prolonged hospital stays.

(a) Folic acid should be supplemented at a dose of 1 mg/day orally to counteract the increased utilization that results from chronic hemolysis.

(b) Pneumococcal vaccine should be given to functionally asplenic patients, although the antibody response is poor after autosplenectomy has occurred.

(c) Pregnancy in sickle cell patients increases the rates of crises; spontaneous abortions and stillbirths are increased. The pregnancy should be managed with folate and iron replacement and exchange transfusions if fetal distress occurs.

(i) Patients with Hb SC or Hb S–β thalassemia fare better during pregnancy.

(ii) Contraception is advised because pregnancy poses a high risk to both the mother and fetus. Tubal ligation or mechanical barriers are preferred to birth control pills because of their thrombogenic effects.

(d) General anesthesia for surgery and invasive diagnostic procedures **can precipitate a vaso-occlusive crisis;** this can be avoided by increasing the Hb A concentration by exchange transfusion to 60% before the procedure.

(i) Careful hydration and oxygenation is still required despite other measures.

(ii) Angiographic contrast materials that can cause sickling should be avoided.

STUDY QUESTIONS

Directions: Each of the numbered items or incomplete statements in this section is followed by answers or by completions of the statement. Select the **one** lettered answer or completion that is **best** in each case.

1. All of the following hemoglobins are present in the normal person EXCEPT

(A) Hb Gower I
(B) Hb Portland
(C) Hb F
(D) Hb A_2
(E) Hb D

2. All of the following tests are useful in the diagnosis of unstable hemoglobin EXCEPT

(A) Heinz bodies test (methyl violet supravital stain)
(B) isopropanol stability test
(C) hemoglobin electrophoresis
(D) heat stability test
(E) history and blood smears

3. All of the following statements about methemoglobinemia are true EXCEPT

(A) the acquired form of methemoglobinemia may be due to accidental ingestion of nitrite-contaminated water from wells
(B) homozygous methemoglobin reductase deficiency often results in death in utero
(C) in Hb M, a mutant α or β chain has lost its ability to stabilize the heme iron in the reduced state because of an amino acid substitution in the vicinity of the metal
(D) a methemoglobin level of 60% is a medical emergency, and the patient should receive an exchange transfusion immediately
(E) methemoglobin reductase deficiency can easily be treated by the administration of ascorbate and methylene blue

4. All of the following statements about unstable hemoglobins are true EXCEPT

(A) unstable hemoglobins are due to mutations in the β-globin chains only
(B) mutations in unstable hemoglobin can cause changes in hemoglobin solubility because of an instability of the quaternary structure; the hemoglobin precipitates spontaneously or in the presence of oxidative drugs
(C) mutations in unstable hemoglobin can affect oxygen affinity and present as familial polycythemia or pseudoanemia
(D) unstable hemoglobin is inherited in an autosomal dominant fashion
(E) unstable hemoglobin presents during childhood with hemolytic conditions such as jaundice, gallstones, and splenomegaly

---

1-E
2-C
3-B
4-A

Directions: The item below contains four suggested answers, of which **one or more** is correct. Choose the answer

A if **1, 2, and 3** are correct
B if **1 and 3** are correct
C if **2 and 4** are correct
D if **4** is correct
E if **1, 2, 3, and 4** are correct

5. The sickle shape of red cells in a patient with sickle cell anemia is due to the

(1) deoxygenation of the hemoglobin
(2) concentration of total Hb S in the erythrocyte
(3) amount of Hb F in the red blood cell
(4) presence of Hb S in red cells in the alignment phase

Directions: Each group of items in this section consists of lettered options followed by a set of numbered items. For each item, select the **one** lettered option that is most closely associated with it. Each lettered option may be selected once, more than once, or not at all.

Questions 6–14

Match the pathophysiological mechanism of sickle cell disease (Hb SS) with the appropriate clinical manifestation.

(A) Vaso-occlusion in the microcirculation and tissue infarction
(B) Hemolysis and shortened red cell survival
(C) Suppression of bone marrow erythropoiesis due to parvovirus infection
(D) Unstable structure of hemoglobin causing precipitation
(E) Impairment of antibody response and complement activation

6. Sickle cell crisis (painful infarctive crisis)

7. Aplastic crisis

8. Acute chest syndrome

9. Gallstones

10. Growth and development retardation in affected children

11. Infections caused by encapsulated organisms

12. Painless hematuria and papillary necrosis

13. Aseptic necrosis of the hip

14. Retinal detachment and blindness

Questions 15–18

Match each clinical manifestation of a mutant hemoglobin combination with the associated mutation.

(A) Hb AC
(B) Hb SS
(C) Hb SO and Hb SC
(D) Hb SS with 20% Hb F

15. Severe sickle cell disease

16. Moderate sickle cell disease

17. Mild form of sickle cell disease with splenomegaly

18. No symptoms of disease

5-E	8-A	11-E	14-A	17-C
6-A	9-B	12-A	15-B	18-A
7-C	10-B	13-A	16-D	

ANSWERS AND EXPLANATIONS

1. The answer is E *[II E 2 c].*
Hemoglobin D (Hb D) is an abnormal mutation that migrates in electrophoretic gel in the hemoglobin S (Hb S) area and can be confused with Hb S, although this mutation does not sickle and can be differentiated by the sickling test. The different embryonal and fetal hemoglobins are Gower I and II, Portland, and hemoglobin F (Hb F). Hemoglobin A_2 (Hb A_2) represents only a small amount of total hemoglobin in the adult.

2. The answer is C *[II B 2 c, E 3 b (2)].*
Hemoglobin electrophoresis is not a useful test in the diagnosis of unstable hemoglobin. The amino acid substitution that results in unstable hemoglobin involves neutral amino acids; thus, a normal pattern will be seen in the electrophoresis gel. In hemoglobin S (Hb S), hemoglobin C (Hb C), and thalassemia, the mutation causes a loss of electrons that will affect the electrophoretic gel pattern. The tests that are helpful in establishing a diagnosis of unstable hemoglobin is a history of hemolysis and blood smear, indicating red cell destruction; the presence of Heinz bodies; and the unstable behavior of the patient's hemoglobin in isopropanol and heat (50° C) compared with normal controls.

3. The answer is B *[II D].*
Homozygous methemoglobin reductase deficiency does not necessarily result in death in utero. Patients affected can manifest levels of hemoglobin M (Hb M) of 10%–40%, indicating that other reduced nicotinamide–adenine dinucleotide phosphate (NADPH)–dependent reducing systems are used when the red cell system fails. Thus, most patients are only mildly affected; however, their condition can become severe if they are exposed to oxidative drugs and agents, as occurs when nitrites are ingested (a common source of which is contaminated well water). An increase in methemoglobin level to 60% is a medical emergency that can be treated by exchange transfusion. Reductase deficiency can be treated by the administration of ascorbate and methylene blue. An amino acid substitution near the iron of hemoglobin creates the methemoglobin, and the mutant globin chain loses its ability to stabilize the heme iron in its reduced state.

4. The answer is A *[II B 2, C].*
Mutations in unstable hemoglobin can affect either α- or β-globin chains, although most frequently they affect β chains. The condition is inherited in an autosomal dominant fashion, and it affects oxygen affinity. The unstable hemoglobins precipitate and are removed by the spleen, causing hemolysis and all of its consequences.

5. The answer is E (all) *[II E 1, 3 c (1)].*
Sickle cell anemia is due to a mutation of the β-globin chain (a substitution of valine for glutamate at position 6) that causes an exaggeration of the normal tendency of deoxyhemoglobin to polymerize. The formation of sickled cells is dependent on the phase of polymerization [i.e., alignment phase, which forms the stiff bundles of hemoglobin S (Hb S)], the total concentration of Hb S (sickling does not occur in sickle cell trait), and the presence of hemoglobin F (Hb F), which does not contain β-globin chains.

6–14. The answers are: 6-A *[II E 3 a (2) (a)],* **7-C** *[II E 3 a (1) (d)],* **8-A** *[II E 3 a (2) (e)],* **9-B** *[II E 3 a (1) (c)],* **10-B** *[II E 3 a (1) (a)],* **11-E** *[II E 3 a (2) (c)],* **12-A** *[II E 3 a (2) (g)],* **13-A** *[II E 3 a (2) (h) (iii)],* **14-A** *[II E 3 a (2) (d)].*
The normal deformation of red cells as they move through the microcirculation to release oxygen is not possible for sickle cells, which become trapped and block the vessels. As adjacent cells attempt to compensate for the resultant tissue anoxia, they also become plugged, which starts a cycle of vaso-occlusion and tissue anoxia. Tissue necrosis results and is the source of the chronic and acute pain of sickle cell anemia. Sickle cells also become trapped in the cords of the spleen when their inclusions grow in response to the relatively anoxic environment, preventing them from squeezing through into the sinuses. These patients lose their splenic function by late infancy because of infarction and anemia, resulting in predisposition to infection by encapsulated organisms. Gallstones result in precipitation of excess bile from the metabolism of heme, which is increased due to hemolysis.

15–18. The answers are: 15-B *[II E 3],* **16-D** *[II E 3 c (1)],* **17-C** *[II E 2 a (1), c],* **18-A** *[II E 2 d].*
Severe sickle cell disease is characteristic of most sickle cell anemia (Hb SS) patients with about 96% hemoglobin S (Hb S) but may be milder in Hb SS patients with 20% hemoglobin F (Hb F). Combinations of Hb S with hemoglobin O (Hb O) or hemoglobin C (Hb C) will result in a mild form of the disease and splenomegaly, which is due to more prominent hemolysis rather than to vaso-occlusive disease in these forms of hemoglobinopathy. Hb C trait [hemoglobin AC (Hb AC)] is an asymptomatic condition similar to hemoglobin AS (Hb AS) without the concomitant hematuria that can occur in sickle cell traits.

10
Approach to Patients with Red Cell Disorders

Emmanuel C. Besa

I. ANEMIA AND THE APPROACH TO ITS EVALUATION. Anemia is defined as the lowering of the circulating red cell mass below the established normal levels. It is a clinical sign and not a diagnostic entity. There are two basic physiologic mechanisms that cause anemia: Anemia is due to either decreased production of red blood cells (see I D) or to increased destruction of red blood cells (see I E).

A. Significance of anemia. Determination of the significance of anemia depends on the concomitant clinical picture of the patient relative to the following factors.

1. **Magnitude of the anemia.** Anemia is defined as **mild** in men with hemoglobin concentrations of 10–12 g/dl and mild in women with hemoglobin concentrations of 9–11 g/dl. Anemia is **moderate** when hemoglobin levels are 8–10 g/dl in men and 7–9 g/dl in women. **Severe** anemia exists when hemoglobin concentrations are below these levels.

2. **Rate of development of the anemia.** Symptoms of weakness and fatigue are associated with slowly developing anemias; overt heart failure and coma are symptoms of rapidly developing anemias.
   a. Anemia may remain asymptomatic when its development is gradual because the patient's cardiovascular adaptive mechanisms and the shift in oxygen affinity of hemoglobin ($Hb–O_2$ affinity) through the action of 2,3-diphosphoglycerate (2,3-DPG) compensate for the low red cell mass.
   b. Duration of the anemia (i.e., acute and recent versus slow and chronic) should be determined so that the anemia can be classified as acquired or congenital.

3. **Presence of an underlying pathologic process** that would explain the anemia and its detection is often the reason for a major workup.
   a. An asymptomatic patient with chronic disease and anemia of 9 g/dl would not require workup or therapy.
   b. Obviously, a young woman with menorrhagia and iron deficiency would not warrant a workup for an occult source of bleeding as would a male patient or a postmenopausal woman with unexplained iron deficiency.

4. **Presence of other medical conditions** that are aggravated by anemia often are major reasons for therapy. A mild anemia may be tolerated by some patients but may be critical in a patient with coronary artery disease.

B. Clinical history and physical examination. A logical and considered use of a careful history and physical examination with the help of a variety of laboratory tests is essential in the determination of the particular mechanism and specific etiology of an undefined anemia (Figure 10-1).

1. **History**
   a. A detailed **nutritional history** should be taken for vitamin deficiencies and dietary causes of the anemia.
   b. The **family history** is necessary in patients whose anemia is chronic and in patients with some forms of acute anemia to detect a congenital or inherited disorder.
   c. **Exposure to medications and potentially harmful industrial or household toxins** should be determined. The nature of the hematinic or drugs the patient may have ingested must be assessed to understand which anemic mechanisms are at work:
      (1) Direct suppression of erythropoiesis (chloramphenicol, phenylbutazone)

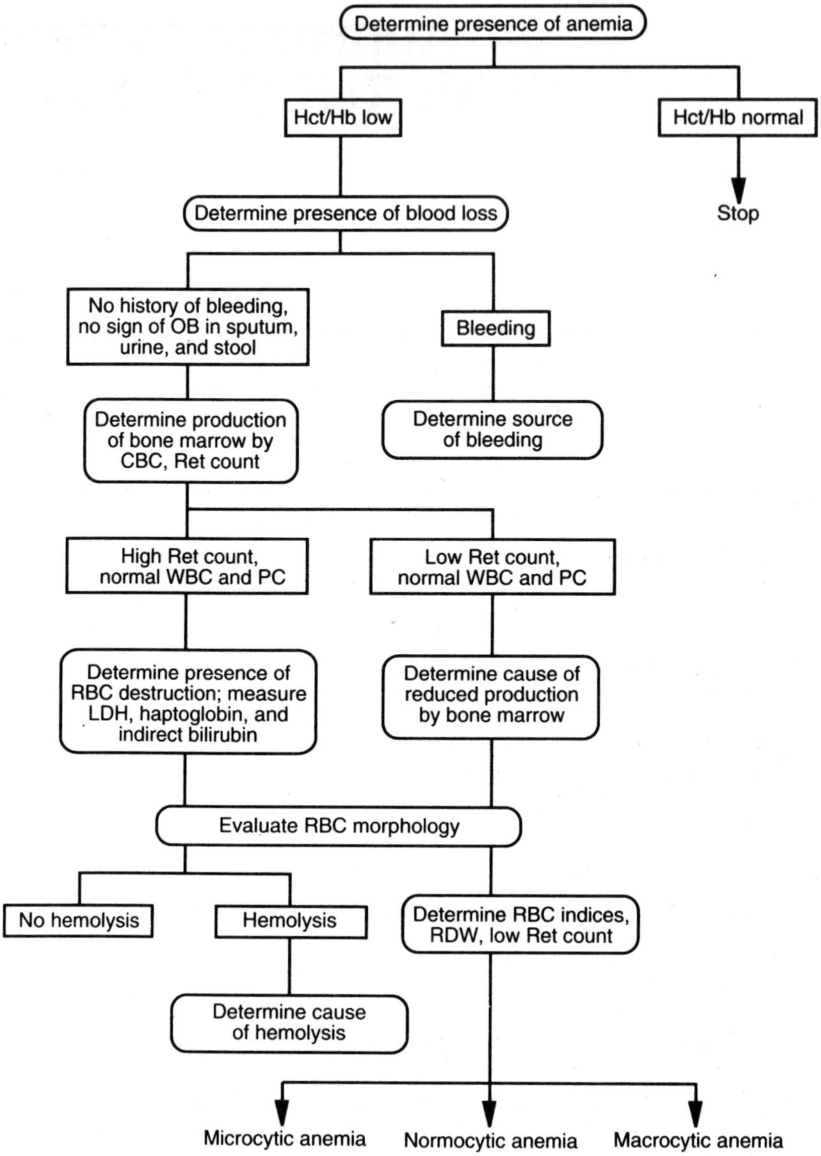

Figure 10-1. A sequential approach to the evaluation of anemia should identify which of three common pathophysiologic mechanisms is involved: blood loss, a marrow production defect, or hemolysis. This approach helps to classify the anemia as hemolytic or nonhemolytic and allows further differentiation into microcytic, normocytic, or macrocytic anemia based on the mean corpuscular volume (MCV). *Hb* = hemoglobin; *Hct* = hematocrit; *LDH* = lactate dehydrogenase; *OB* = occult bleeding; *PC* = platelet count; *RBC* = red blood cell; *RDW* = red cell distribution width; *Ret* = reticulocyte; *WBC* = white blood cell count.

(2) **Disturbance of normal red cell maturation** (phenytoin, alcohol)
(3) **Accelerated hemolysis** (sulfonamides, methyldopa)

2. Signs and symptoms

a. Presenting signs and symptoms of anemia will vary from those in the asymptomatic patient who is discovered to be anemic by routine screening blood examination to those in the patient who presents with weakness, fatigue, and other signs and symptoms listed in Table 10-1.

Table 10-1. Signs and Symptoms of Anemia

Cardiovascular and respiratory	
	Exertional dyspnea, tachycardia and palpitations, orthopnea, angina, claudications
	Bounding peripheral pulses, cardiomegaly, pedal edema, murmurs, vascular bruits
	Increased respiratory rate
Neurologic	
	Headaches, tinnitus, dizziness, faintness, loss of concentration, fatigue, cold sensitivity
Skin	
	Pallor of skin, mucous membranes, nailbeds, and palms
Gastrointestinal	
	Anorexia, nausea, constipation, diarrhea
Genitourinary	
	Menstrual irregularity, amenorrhea, menorrhagia, loss of libido or potency

b. **Presence of excessive blood loss** should be determined. This would include a detailed menstrual history, inquiries regarding stool character and color, the examination of sputum or vomitus when present, and observation of the color of the urine.

C. **Laboratory studies.** The following logical sequence for the laboratory workup of anemia is suggested.

1. **Make sure that the anemia is real.** In certain cases, a repeat confirmatory hematocrit must be performed and an estimate made of possible acute fluid overload.
2. **Determine if an occult blood loss is present** in patients without obvious hemorrhage.
   a. Examination of the stools for blood (Hematest) is a necessary part of the routine physical examination.
   b. Acute blood loss will not present as anemia but as hypovolemia, since after the equal loss of red cells and plasma, hours will pass before the plasma volume can be expanded by the normal compensatory mechanisms, causing a lowering of the hematocrit and hemoglobin levels.
3. **Determine the degree of bone marrow response to the anemia** by measuring the reticulocyte count.
4. **Evaluate the red cell morphology,** looking for variations in size, shape, and hemoglobin content, examining the blood smear using red cell indices. The type of anemia can be classified according to the mean corpuscular volume (MCV) as **normochromic, normocytic anemia; hypochromic, microcytic anemia; and hyperchromic, macrocytic anemia** (see I D).
5. **Determine the presence of hemolysis** (short red cell survival) **or ineffective erythropoiesis** by measuring serum lactate dehydrogenase (LDH), unconjugated bilirubin, and haptoglobin (see I E).

D. **Approach to a patient with hypoproliferative anemia**

1. **Normochromic, normocytic anemia** should be approached by looking for **bone marrow suppression of erythropoiesis** (Figure 10-2) using the following sequence of tests.
   a. When **serum erythropoietin levels** are suppressed, systemic factors should be sought.
      (1) **Increased serum creatinine and blood urea nitrogen (BUN) levels** would indicate poor renal function due to renal disease, which leads to poor secretion and lower serum levels of erythropoietin.
      (2) **Endocrine function abnormalities** should be explored.
         (a) **Hypothyroidism.** Lack of thyroxine leads to a decreased need for oxygen and a decreased level of erythropoietin. Hypothyroidism has been associated with pernicious anemia (PA), macrocytic anemia, and iron deficiency.

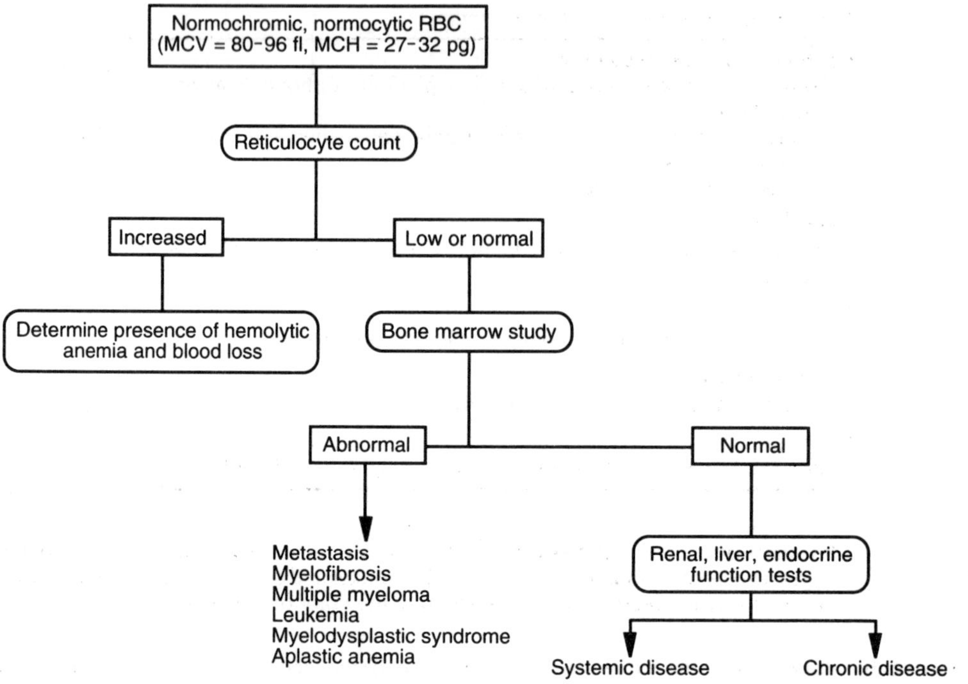

Figure 10-2. A sequential approach to the analysis of normochromic, normocytic anemia should include a reticulocyte count. A low reticulocyte count should be analyzed by bone marrow examination and the evaluation of systemic disorders that can influence the normal marrow response (e.g., endocrine, renal, and liver dysfunctions). *RBC* = red blood cell; *MCV* = mean corpuscular volume; *MCH* = mean corpuscular hemoglobin.

(b) **Hypopituitarism.** Decreased levels of growth factor reduce erythropoiesis since growth factor is a minor hormone promoting erythropoiesis.

(c) **Hypogonadism.** Decreased androgen serum levels will lead to a mild decrease in hemoglobin levels in males.

(3) The presence of **chronic inflammatory or distant malignant disease** leading to interleukin 1 (IL-1) secretion, which inhibits iron reutilization and lowers erythropoietin levels, can cause either a normocytic or a microcytic anemia.

b. **Bone marrow study** will **show direct damage to or involvement of the cellular marrow by:**

(1) **Metastatic carcinomas,** such as those from the prostate, breast, lung, and kidneys

(2) **Primary or secondary myelofibrosis**

(3) **Malignancies of the hematopoietic tissues,** such as lymphomas, multiple myeloma, and leukemia

(4) **Exposure to drugs,** toxic chemicals, or radiation

(5) **Idiopathic causes** such as aplastic anemia and myelodysplastic syndrome

2. **Hypochromic, microcytic anemias** are caused by decreased hemoglobin synthesis. They can be approached in the sequence shown in Figure 10-3 and can be diagnosed by performing the following tests.

a. **Storage iron.** Measurement of the level of ferritin in the serum or performance of an iron stain of the bone marrow will differentiate the following conditions, which can lead to decreased heme synthesis:

(1) **Low serum ferritin or absent iron stores in the bone marrow cells,** indicating iron deficiency

(2) **Increased serum ferritin or iron stores in the reticuloendothelial (RE) cells of the marrow,** indicating iron reutilization abnormalities such as chronic diseases

(3) **Presence of abnormal ringed sideroblasts in the bone marrow erythroid precursors,** indicating acquired porphyrin synthesis abnormalities such as sideroblastic anemias

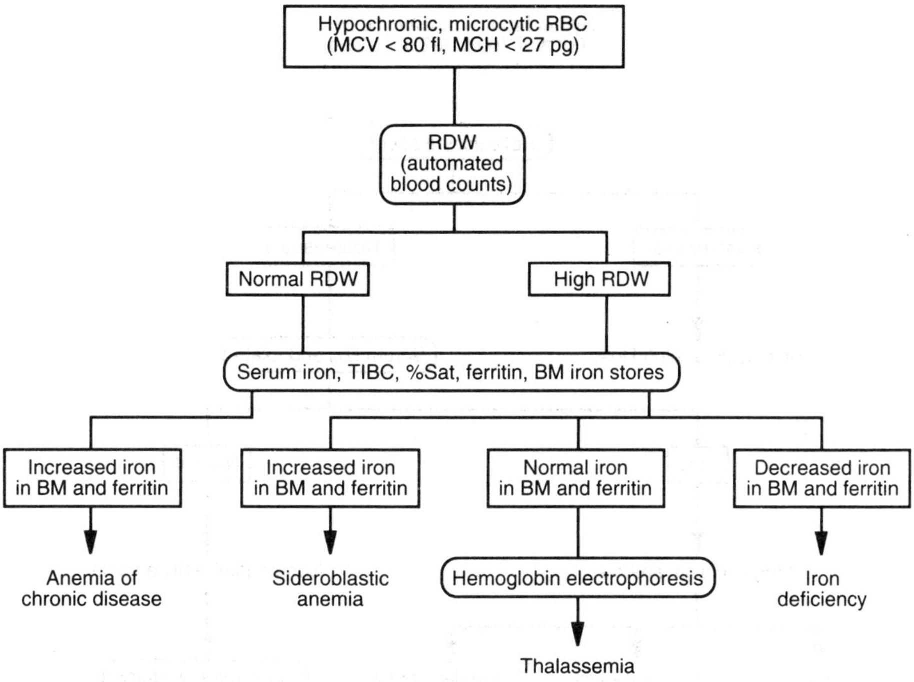

Figure 10-3. A sequential approach to the analysis of hypochromic, microcytic anemia is based on eliminating the most common causes initially (i.e., iron deficiency anemia and anemia of chronic disease), which can be differentiated easily by iron studies. Bone marrow evaluation is essential in the diagnosis of sideroblastic anemia; hemoglobin electrophoresis is essential in the diagnosis of thalassemia. *RBC* = red blood cell; *MCV* = mean corpuscular volume; *MCH* = mean corpuscular hemoglobin; *RDW* = red cell distribution width; *BM* = bone marrow; *%Sat* = percent saturation; *TIBC* = total iron-binding capacity.

b. **Globin synthesis abnormalities,** presenting as different forms of thalassemia, **can be detected by**:
   (1) **Hemoglobin electrophoresis,** demonstrating increased levels of hemoglobin (Hb) A_2 and Hb F resulting from the replacement of β chains with δ and γ chains in β thalassemias
   (2) **Heinz bodies test,** demonstrating unstable hemoglobin

3. **Hyperchromic, macrocytic anemias** should be approached initially to determine whether the large red cells are young and newly released into the circulation or whether they are abnormal.
   a. **Abnormalities in DNA synthesis and maturation defects in erythropoiesis** can cause hyperchromic, macrocytic anemias. Differentiation of a megaloblastic anemia from a nonmegaloblastic anemia should proceed as shown in Figure 10-4. The **reticulocyte count** directs the workup when looking for a macrocytic cause or a hemolytic or blood loss cause for the anemia.
      (1) A **high reticulocyte count** indicates either hemolysis or bleeding.
      (2) A **low reticulocyte count** indicates that the levels of serum folate and vitamin B_{12} should be measured. The results distinguish between the two most common causes of megaloblastic anemia.
         (a) **Low levels of vitamin B_{12}** indicate that a **Schilling test** [see Ch 6 III D 3 d (4)] should be performed.
            (i) A **normal part I** indicates low intake because of a vegetarian diet.
            (ii) An **abnormal part I and** a **normal part II** indicate PA.
            (iii) **Abnormal parts I and II** indicate malabsorption, and, after 1 week of oral antibiotics, a **normal part III** indicates a blind-loop syndrome or bacterial overgrowth in an area of stasis in the gastrointestinal tract.
            (iv) If the condition is not corrected by antibiotics and an **abnormal part III** persists, mucosal damage at the site of absorption is indicated.

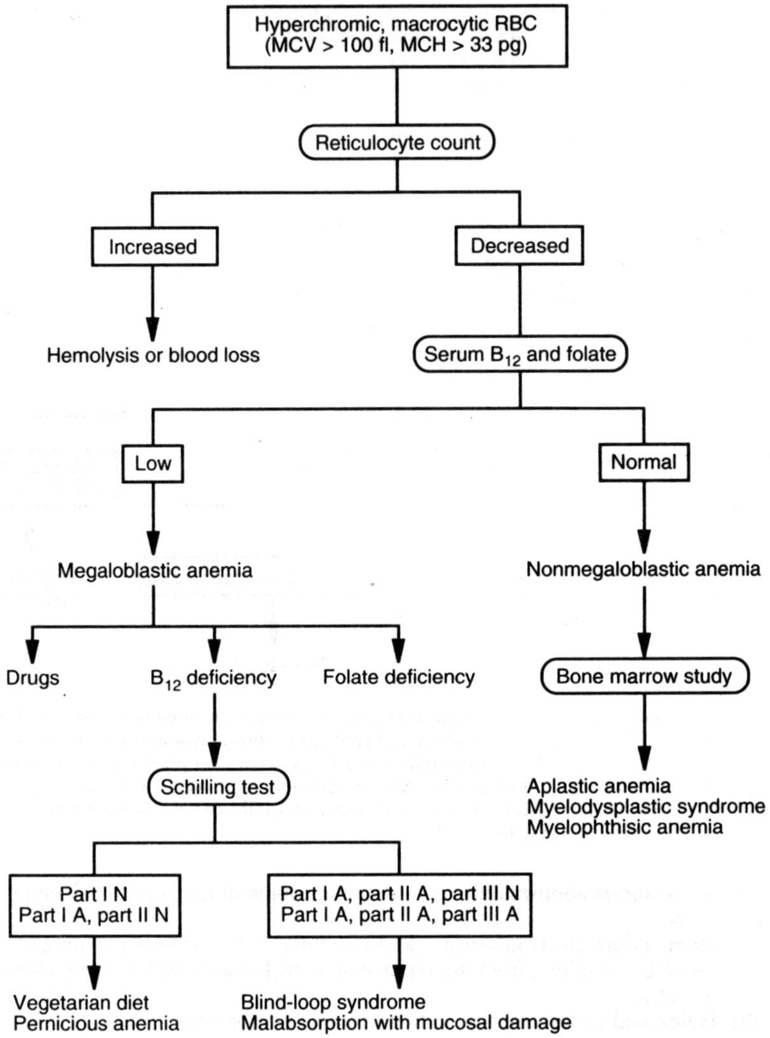

Figure 10-4. A sequential approach to the analysis of macrocytic anemia initially rules out large red cells caused by reticulocytosis in hemolysis. A low reticulocyte count indicates a bone marrow abnormality that can have characteristically megaloblastic or nonmegaloblastic causes. Megaloblastoid changes in the bone marrow can be seen in myelodysplastic syndrome, but these patients would have normal serum B_{12} and folate levels. *RBC* = red blood cell; *MCV* = mean corpuscular volume; *MCH* = mean corpuscular hemoglobin; *A* = labeled B_{12} is absorbed; *N* = labeled B_{12} is not absorbed.

(b) **Normal serum levels of vitamin B_{12} or folate** indicate that a bone marrow study should be performed.

(i) Megaloblastoid changes in the hematopoietic cells indicate myelodysplastic syndrome.

(ii) A hypoplastic marrow indicates aplastic anemia may be producing the macrocytic red cells.

(iii) Malignant cells, granulomas, and fibrosis indicate a myelophthisic process that is destroying the hematopoietic tissue because of direct marrow injury, causing the early release of nucleated erythroid cells.

b. Drugs can also cause a macrocytic anemia, which is usually mild, occurring as a harmless part of the therapeutic action. This anemia generally does not require treatment but possibly becomes significant in a complex illness such as acquired immune deficiency syndrome (AIDS). These drugs include:

(1) Inhibitors of DNA synthesis, such as hydroxyurea

(2) **Folate antagonists,** such as the antiprotozoal drug pentamidine and the pyrimethamine antibiotics trimethoprim and zidovudine, which is also known as AZT and is used for the treatment of AIDS

(3) **Vitamin B_{12} inactivators,** such as nitrous oxide, an anesthetic agent

E. Approach to a patient with hemolytic anemia. The location of the red cell destruction should be sought as either extravascular or intravascular (Figure 10-5).

1. **Extravascular hemolysis.** The sign of extravascular hemolysis is **splenomegaly,** although hemolysis of this type may not manifest early in the disease with an enlarged or palpable spleen. The spleen, which contains the active RE cells that remove the red cells from the circulation, hypertrophies during acute and chronic forms of extravascular hemolysis. The exception occurs, perhaps, in sickle cell disease, where the spleen itself atrophies after multifocal infarction because of obstruction of the capillaries by the deformed erythrocytes. The most common causes of this type of hemolysis are immunologically mediated, and performing the **Coombs' test** is important.

   a. A **positive direct Coombs' test** indicates that an immune process is involved with the hemolysis that can be further characterized by the following.

      (1) **Warm-type autoantibodies** can be idiopathic or can occur secondary to:

         (a) Drugs such as methyldopa

         (b) A connective tissue disease such as systemic lupus erythematosus or rheumatoid arthritis

         (c) A lymphoproliferative disorder such as chronic lymphocytic leukemia (CLL), Hodgkin's lymphoma, or non-Hodgkin's lymphoma

      (2) **Cold-type autoantibodies** may be idiopathic or secondary to infections such as mycoplasmal pneumonia or infectious mononucleosis or secondary to an underlying lymphoma.

   b. A **negative Coombs' test** indicates that further studies should be performed.

      (1) The **peripheral blood smear** may show findings of abnormal red cells.

         (a) **Sickled red cells.** Hemoglobin electrophoresis should be performed for a specific diagnosis of sickle cell anemia.

         (b) **Spherocytes.** The osmotic fragility test, along with family history, is used to support a diagnosis of hereditary spherocytosis.

         (c) **Spur cells.** Liver function tests and evaluation of serum lipids may support a diagnosis of hypercholesterolemia.

      (2) Hemolysis in association with oxidative agents should lead to a Heinz bodies test to look for unstable hemoglobin or glucose-6-phosphate dehydrogenase (G6PD) deficiency.

2. **Intravascular hemolysis** occurs when excess hemoglobin in the serum (**hemoglobinemia**) and urine (**hemoglobinuria**) overwhelms the normal physiologic mechanisms of haptoglobin, which disappears from the plasma.

   a. The **absence of haptoglobin** is a positive sign of hemolysis.

   b. **Paroxysmal nocturnal hemoglobinuria** presents classically with hemoglobinuria or a thrombotic condition associated with a hypercoagulable state. Time of day is not necessarily relative to the condition. The Ham test and the sugar water test aid in the diagnosis.

   c. **Etiology** of intravascular hemolysis can be either **mechanical** or **immunologic**.

      (1) The cause of the red cell destruction may be **mechanical** when the smear shows a prominent increase in red cell fragments and schistocytes. Potential sources of red cell damage are:

         (a) **Artificial heart valves** or dysfunctions such as a "leak" or insufficiency

         (b) **Coagulopathy,** as occurs in disseminated intravascular coagulation (DIC)

         (c) **Malignant hypertension** due to severe vascular constriction

         (d) **Malignancies,** which form tortuous blood vessels, leading to abnormal flow

      (2) The cause of the red cell destruction may be **immunologic,** such as:

         (a) Isoimmune hemolytic anemia

         (b) ABO or Rh incompatible transfusion reaction

         (c) Delayed hemolytic transfusion reactions

II. ERYTHROCYTOSIS AND POLYCYTHEMIA. The terms erythrocytosis and polycythemia have been used interchangeably to indicate a pathologic increase in total red cell mass; however, **polycythemia** specifically refers to an increase in two or more hematopoietic lines. Increases in the

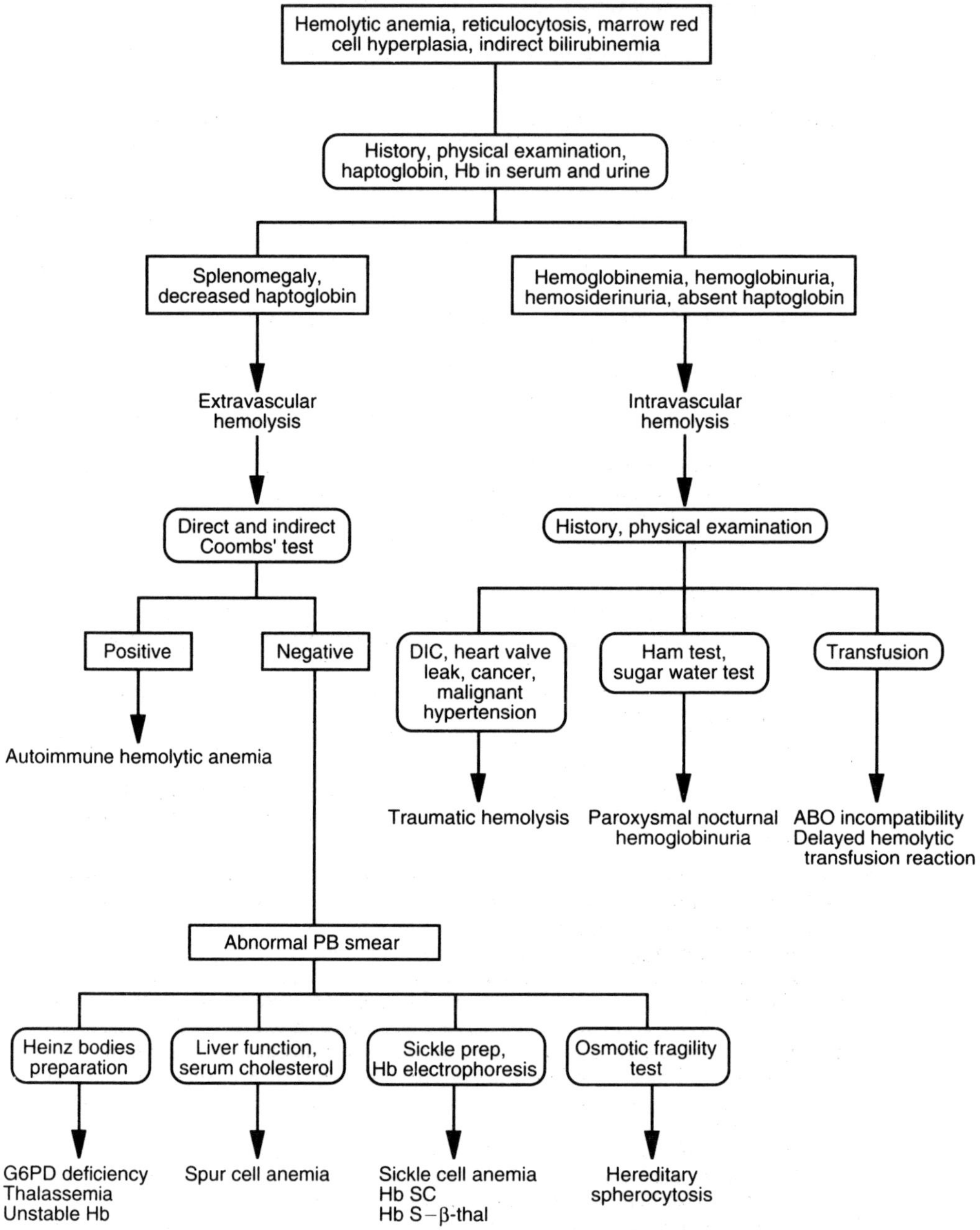

Figure 10-5. A sequential approach to the diagnosis of hemolytic anemia is based on initially establishing the prominent features of the hemolytic process (i.e., intravascular versus extravascular). Patient history and the findings on physical examination are important and, with the aid of special laboratory tests, help to narrow the possibilities and to establish the diagnosis. *Hb* = hemoglobin; *DIC* = diffuse intravascular coagulation; *G6PD* = glucose-6-phosphate dehydrogenase; *PB* = peripheral blood; *Hb SC* = hemoglobin SC disease; *Hb S-β thal* = sickle cell-thalassemia disease.

hematocrit and hemoglobin levels are the presenting signs and may be secondary to an increase in red cell mass (true erythrocytosis) or a decrease in plasma volume (pseudoerythrocytosis). The approach to a patient with an elevated hematocrit is shown in Figure 10-6.

A. **Normal red cell mass and its measurement.** Since the measurements of the hematocrit and hemoglobin depend on the ratio of the red cells and the plasma, direct measurement of total blood volume and red cell mass is important.

1. **Technique.** The patient's red cells must be labeled with chromium 51 (^{51}Cr). The total red cell mass is then calculated by measuring the total blood volume from dilution of the label. Total plasma volume can also be measured directly by iodine 125 (^{125}I)-labeled albumin or calculated from the total blood volume and red cell mass.

2. **Normal values,** which are based on people living at sea level (higher values are observed in residents of elevated locations), are as follows:
   a. **^{51}Cr technique**
      (1) Men have a normal red cell mass between 25 and 35 ml/kg.
      (2) Women have a normal red cell mass between 22 and 32 ml/kg.
   b. **^{125}I technique.** Normal plasma volume values range between 40 and 50 ml/kg.

B. **Pseudoerythrocytosis** is the condition in which an elevated hematocrit is due to a pathologic contraction of the plasma volume. Clinically, a high hematocrit caused by either an expanded red cell mass or a contracted plasma volume results in **hyperviscosity** and can cause damage by impairing the circulation in highly oxygen-dependent tissues.

1. **Stress (spurious) polycythemia** is frequently seen in young men under stress.

2. **Gaisböck syndrome** is related to hypertension, obesity, and a hard-driving personality. Patients should not be started on diuretics to control their blood pressure due to aggravation of the hyperviscosity by a further decrease of plasma volume.

3. **Dehydration** leads to a temporary contraction of the plasma volume until fluid replacement occurs.

C. **True erythrocytosis** is a condition associated with an expanded red cell mass that can be due to the following conditions.

1. **Primary causes** of increased erythropoiesis, resulting in an expansion of the circulating red cell mass, are due to an **abnormal erythroid precursor cell** that proliferates and matures in the absence of normal growth factors and regulatory mechanisms.
   a. **Polycythemia vera (PV)** is a stem cell defect resulting in abnormal myeloproliferation. The signs and symptoms of multi–cell line involvement, such as increased numbers of white cells and platelets, splenomegaly, and elevated serum levels of uric acid, help differentiate this condition from secondary causes of erythrocytosis. If there are no signs of myeloproliferation, secondary causes of erythrocytosis must be eliminated.
   b. **Primary erythrocytosis** is a rare condition in which signs of involvement of other cell lines and secondary causes are both absent. Familial cases have been described, although the condition is often sporadic, skipping generations. Follow-up may demonstrate an early form of PV.

2. **Secondary causes** of erythrocytosis may be due to a compensatory mechanism for tissue hypoxia or inappropriate secretion of erythropoietin. Serum levels of erythropoietin will be elevated or normal (but high for the existing hematocrit level).
   a. **Compensatory increase in erythropoietin**
      (1) A compensatory increase in the erythropoietin level may be secondary to a physiologic response to **tissue hypoxia**. The impaired oxygen release at the tissue level may be due to:
         (a) High levels of carboxyhemoglobin (smoker's erythrocytosis)
         (b) Hemoglobins with a high oxygen affinity
      (2) A compensatory increase in the erythropoietin level may be due to **chronic hypoxemia** with decreased arterial saturation caused by:
         (a) Alveolar hypoventilation in the lungs, due to chronic obstructive pulmonary disease or pickwickian syndrome (i.e., sleep apnea, hypoventilation, obesity, erythrocytosis)

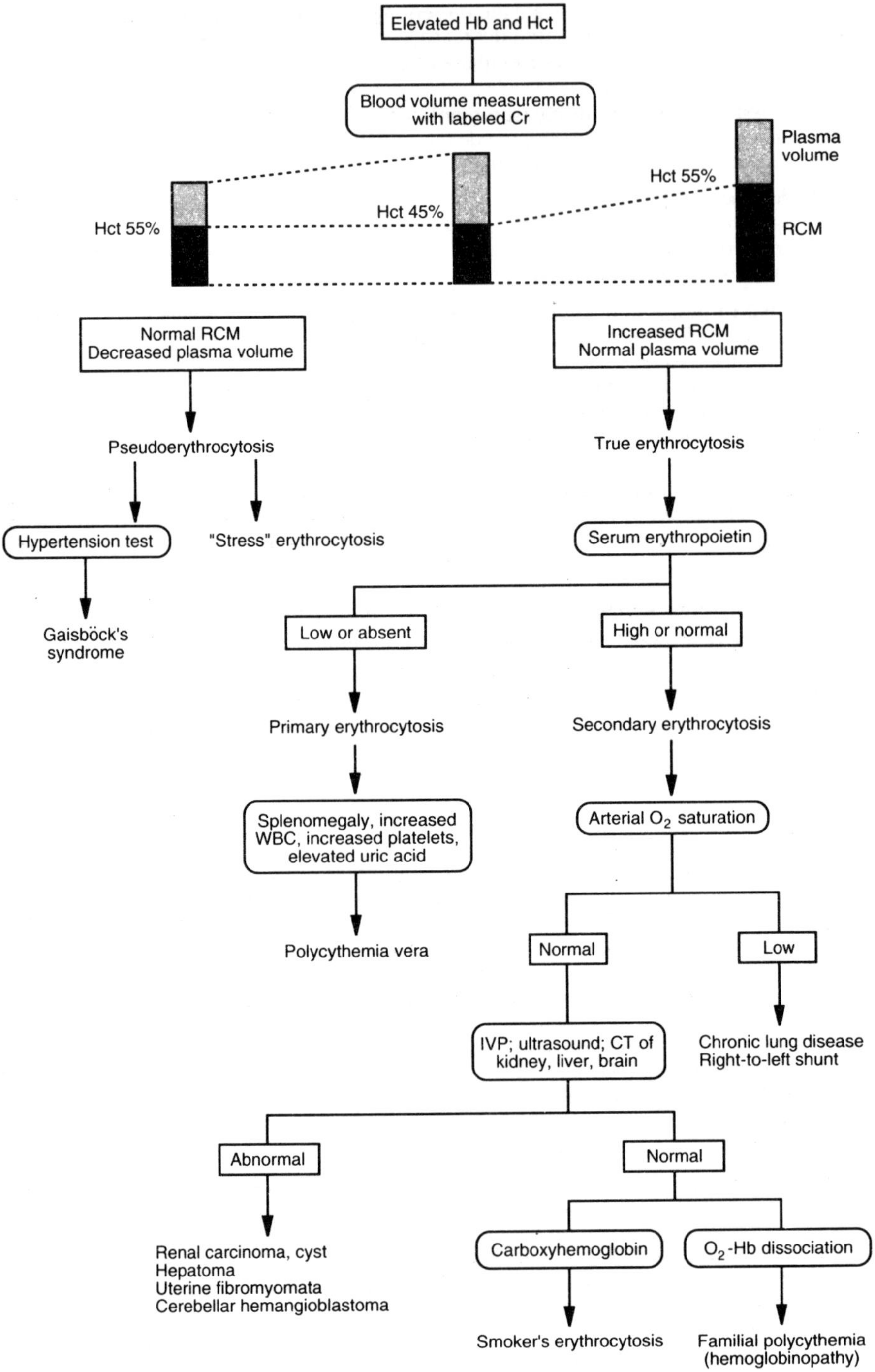

Figure 10-6. A sequential approach to the diagnosis of erythrocytosis is based on initially establishing the presence or absence of an elevated red cell mass (i.e., erythrocytosis versus pseudoerythrocytosis). The sequence of tests in a patient with high hematocrit (*Hct*) and hemoglobin (*Hb*) levels are best done in a logical manner to eliminate performing unnecessary tests. Secondary causes are best characterized by a level of serum erythropoietin that is elevated for the level of hemoglobin. *Cr* = chromium; *CT* = computed tomography; *RCM* = red cell mass; *WBC* = white blood cell count; *IVP* = intravenous pyelogram.

(b) Congenital cyanotic heart disease, which is due to anomalies that allow the mixture of venous with arterial blood (e.g., right-to-left shunts)

b. Inappropriate secretion of erythropoietin may be caused by:

(1) Renal diseases associated with increased erythropoietin secretions, such as:

(a) Renal cell carcinoma (hypernephroma), in which the malignant cells can secrete erythropoietin autonomously, unregulated by normal physiologic mechanisms

(b) Renal cysts that occupy space in the kidney tissue and exert pressure on the surrounding cells, causing focal renal tissue hypoxia and stimulating erythropoietin secretion

(c) Hydronephrosis, which may exert pressure on the major renal vessels as the condition worsens and cause mechanical obstruction of or interference with the arterial blood supply of the kidney

(d) Renal graft rejection, which may cause erythrocytosis with increased levels of erythropoietin (however, the mechanism is undetermined)

(2) Tumors outside the kidney associated with erythrocytosis, such as:

(a) Hepatocellular carcinoma (hepatoma), which can secrete erythropoietin

(b) Pheochromocytoma, which has been reported in some cases to secrete erythropoietin

(c) Cerebellar hemangioblastoma (Hippel-Lindau disease), which can autonomously produce erythropoietin

(d) Large uterine leiomyomata, which are benign tumors that may stimulate erythropoietin by depriving the kidneys of their blood supply through mechanical means

(3) Endocrinopathies, such as adrenal cortical hypersecretion and the effects of exogenous androgens, which are associated with increased erythropoietin levels and have a direct stimulatory effect on the erythroid marrow

STUDY QUESTIONS

Directions: Each of the numbered items or incomplete statements in this section is followed by answers or by completions of the statement. Select the **one** lettered answer or completion that is **best** in each case.

1. All of the following statements regarding a hypochromic, microcytic anemia are true EXCEPT

(A) production of small red cells is due to the low levels of hemoglobin from an abnormality in the different stages of heme and globin synthesis
(B) iron deficiency in asymptomatic patients with increased demands for iron, as occurs in infancy, adolescence, and pregnancy, does not require an extensive workup for occult bleeding
(C) thalassemias are the result of globin synthesis defects and cause hemoglobinopathies
(D) iron deficiency and anemia of chronic disease resulting from a relative iron deficiency cause anemias that are indistinguishable from each other
(E) sideroblastic anemias can result in both macrocytic and microcytic red cells in different patients

2. A 54-year-old man with a diagnosis of chronic lymphocytic leukemia (CLL) on intermittent treatment with chlorambucil and prednisone presents at the hospital with chest pains, dark urine, a palpable spleen, and the following blood counts: hematocrit of 26%, hemoglobin of 7 g/dl, white blood count of 122,000 with 86% lymphocytes, platelet count of 125,000/μl, a reticulocyte count of 12%, and spherocytes in the peripheral blood smear. His hematocrit 1 week ago was 36%. The next test for this patient should be the

(A) Schilling test
(B) osmotic fragility test
(C) Ham test
(D) Coombs' test
(E) Heinz bodies test

3. A 45-year-old woman who underwent mitral valve replacement 10 years ago presents with congestive heart failure and anemia. Her hemoglobin is 8 g/dl, her reticulocyte count is 5%, and her peripheral blood smear shows red cell fragments. She has developed a new mitral diastolic murmur. The appropriate therapy for this patient is

(A) vitamin B_{12} supplementation
(B) iron supplementation
(C) splenectomy
(D) mitral valve and folate replacement

4. An asymptomatic 54-year-old woman with diabetes is shown to have a mild anemia, with hemoglobin of 10 g/dl and a mean corpuscular volume (MCV) of 76; a smear shows cigar-shaped red cells and small red cells with pale cytoplasms. Her serum total iron-binding capacity was increased, and she had low serum levels of ferritin and absent iron in the bone marrow. What is the best procedure for this patient?

(A) Start oral administration of ferrous sulfate three times a day
(B) Distribute three occult blood screening cards to the patient and schedule her for a barium enema
(C) Follow up in 6 months
(D) Discharge from clinic

5. A 22-year-old black woman with a diagnosis of sickle cell anemia presents to the emergency room with abdominal pain and an enlarged spleen with a complete blood count showing a hematocrit of 27%, a reticulocyte count of 7%, a white blood count of 14,000 with 64% neutrophils and 6% band forms, and red cells that show sickle and oak-leaf shapes. The most likely explanation for the enlarged spleen is

(A) hemoglobin (Hb) SC or S-thal
(B) splenic crisis
(C) abscess of the spleen
(D) amyloidosis of the spleen
(E) hypernephroma mimicking an enlarged spleen

1-D
2-D
3-D
4-B
5-A

6. A 65-year-old man who is a known hypertensive patient and who has been on methyldopa for the last 5 years was examined by his physician because of pallor and fatigue. His physical examination was unremarkable except for pallor, and his complete blood count showed a hemoglobin of 10 g/dl, a reticulocyte count of 8%, low haptoglobin, a positive direct Coombs' test, an elevated serum lactate dehydrogenase (LDH), and indirect bilirubin. The most likely mechanism for this patient's drug-related hemolysis is

(A) hapten-related mechanism with antibodies formed against the drug that bind to the patient's red cells
(B) innocent bystander mechanism resulting from the formation of an IgM antibody that reacts with the drug in an antigen–antibody complex, which attaches to the red cell membrane where it activates and fixes complement, causing hemolysis
(C) true drug-induced autoimmune hemolytic anemia that results from the long-term effects on the suppressor T cells
(D) oxidant hemolysis from the denaturation of hemoglobin and precipitation, forming Heinz bodies
(E) a deficiency in a red cell enzyme that is aggravated by the drug

6-C

ANSWERS AND EXPLANATIONS

1. The answer is D *[I D 2 a (2)].*
The anemia of chronic disease may be hypochromic, microcytic in some cases and may be differentiated from iron deficiency by the increased iron stores in the macrophages in the bone marrow, increased serum ferritin, and decreased total iron-binding capacity. Chronic disease anemia is also associated with low serum levels of erythropoietin and may be a normocytic anemia in the presence of relative iron deficiency.

2. The answer is D *[I E 1].*
The clues for a diagnosis of hemolysis are dark urine and a sudden drop in hematocrit with a high reticulocyte count. Autoimmune hemolytic anemia is usually associated with drugs, connective tissue diseases, and lymphoproliferative diseases such as chronic lymphocytic leukemia (CLL) or idiopathic leukemia and is best diagnosed by demonstrating antibodies in the surface of the patient's red cells through the Coombs' test.

3. The answer is D *[I E 2 c (1) (a)].*
This patient is presenting with traumatic hemolytic anemia due to turbulent blood flow through a tight or insufficient valve, as indicated by the appearance of a new murmur. Since this is a chronic process, an increased demand for folic acid would require replacement, but removing the cause of the hemolysis by replacing the mitral valve is imminently more important because of the danger of congestive heart failure.

4. The answer is B *[I B 2 b].*
A postmenopausal patient has no reason to become iron deficient and deserves a workup to identify the source of occult bleeding. In such a patient, the gastrointestinal tract is the most frequent source. Although sampling the stools three times for occult blood is a good screen, an intermittently bleeding lesion may be missed, so a gastrointestinal workup should be performed.

5. The answer is A *[I E 1; Figure 10-5].*
The most likely explanation for a patient with a typical clinical presentation of sickle cell disease and an enlarged spleen is a combination of hemoglobin (Hb) S with Hb C or thalassemia. Splenic crisis is most often seen in infants, and by the second year of age, most sickle cell anemia patients with Hb SS would have an atrophied spleen because the multiple small infarctions result in autosplenectomy. Splenic crisis, an abscess of the spleen, amyloidosis of the spleen, or hypernephroma are remote possibilities.

6. The answer is C *[I E 1 a (1)].*
The drug-induced hemolysis associated with long-term use of methyldopa is caused by a true autoimmune hemolytic anemia since the drug itself is not directly responsible for the positive Coombs' test and the antibody lacks any antidrug activity.

11 Normal Physiology and Non-neoplastic Disorders of Granulocytes, Monocytes, and Lymphocytes

Jeffrey A. Kant

I. NORMAL PHYSIOLOGY OF GRANULOCYTES AND MONOCYTES

A. Granulo-monocytopoiesis (see also Ch 2 II). In hematopoiesis, stem cells commit to differentiation along a particular pathway. The signals that induce such commitment are poorly understood but are thought to involve, at least to some extent, **stromal cells of the bone marrow,** which are sometimes referred to as the hematopoietic microenvironment.

1. **Hematopoietic growth factors** for granulo-monocytopoiesis [sometimes called **colony-stimulating factors** (CSFs)] contribute to the maturation of committed precursors and probably also initiate their self-renewal to satisfy the next demand for cells of that lineage. These factors, which are produced by T cells and by endothelial and mesenchymal cells, include the following.
   a. **Granulocyte/macrophage colony-stimulating factor (GM-CSF)** stimulates production and function of neutrophils, monocytes, and eosinophils.
   b. **Granulocyte colony-stimulating factor (G-CSF)** stimulates production and maturation of neutrophils.
   c. **Macrophage colony-stimulating factor (M-CSF)** stimulates production and maturation of monocytes.
   d. **Interleukin-3 (IL-3)** [also known as **multi–colony-stimulating factor (multi-CSF)**] is a multipotential hematopoietic growth factor.
   e. **Interleukin-1 (IL-1)** and **interleukin-5 (IL-5)** also are involved in the proliferation and differentiation of granulocytes. IL-1 affects basophils and, possibly, eosinophils; IL-5 affects eosinophils.

2. **Other mediators.** Although the events that initiate myelopoiesis are beginning to be understood, the mechanisms or mediators that may downregulate production—including lactoferrins, acidic isoferritin, other chalones, and CSFs themselves—are poorly understood.

3. **Differentiation**
   a. **Neutrophils and monocytes** arise from a single precursor cell type—granulocyte/macrophage colony-forming unit (CFU-GM)—depending on the differentiation signals received. CFU-GM is thought to arise from multipotential precursors capable of differentiating into granulocytes, erythrocytes, macrophages, and megakaryocytes (CFU-GEMM).
      (1) Neutrophils mature over 1–2 weeks in the bone marrow to yield fully differentiated forms. There are five stages of maturation: **myeloblast, promyelocyte, myelocyte, metamyelocyte,** and **band neutrophil** (see I B 1 a).
      (2) Differentiation of monocytes proceeds through **promonocytes** to the mature **circulating blood monocyte**. Two growth factors, M-CSF and GM-CSF, are important for growth and maturation. These factors are produced by endothelial and other mesenchymal cells as well as by monocytes themselves.
   b. **Eosinophils and basophils.** Separate precursors for eosinophils (CFU-Eo) and basophils (CFU-Baso) are also thought to derive from the CFU-GEMM cell (see Figure 2-1).
      (1) The mechanisms by which growth factors affect eosinophil proliferation and differentiation are not well understood, but these factors probably are produced by T cells.
      (2) Little is known about the growth factor requirements of basophils or mast cells.

B. Neutrophils

1. **Morphology.** The mature neutrophil is characterized by a light orange–pink cytoplasm that contains granules and a nucleus with three or four segments connected by thin chromatin filaments. In females, a drumstick-like nuclear chromatin appendage equivalent to the Barr body is seen in tissue cells (e.g., fibroblasts) and marks the inactivated X chromosome.
   a. **Maturation stages.** The maturation stages of neutrophils (Figure 11-1) are as follows.
      (1) **Myeloblasts** are derived from CFU-GEMM, a multipotential progenitor that is believed to give rise also to basophilic, eosinophilic, megakaryocytic, and erythroid blasts. The nuclear chromatin is fine with one or more nucleoli, and there is a small rim of light blue cytoplasm with very few or no granules.
      (2) **Promyelocytes** are slightly larger than myeloblasts. The nucleus exhibits slightly condensed chromatin, often with nucleoli. There is somewhat more cytoplasm, which features purple–red azurophilic **primary granules**.
      (3) **Myelocytes** have nuclei that usually are pushed to one side of the cell and that display increased chromatin condensation relative to the promyelocyte; there are no nucleoli. Half of the cell is orange–pink cytoplasm, which reflects the presence of increasing numbers of **secondary granules**. The myelocyte is the **last mitotically active stage in the granulocyte series**.
      (4) **Metamyelocytes** have nuclei that are indented (less than half the diameter of the entire nucleus), and the cytoplasm is completely orange–pink with granules.
      (5) **Band neutrophils** have nuclei that are indented more than half its greatest diameter but that contain no identifiable nuclear segments connected by filaments. Band neutrophils are the immediate precursors of mature neutrophils.
   b. **Constituents of mature cells**
      (1) **Granules.** Two major classes of granules are found in neutrophils. To a large extent, the release of primary and secondary granules can be controlled separately, although some stimuli cause the release of both.
         (a) **Primary (azurophilic) granules** (approximately 0.2–1.0 μm) contain myeloperoxidase, lysozyme, neutral proteases, and acid hydrolases as well as other polypeptides including cationic proteins, defensins, and toxic or permeability-inducing proteins for microorganisms.
         (b) **Secondary (specific) granules** (approximately 0.1–0.3 μm) contain collagenase, lysozyme, lactoferrin, vitamin B_{12}–binding proteins, and other substances that activate complement (e.g., C5a cleaving enzymes) and plasminogen.
         (c) **Tertiary granules** (approximately 0.1–0.2 μm) that contain gelatinase and other proteins exist as a minor population.
      (2) **Surface membrane receptors** for complement components C3 and C5a, Fc regions of IgG, inflammatory peptides, and cytokines in addition to adherence proteins and other molecules provide the neutrophil with numerous ways in which to respond to inflammatory stimuli and changes in its environment.

2. **Functions**
   a. **Chemotaxis**
      (1) Neutrophils are attracted to sites of inflammation in response to various substances, or **chemotactic factors,** for which they bear surface receptors. Among these substances are:
         (a) Complement components C5a and C3
         (b) Arachidonic acid metabolites [e.g., hydroxyeicosatetraenoic acid (HETE), leukotriene B_4 (LTB_4)], which are generated exogenously or through the action of neutrophilic granular constituents

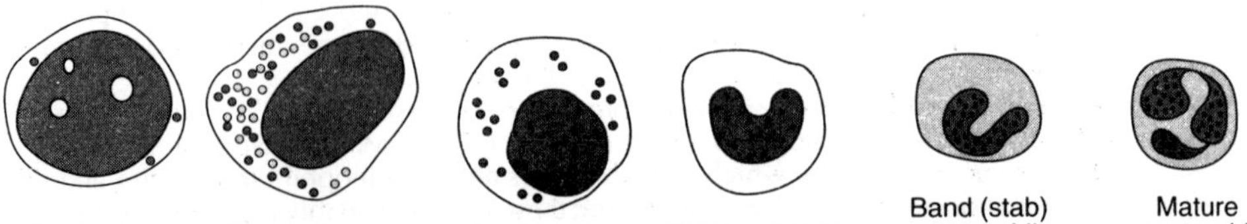

Figure 11-1. Granulocyte differentiation: the neutrophil pathway.

(c) Peptides (e.g., fMet-Leu-Phe)

(2) Neutrophils move via **pseudopodia**. These foot-like extensions of the cell extend forward by polymerization and depolymerization of cytoskeletal proteins, propelling neutrophils toward areas of inflammation.

(3) Not only do neutrophils actively migrate toward the site of inflammation in this fashion, they are also extracted from the blood by **diapedesis** (squeezing) between capillary endothelial cells and enter tissues.

b. Cytotoxic activities

(1) **Phagocytosis** is the engulfment and subsequent destruction of exogenous organisms or particles. **Neutrophils** and **monocytes** are the major phagocytic cells of the blood; eosinophils may also demonstrate phagocytosis. When neutrophils or monocytes contact bacteria, which often are covered with antibody, complement, or other **opsonins** (i.e., serum substances that enhance interaction with phagocytes), the cell membrane envelops the organism to form a **phagosome**.

(2) **Granule toxicity**

(a) The contents of primary and secondary granules fuse with the phagosome, killing the microorganisms and degrading other materials. To accomplish this, surface receptors for fMet-Leu-Phe, LTB_4, and platelet-activating factor (PAF) couple with membrane-bound G proteins, activating phospholipase C and producing inositol triphosphate (IP_3) and calcium influx.

(b) Granule release and fusion follows, delivering the following to phagosomes:

(i) Microbicidal defensins

(ii) Cationic proteins, which lyse gram-negative bacteria

(iii) Myeloperoxidase, which interacts with hydrogen peroxide (H_2O_2) and hydrogen chloride (HCl) to generate toxic hypochlorous acid (HOCl)

(iv) Lysozyme, which hydrolyzes mucoproteins that comprise bacterial cell walls

(v) Superoxide (O_2^-) and hydroxyl (OH^-) radicals, which are generated via nicotinamide-adenine dinucleotide phosphate (NADPH) oxidase

(c) The toxic contents of granules can damage normal tissues if they leak out during phagocytosis or locomotion.

3. Metabolic pathways

a. Cytoplasmic **glycogen** provides an important source of energy, allowing neutrophils to function at low oxygen tensions (Po_2) using glycolysis.

b. The hexose monophosphate shunt generates **NADPH,** an important source of electrons for microbicidal activities dependent on H_2O_2, O_2^-, and free OH^- radicals. Cytoplasmic catalase, superoxide dismutase, glutathione peroxidase, and oxidase help maintain an appropriate balance of molecules.

c. Enzymes of arachidonic acid metabolism (e.g., **cyclooxygenase** and **lipoxygenase**) are essential for the generation of biologically active metabolites, including **prostaglandins** and **leukotrienes** (Figure 11-2).

4. Life span and circulation

a. Transit time in blood for mature neutrophils is 1 day or less. Neutrophils leave the circulation and probably survive 1–2 days in tissue. Good tests of neutrophil longevity are not available.

b. Normal peripheral blood levels of neutrophils are $4.0–11.0 \times 10^9$/L ($10^3/\mu l$). Actual peripheral blood neutrophil levels probably are double the white cell count, since half are in a noncirculating marginated pool along blood vessels.

C. Eosinophils

1. Morphology

a. General features. Mature eosinophils are easily recognized cells with refractile orange–red granules and segmented nuclei on stained peripheral blood smears. In contrast to neutrophils, many eosinophils exhibit a bilobed nucleus. Maturation is similar to that for neutrophils (see Figure 11-1).

b. Granules first appear at the myelocyte stage of differentiation. The large granules have a central crystalloid containing **major basic protein (MBP),** hydrolytic enzymes, peroxidase, and other proteins such as eosinophil-cationic protein.

c. Surface membrane receptors. Eosinophil cell membranes contain Fc receptors for IgE, IgG, and IgM, along with C3b and C4 receptors.

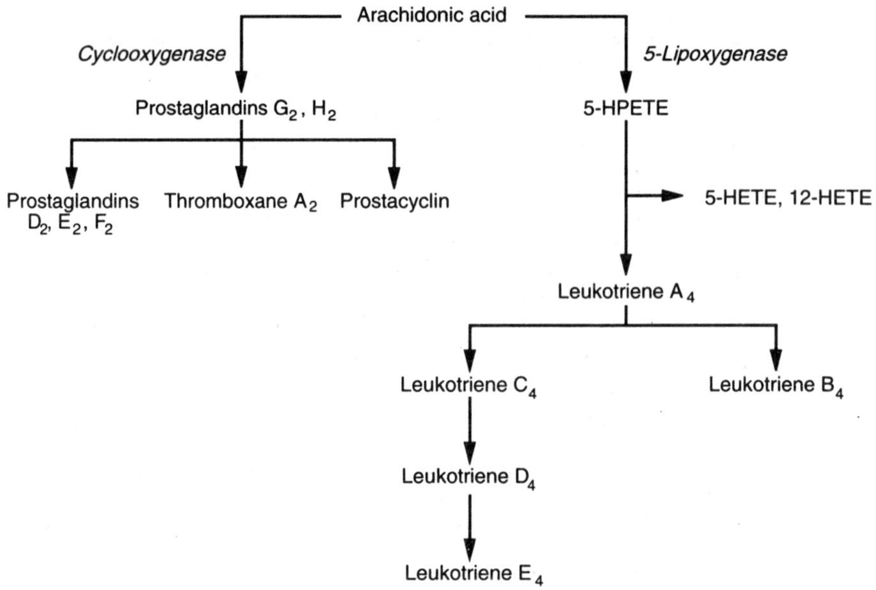

Figure 11-2. Arachidonic acid metabolism. *5-HPETE* = 5-hydroperoxyeicosatetraenoic acid; *5-, 12-HETE* = 5-, 12-hydroxyeicosatetraenoic acid.

2. Functions

a. Eosinophils are a **first line defense against parasites** (e.g., helminth larvae); they participate in killing these agents by releasing their granular contents after activation by antibody and complement. Activation is associated with fusion and release of granules as well as an increase in cell metabolic rate and expression of Fc and complement receptors.

b. Eosinophils also **modulate hypersensitivity reactions;** their granular contents neutralize histamine and inhibit mast cell degranulation.

c. Eosinophils **migrate to inflammatory sites** in response to factors such as histamine.

3. Life span and circulation

a. Eosinophils usually exist in concentrations of 100–400/μl in peripheral blood and appear to reside there for less than 12 hours.

b. Their patterns of circulation and survival outside the blood is poorly understood, but they are known to target such organs as the skin, lungs, and gastrointestinal tract. The presence of eosinophils in lymph nodes and thoracic duct lymph supports a circulation pattern different from that of neutrophils.

D. Basophils and mast cells

1. Morphology

a. General features. Despite similar appearance on Wright's-stained smears with prominent purple-blue cytoplasmic granules, basophils and mast cells are distinctly different morphologically and functionally (Table 11-1).

(1) Basophils derive from granulocytic precursors and exhibit segmented nuclei. The cytoplasm contains a few large granules.

Table 11-1. General Features of Basophils and Mast Cells

Feature	Basophils	Mast Cells
Distribution	Blood; bone marrow	Tissue
Life span	Short	Long
Self-replication	No	Yes
Morphology	Segmented nucleus; few large granules	Round nucleus; numerous small granules

(2) **Mast cells.** The nucleus is round, and the cytoplasm is filled with an abundance of small basophilic granules that usually do not cover the nucleus. Current evidence suggests that mast cells are not derived from basophils but from a separate bone marrow-derived precursor.

b. Granules in both basophils and mast cells contain **proteoglycans,** including heparin, vasoactive histamine, neutral proteases, and other enzymes.

2. Functions

a. Basophil degranulation is involved in **immediate hypersensitivity** reactions (e.g., asthma, urticaria, anaphylaxis) and may be associated with **flushing**.

b. IgE Fc receptors trigger **anaphylactic degranulation** via cross-bridging of two or more IgE molecules and resultant granule-membrane fusion.

c. Like neutrophils, basophils and mast cells form biologically **active arachidonic acid metabolites** (e.g., leukotrienes, prostaglandins).

3. Life span and circulation

a. Basophils. Clinically, basophils are most commonly noted in the peripheral blood and bone marrow, where the high solubility of granule constituents in alcohol sometimes yields only a few large basophilic granules on stained peripheral blood smear. Their short peripheral blood transit time is similar to that of neutrophils (i.e., about 1–2 days).

b. Mast cells, by contrast, are found relatively infrequently, primarily in connective tissue adjacent to blood vessels and beneath epithelial surfaces; they are present in blood only in pathologic conditions. Human mast cell life span is not clearly defined; murine studies suggest mast cells survive several weeks to several months in tissue.

E. Monocytes. It is now clear that bone marrow monocytes give rise not only to circulating monocytes but also to an extensive network of macrophages referred to as the mononuclear phagocyte system.

1. Cells of the mononuclear phagocyte system are distributed throughout the body and are named differently depending on their location. Components of the system include:

a. Pulmonary alveolar macrophages

b. Pleural and peritoneal macrophages

c. Kupffer's cells of the liver

d. Histiocytes of mesenchymal and connective tissue, including cutaneous Langerhans' cells

e. Mesangial cells of the kidney

f. Fixed and mobile macrophages in the lymph nodes, spleen, and bone marrow

2. Morphology

a. General features

(1) As seen on Wright's-stained peripheral blood smear, monocytes vary in size from 10–20 μm. Macrophage cell size ranges up to 50 μm in tissue where monocytic cells may fuse under conditions of inflammation to form large multinucleated Langerhans' giant cells.

(2) Nuclei often are slightly indented and have reticular chromatin that is less clumped than in lymphocytes. The relatively abundant cytoplasm is gray to blue–gray and contains small orange–red granules. Cytoplasmic vacuoles are common.

b. Granules. Monocytes contain two functional sets of granules.

(1) One set is a lysosomal group of granules that contain acid phosphatase, arylsulfatase, and peroxidase analogous to neutrophil primary granules. These granules fuse with phagosomes to form secondary lysosomes.

(2) The function of the other set of granules is not well understood.

c. Cell membrane receptors. Many functions of monocytes are mediated through the interaction of immune complexes and antigens with cell membrane receptors for immunoglobulins (Fc receptors), complement (especially C3), and human leukocyte antigen–DR (HLA-DR) [Ia-like] antigens. Monocytes also express the CD4 antigen (see II A 2, Table 11-2), originally thought to be restricted to helper-inducer T cells.

3. Functions

a. Activating stimuli. Monocytes and macrophages can be activated by various stimuli that cause an increase in cell size, metabolic rate, lysosomal enzyme levels, and production of mediators (e.g., IL-1, prostaglandins, interferons, chemotactic factors for neutrophils, M-CSF, GM-CSF).

b. **Chemotaxis.** As with neutrophils, monocytes display active chemotaxis toward sites of inflammation and necrosis.

c. **Phagocytosis.** Chemotaxis serves primarily to recruit monocytes for phagocytosis. Receptors for antibody or complement-coated organisms and cytoplasmic lysosomal granules play a major role in this function as does the generation of toxic oxidative metabolites (e.g., H_2O_2, O_2^-, O_2 radicals) much the same as in neutrophils.

(1) **Red cell removal.** Monocytes remove senescent red cells in the liver and spleen and serve as the primary cells for **iron processing** and **storage** in the bone marrow and other organs.

(2) **Resistance to phagocytosis.** Some microorganisms (e.g., certain *Mycobacteria* or *Leishmania* species) may escape destruction after phagocytosis by intrinsic resistance or interference with normal lysosomal function.

(3) **Antigen presentation.** Cells of the mononuclear phagocyte system play an important role in the generation of both humoral and cell-mediated immunity by presenting antigen to T cells via HLA-DR class II molecules.

(4) **Tissue destruction.** Macrophages at sites of inflammation produce and secrete various mediators that may contribute to tissue destruction including **collagenase,** other **lysosomal enzymes,** and **oxidative metabolites**.

(a) **Complement components** opsonize organisms and serve as sources of chemotactic and inflammatory peptides.

(b) **Tissue plasminogen activator (TPA)** helps degrade clots at sites of inflammation to facilitate tissue repair and remodeling.

(c) **Cytokines** [e.g., IL-1, tumor necrosis factor (TNF)] facilitate the response to inflammation by promoting other cells to secrete growth factors that stimulate production of more monocytes and by contributing to systemic symptoms such as fever.

(5) **Neoplastic cell destruction.** Activated macrophages may also play a role in destruction of neoplastic cells, although this function is not well studied.

II. NORMAL PHYSIOLOGY OF LYMPHOCYTES AND PLASMA CELLS.

Lymphocytes form the core of the human immune system, which functions to protect the body against infection or engraftment by foreign organisms or tissue and, possibly, against tumor development. There are three major functional classes of lymphocytes: B lymphocytes (B cells), T lymphocytes (T cells), and natural killer (NK) cells. Plasma cells are fully differentiated B cells that produce and secrete immunoglobulins.

A. Lymphopoiesis.

Lymphoid stem cells give rise to the major functional classes of lymphocytes.

1. **Lymphoid stem cells,** which morphologically resemble small lymphocytes, are **derived from pluripotential hematopoietic stem cells,** which also give rise to progenitor cells responsible for the production of granulocytes, monocytes, red cells, and platelets.

2. **Differentiation.** As lymphocytes differentiate from precursors into functionally mature forms, there is a complex programmed expression involving both acquisition and loss of a series of surface antigens, which can be defined by **monoclonal antibodies**. Because antibodies from different sources often recognize identical antigens, **cluster designations (CD)** have been defined for most major surface determinants. CD groups associated with B and T cells are defined in Table 11-2.

a. **B cells** are derived from stem cells that have undergone conditioning to establish that their progeny will produce immunoglobulins. In birds, conditioning occurs in a specific organ, the **bursa of Fabricius** (hence "B" cells). In humans, this function is thought to be served by the **bone marrow**. A discrete series of steps leads to a mature B cell capable of producing immunoglobulin.

(1) The initial commitment to B cell development is manifested by rearrangement of the immunoglobulin heavy chain gene in the **pre-pre (or pre-pro) B cell**.

(2) Shortly thereafter, in the **pre-B cell,** monoclonal cytoplasmic IgM can be detected.

(3) **Mature B cells** express monoclonal surface, but not cytoplasmic, IgM (and often IgD).

(4) Stimulation of mature B cells through cross-linkage of surface immunoglobulin or via effector T cells causes differentiation to **plasma cells,** with cytoplasmic synthesis and secretion of the specific immunoglobulin for which the B cell is programmed. This differentiation sequence is accompanied by sequential expression of a variety of other B cell membrane antigens (e.g., CD19, CD20) as well as receptors for complement and Fc regions of immunoglobulin heavy chains.

Table 11-2. Important Cluster Designation (CD) Antigens Associated with Lymphocyte Classes

Antigen	Distribution	Identity or Function
CD1	Thymocytes, Langerhans' cells	. . .
CD2	T cells, NK cells	T cell differentiation antigen; sheep RBC receptor
CD3	T cells	T cell antigen receptor–associated antigen
CD4*	Helper-inducer T cell subset	MHC class II–restricted immune recognition
CD5	T cells, B cell subset†	. . .
CD7	T cells, NK cells	Possible IgM Fc receptor
CD8*	Cytotoxic suppressor T cell subset	MHC class I–restricted immune recognition
CD10 (CALLA)	Pre-B cells	Endopeptidase
CD11c	NK cells	Receptor for C3bi
CD16 (Leu 11)	NK cells	Fc_{γ} receptor III
CD19 (B4)	B cells	. . .
CD20 (B1)	B cells	. . .
CD21 (B2)	B cells	Receptor for C3d and EBV

NK cells = natural killer cells; RBC = red blood cell; MHC = major histocompatibility complex; CALLA = common acute lymphocytic leukemia antigen; EBV = Epstein-Barr virus. (Adapted from Lydyard PM, Grossi CE: Cells involved in the immune response. In *Immunology,* 2nd edition. Edited by Roitt IM, Brostoff J, Male DK. London, Gower Medical Publishing, 1989, p 2.5).

*Analysis of the molecular structure of CD4 and CD8 antigens places them in the "immunoglobulin supergene family" with immunoglobulins, MHC molecules, and T cell antigen receptors.

†CD5 antigen is present on B cell chronic lymphocytic leukemia.

b. **T cells** (Figure 11-3) are derived from stem cells that undergo maturation in the **thymus,** where T cells acquire the capacity for specific immunologic roles.

(1) **Morphologic polarity** is associated with the maturation of T cells.

(a) Immature T cells that lack CD3, CD4, or CD8 antigens localize preferentially in the **thymic cortex**. These cells also express other pan–T cell antigens (e.g., CD2, CD5, CD7) as well as antigens characteristic of immature cells (e.g., CD1).

(b) As functional maturation proceeds, T cells lose CD1 and acquire CD3, CD4, and CD8 antigens in the **inner cortex**.

(c) This is followed by the loss of either the CD4 or CD8 antigen to yield two major mature T cell subsets—$CD3^+/CD4^+$ cells and $CD3^+/CD8^+$ cells—in the **thymic medulla**. Each T cell subset has distinctly different functions (see II E 2).

(2) **Inappropriate expression** of early differentiation antigens or deviations from these well-defined patterns of differentiation is a feature of many T cell neoplasms that may be useful in diagnosis.

B. Morphology

1. **Lymphocytes** are small (6–10 μm) to medium-sized (10–15 μm) **mononuclear cells** with relatively high nuclear–cytoplasm ratios, scant to moderate light blue cytoplasm, and relatively few cellular organelles. Some lymphocytes, particularly NK cells, display scattered prominent cytoplasmic granules. Activated lymphocytes, by contrast, are larger (15–30 μm) cells with moderately abundant blue cytoplasm and nuclei featuring less condensed chromatin and occasional prominent nucleoli.

2. **Plasma cells** have eccentric nuclei, often with condensed chromatin along the nuclear rim to form a "clock-face" pattern and basophilic cytoplasm reflecting abundant RNA. A perinuclear cytoplasmic clear zone, the **hof,** reflects an active Golgi complex.

C. Distribution. Many lymphocytes are mobile and circulate throughout the lymphoid organs, blood, and body tissues. In adult peripheral blood, small lymphocytes and less frequent medium-sized lymphocytes constitute 20%–50% of white cells; the levels are a bit higher in young children. Lymphocytes also comprise most of the cells in lymphoid organs. The specific distribution of lymphocytes is determined by immunologic function.

1. **B cells.** Recent evidence suggests that B cells are drawn to particular regions of the lymphoid system in response to interactions between specific surface receptors of the lymphocyte function–associated (LFA) class on B cells and endothelial cells of high endothelial venules in these regions. B cells localize primarily to the:

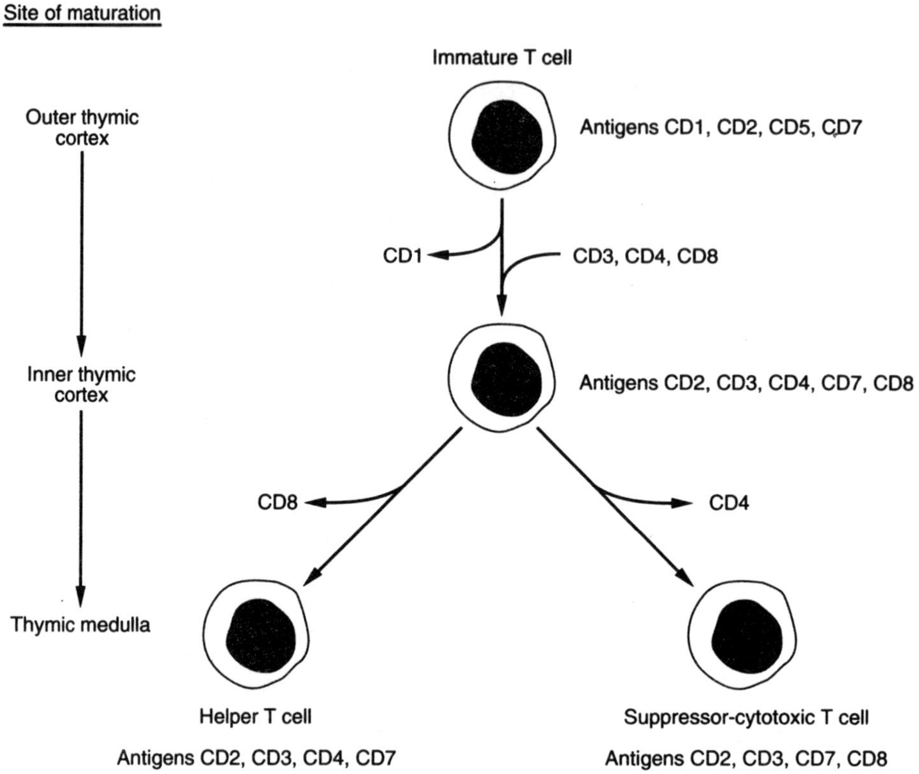

Figure 11-3. T cell maturation in the thymus.

- **a.** Primary and secondary follicles (germinal centers) of the lymph nodes
- **b.** Periarteriolar splenic white pulp, where they form follicles
- **c.** Submucosa of the oropharynx and nasopharynx (tonsils) and Peyer's patches of the small bowel
- **d.** Peripheral blood, where they constitute a minority (< 10%) of circulating lymphocytes

2. T cells. Normally, there is roughly a 2:1 ratio of $CD4^+$ cells to $CD8^+$ cells. Like B cells, T cells localize to specialized regions of the lymphoid system, including the:

- **a.** Interfollicular (paracortical) regions of lymph nodes
- **b.** Periarteriolar splenic white pulp along vessels and surrounding follicles
- **c.** Thymus
- **d.** Peripheral blood, where they constitute the majority (> 85%) of circulating lymphocytes

3. NK cells comprise approximately 5%–10% of circulating lymphocytes.

4. Plasma cells are not seen normally in peripheral blood but may be present in response to inflammatory stimuli.

D. B cell function. B cells are primarily responsible for **humoral immunity** (i.e., antibody production). Antibodies (immunoglobulins) are the major product of B cells; an enormous diversity is required to combine specifically with the range of foreign antigens a host may encounter. Each B cell produces immunoglobulins with a single antigenic specificity, or idiotype.

1. Antibody production requires activation of resting B cells, proliferation of activated B cells, and differentiation of B cells into immunoglobulin-secreting plasma cells.

a. B cell activation

(1) T cell–independent activation involves the binding of large antigens with multiple copies of the recognized epitope (e.g., polysaccharides in the capsules of bacteria), with resultant cross-linkage of surface immunoglobulin molecules.

(2) **T cell–dependent activation** is more frequent and involves the presentation to B cells of processed antigens (probably polypeptide antigens) in combination with the host's major histocompatibility complex (MHC) class II molecules.

b. Biochemical changes following activation

(1) The interaction of antigen with surface immunoglobulin triggers a cascade of biochemical events involving increased synthesis of **IP_3** and **diacylglycerol** with subsequent activation of **protein kinase C,** phosphorylation of membrane proteins, and an influx of **free calcium** into the cell. These events trigger increases in the expression of various genes in the B cell nucleus, including growth-related proto-oncogenes such as c-*myc,* c-*myb,* and c-*fos.*

(2) During activation, **memory lymphocytes** arrested at the G_0 stage of the cell cycle are promoted to G_1 and then go into full DNA synthesis with clonal expansion.

c. B cell proliferation and differentiation is under the influence of a variety of interleukins such as IL-1, IL-4, IL-5, IL-6, and even IL-2, presumably through interactions with cell surface receptors for these molecules.

(1) Individual resting lymphocytes normally express surface IgM.

(a) Following activation, as B cell differentiation proceeds, these cells usually express increased surface IgD followed by a heavy chain class switch to surface IgG or IgA [see II D 2 b (4)] .

(b) This stage is followed by the secretion of antibodies as maturation proceeds through activated lymphocytes and immunoblasts to the plasma cell stage.

(2) Some cells secrete only IgM and are more evident early in humoral responses.

(3) In addition to functional antibody-secreting cells, **long-lived memory B cells** also are produced during this cycle of activation, proliferation, and differentiation. These cells are capable of a more rapid and higher titer response if the host encounters the same antigen again.

d. Regulation of antibody production is not fully understood but probably involves effects from helper T cells, withdrawal of the antigen through entrapment by the immunoglobulin produced, and generation of activity against immunoglobulin-producing cells in the form of **anti-idiotypic** antibodies or T cells directed against those idiotypes.

2. B cell products: immunoglobulins (Table 11-3)

a. Structure (Figure 11-4). The basic structural unit of immunoglobulins consists of two identical heavy polypeptide chains and two identical light polypeptide chains covalently linked by disulfide bonds. There are five heavy chain classes—mu (μ), gamma (γ), alpha (α), delta (δ), and epsilon (ϵ)—and two light chain classes—lambda (λ), and kappa (κ). Each heavy and light chain of the immunoglobulin molecule is divided into two regions.

(1) The **variable (V) regions** are highly heterogeneous and are the sites responsible for antigen recognition. These regions are contained within the **Fab fragments** that are produced following pepsin degradation of the molecule.

(2) The **constant (C) regions** control other functions (e.g., binding of complement). The constant regions of the heavy chains are found in the **Fc fragment** that is produced following papain degradation of the molecule. (The constant regions of light chains are in the Fab fragment.)

Table 11-3. Properties of Immunoglobulin Classes

Property	IgG	IgA	IgM	IgD	IgE
Heavy chain	γ	α	μ	δ	ϵ
Heavy chain subclasses	$\gamma_1, \gamma_2, \gamma_3, \gamma_4$	α_1, α_2	μ_1, μ_2	No	No
Molecular weight (kD)	~150	~150–400*	~900	~175	~190
J chain	No	Yes	Yes	No	No
Serum concentration (mg/dl)	800–1800	110–500	60–220	< 3	< 0.05
Serum half-life (days)	21†	6	10	3	2
Functions					
Complement activation	Yes‡	Rare	Yes	No	No
Opsonization	Yes	Weak	No	No	No
Anaphylaxis	No	No	No	No	Yes

Adapted from Hyde RM: *Immunology,* 2nd edition. Baltimore, Williams & Wilkins, 1991, p 29.

*Secretory IgA.

†Subclass IgG3 has a half-life of 7 days.

‡Subclasses IgG1 and IgG3.

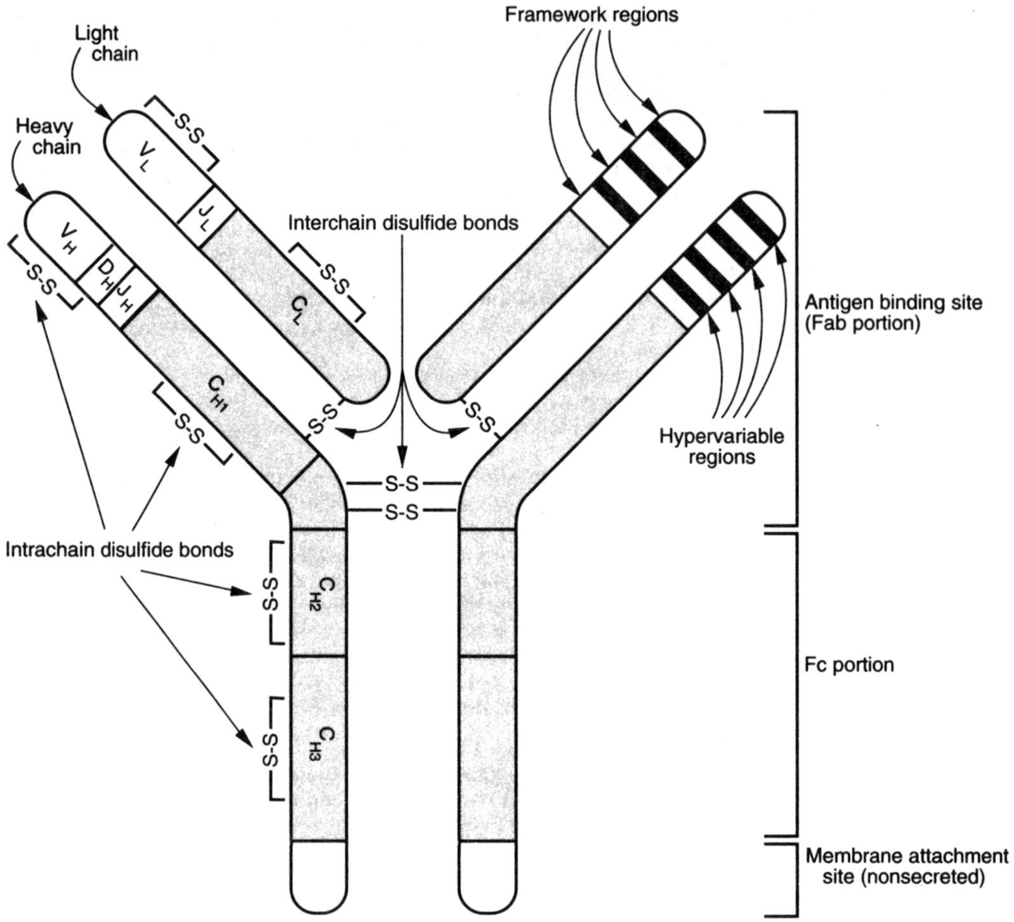

Figure 11-4. The basic structural unit (monomer) of immunoglobulin molecules consists of two identical heavy polypeptide chains and two identical light polypeptide chains linked covalently by disulfide bonds. In two immunoglobulin subclasses, IgM and IgA, the basic units are linked by a short polypeptide, the J chain, to form pentamers and dimers, respectively. *V* = variable region; *J* = joining region; *C* = constant region; *D* = diversity region; *H* = heavy chain; *L* = light chain; S-S = disulfide bond.

b. Genetic basis of immunoglobulin diversity. The extraordinary diversity of immunoglobulins, which is demanded by the range of antigens encountered by the immune system, is derived from a unique combinatorial system of joining individual small gene segments (Figure 11-5A).

(1) Heavy chain rearrangement

(a) Structure of heavy chain gene complex. The immunoglobulin heavy chain gene complex on chromosome 14 consists of 200–300 **V genes** that are each about 100 amino acids long. Adjacent to the V region are four or five **diversity (D) genes** of roughly 10 amino acids. Closely adjacent to the D segments are six **joining (J) genes** of about 10 amino acids. The 200,000 nucleotides following the J segments contain the **μ, δ, γ, ε,** and **α** heavy chain C gene segments.

(b) VDJ joining

(i) Through mechanisms that are not fully understood, with commitment to B lymphoid differentiation in the pre-pre B cell, DNA between one D and one J segment of one immunoglobulin heavy chain gene is looped out and lost. The **elimination of DNA places the two coding segments—D and J—directly next to each other**.

(ii) There follows a similar joining of a V segment to the previously rearranged DJ segment, producing a contiguous VDJ segment.

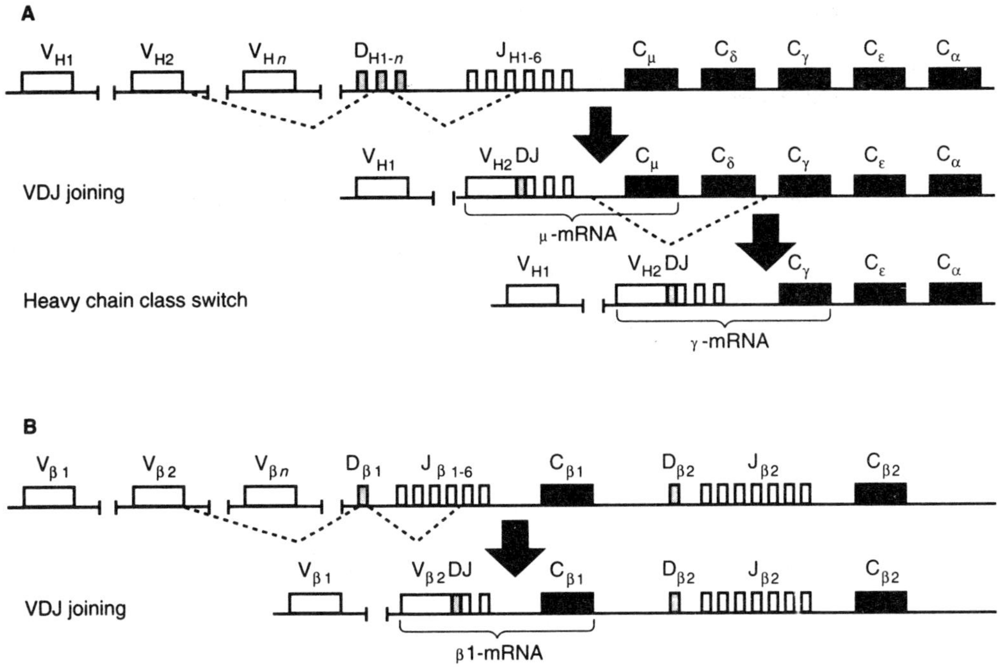

Figure 11-5. (*A*) Immunoglobulin heavy chain gene. VDJ joining allows production of IgM and subsequent class switch to IgG using the identical heavy chain variable/joining/diversity regions. (*B*) T cell β chain antigen receptor gene. *V* = variable genes; D_H = diversity genes; J_H = joining genes; *C* = constant genes. (Note: This illustration is schematic and not to scale.)

(iii) Additional nucleotides may also be added or deleted during the joining of these segments, probably via the enzyme **terminal deoxynucleotidyl transferase (TdT)**.

(iv) If the resulting VDJ nucleotide sequence encodes a functional V region polypeptide, the process stops. If not, the second immunoglobulin heavy chain gene on the other chromosome 14 undergoes similar rearrangement in an attempt to form a functional immunoglobulin V region gene.

(2) **Light chain rearrangement. κ and λ light chains on chromosomes 2 and 22,** respectively, undergo a similar rearrangement process, except these genes lack D segments, so **rearranged VJ segments are produced**. The cell attempts first to rearrange the two κ loci and then the λ genes. This is the reason for the 2:1 κ:λ ratio of B cells. Gene rearrangement stops when a functional light chain gene is produced. Immunoglobulin heavy chain genes are rearranged before light chain genes.

(3) **Somatic mutation.** A unique feature of immunoglobulin molecules is additional amino acid diversity due to somatic point mutations in immunoglobulin genes that occur after VDJ rearrangements.

(4) **Immunoglobulin heavy chain class switch.** In the classic antibody response by B cells, immunoglobulin produced by a single cell initially is IgM; eventually, production switches to IgG. **Light chains are identical for each class as are heavy chain V regions.** Chromosomal rearrangements deleting the μ and δ heavy chain C regions accompany the switch to IgG production, and virtually all of the heavy chain gene locus is deleted in IgA-producing cells (see Figure 11-5A). Cells that produce more than one class of immunoglobulin are presumed to do so by **alternative splicing** of heavy chain messenger RNAs (mRNAs).

E. T cell function. The predominant function of T cells is **cell-mediated immunity,** including delayed hypersensitivity, graft rejection, contact allergic reactions, and cytotoxic responses toward other cells. T cells also facilitate antibody production by B cells. Each T cell has a cell surface receptor molecule that is structurally similar to immunoglobulin and is specific for a particular homologous antigen (see II E 3). A similar cycle of activation, proliferation, and differentiation occurs in T cells when the cell surface receptor recognizes its homologous antigen.

1. **T cell activation, proliferation, and differentiation**
   a. **T cell activation**
      (1) T cell activation occurs primarily through the **T cell antigen receptor**.
         (a) Antigens are presented by monocytes or other T cells, in association with host class I or II MHC molecules; thus, the response is described as **MHC-restricted**.
         (b) The actual antigens presented likely are small peptides processed by these cells from larger complete protein molecules.
      (2) Activation also is possible, in vitro at least, through binding to several alternative T cell surface antigens, specifically the **CD2** and **CD28 classes**. An interesting feature of CD28 activation is its resistance to the immunosuppressant cyclosporine.
   b. **T cell proliferation and differentiation**
      (1) Initial biochemical events at the membrane following T cell activation probably are similar to those described for B cell activation (i.e., alterations in lipid metabolism, protein phosphorylation, and ion fluxes).
      (2) These events are followed by the expression of new proteins, among which are high-affinity membrane receptors for IL-2, and production of IL-2 itself by certain classes of T cells. IL-2 interacts with its receptors to initiate a series of actions resulting in cell division and proliferation of stimulated T cell clones. Memory cells also are produced.

2. **Functional subsets of T cells**
   a. **$CD4^+$ cells,** sometimes known as **helper T cells,** present antigen in the context of **MHC class II molecules**. At least two subsets of $CD4^+$ cells have been defined.
      (1) **Helper-inducer cells** produce IL-4 and IL-5 and assist in antibody production but not in cytotoxicity or delayed type hypersensitivity.
      (2) **Suppressor-inducer cells** suppress antibody responses and may function in cytotoxic and hypersensitivity responses.
   b. **$CD8^+$ cells,** sometimes called **cytotoxic suppressor cells,** present antigen in the context of MHC class I molecules and mediate direct cytotoxic responses toward other cells.

3. **T cell antigen receptors** are the basis for specific immunologic reactions mediated by T cells. They face the extracellular environment from an anchored position in the membrane. **Each T cell produces a single antigen receptor with limited specificity.**
   a. **Structure.** T cell receptors are **heterodimers** of α, β, γ, and δ chains that are similar to immunoglobulin light chains. Each consists of about 200 amino acids divided roughly equally between **V and C regions** that are joined by disulfide bonds. Two major classes are defined.
      (1) **αβ receptors** are found on most mature T cells in association with the CD3 antigen.
      (2) **γδ receptors** are similar in size and structure to αβ receptors and are present on a minority of T cells. Although their function is less well understood than that of the αβ receptors, they are also found in association with CD3 antigen and appear capable of stimulating T cell proliferation.
   b. **Genetic basis for diversity.** T cell antigen receptor genes are genetically similar to immunoglobulins (see Figure 11-5B) and undergo analogous chromosomal rearrangements. The **α** and **β genes** feature V and J regions like immunoglobulin light chains; **β and δ genes** have V, D, and J regions like immunoglobulin heavy chains. Each also has one or two C regions.
      (1) The **α** and **δ chain genes** are located near the centromere on the long arm of chromosome 14. Interestingly, the δ gene uses the same V region segments as the α gene, and its D, J, and C regions are located inside the total expanse of the α chain gene. Consequently, δ chain sequences are lost during rearrangements that occur in the formation of a functional α chain gene.
      (2) The **β** and **γ chain genes** are located far from each other on chromosome 7. The γ chain gene has a more limited number of V region genes (< 15) available for generation of diversity.

4. **Mediators affecting the function of T cells and other lymphocytes**
   a. **Interleukins** are molecules, many of which are secreted by lymphocytes, which affect the function of other leukocytes, particularly other lymphocytes. Interleukins engage in complex interactions with other interleukins, hematopoietic growth factors, and many other proteins such as TNF and lymphotoxins. Table 11-4 lists currently known interleukins and major functions associated with each.

Table 11-4. Interleukins Involved in the Immune Response

Interleukin	Sources	Important Effects
IL-1	Monocytes/macrophages Endothelial cells Other (e.g., epithelial) cells B cells, NK cells	B and T cell activation Pyrexia Induction of IL-6 synthesis Acute-phase reaction*
IL-2	Activated T cells	B and T cell proliferation Enhancement of cytotoxic activity
IL-3	Activated B and T cells	Multilineage hematopoietic growth factor
IL-4	Activated T cells	B and T cell activation Proliferation of B and T cells, mast cells, and (with other cytokines) granulocytes and erythrocytes
IL-5	Activated T cells	Differentiation of B and T cells and eosinophils
IL-6	Monocytes/macrophages Fibroblasts, endothelial cells T cells, cell lines Neoplastic plasma cells	Differentiation of B cells and plasma cells T cell activation function Acute-phase reaction Possible growth factor for myeloma cells
IL-7	B cells, stromal cells	B cell proliferation
IL-8	Fibroblasts, vascular endothelium	Neutrophil and lymphocyte chemotaxis Enhancement of neutrophil function
IL-9	T cells	Growth of T cell, megakaryocyte, and erythroid cell lines
IL-10	T cells (Th2 subset)	Inhibition of cytokine synthesis by other Th1 cells and macrophages; possible role in mast cell proliferation
IL-11	Bone marrow stromal cells	Stimulation of B cell development; stimulation of hematopoiesis (with IL-3)
IL-12	B cells	Facilitates proliferation of activated T (LAK) and NK cells

LAK cells = lymphocyte-activated killer cells; NK cells = natural killer cells.

*Acute-phase reaction refers to the increased concentration of certain serum proteins (C-reactive protein, amyloid A, haptoglobin, ceruloplasmin, and many complement components) that occurs in response to acute inflammation.

b. **LFA adhesion molecules.** As with B cells, T cells have many membrane LFA adhesion molecules whose functions are important for normal T cell immune responses.

F. **NK cells** are lymphoid cells defined by their ability to **lyse cells without regard to HLA restriction**. NK cells also **mediate antibody-dependent cellular cytotoxicity**. In the blood, **large granular lymphocytes (LGLs) account for NK activity**. Whether NK cells are T cells or not has been controversial. There are both $CD3^+$ and $CD3^-$ subsets. Most NK cells express surface receptors for IgG Fc regions (CD16).

III. NON-NEOPLASTIC DISORDERS OF GRANULOCYTES, MONOCYTES, AND LYMPHOCYTES

A. **Classification.** Two major categories of non-neoplastic disorders can be defined.

1. **Disorders of cell number.** An abnormally decreased number of leukocytes of a particular class is indicated by the suffix "-cytopenia." An abnormally increased number of leukocytes of a particular class is indicated by the suffix "-cytosis."
2. **Disorders of function and morphology** may be associated with increases or decreases in cell numbers in one or more classes of leukocytes.

B. **Disorders of neutrophils**

1. **Neutropenia** refers to an absolute neutrophil count (ANC) of less than 1500/μl.
   a. **Etiology**
      (1) **Drug-induced neutropenia** is a common cause of decreased neutrophils.
         (a) **Cancer chemotherapy** often results in significant and prolonged neutropenia.

(b) **Dose-related idiosyncratic neutropenia** associated with shutdown of neutrophil production may occur with drugs such as chloramphenicol and phenothiazines.
(c) Many other drug-related neutropenias probably involve **immunologically mediated destruction of neutrophils** or neutrophilic precursors.

(2) **Immune neutropenia,** in which **antibodies to surface antigens either facilitate destruction or impair the production of neutrophils,** may be sporadic or associated with autoimmune disorders [e.g., systemic lupus erythematosus (SLE), rheumatoid arthritis].
(a) The combination of splenomegaly, rheumatoid arthritis, and neutropenia is known as **Felty's syndrome**.
(b) It is not known if the severe neutropenia associated with **large granular (T_γ) lymphocytosis** [see Ch 12 II C 2 e (2)] is immunologically mediated.

(3) **Myelodysplastic syndromes** frequently include neutropenia as part of the overall defect in hematopoiesis.

(4) **Infectious diseases** (e.g., bacterial, viral, fungal, parasitic, rickettsial) often include neutropenia. Mechanisms include:
(a) Infection and compromise of neutrophil (and other) precursors, as may occur with human immunodeficiency virus (HIV) infection
(b) Increased peripheral utilization of neutrophils, as occurs in bacterial infections
(c) Endothelial damage with increased adherence

(5) **Chronic idiopathic neutropenia** occurs in both children and adults and may represent a **mixture of congenital and acquired diseases**. Other blood elements are normal. Well-defined congenital neutropenic disorders (e.g., Kostmann's syndrome) are very rare.

(6) **Cyclic neutropenia** is an interesting but uncommon disorder with recurring neutropenic nadirs at 3-week intervals. An animal model (the gray collie dog) has shown an intrinsic **defect in regulation of hematopoietic stem cells**.

(7) **Hypersplenism may lead to some degree of neutropenia,** but clinical consequences are rarely severe enough to warrant splenectomy.

b. **Clinical features**
(1) **Moderate neutropenia** (ANC of 500–1,000/μl) is associated with increased likelihood of infection.
(2) **Severe neutropenia** (ANC $< 500/\mu l$) is associated with a markedly increased risk of infection.
(3) **Agranulocytosis** (ANC that approaches 0) is associated with high mortality if prolonged.

c. **Diagnosis.** Good tests of neutrophil kinetics are not available; thus, the ANC with bone marrow evaluation is the best way to discriminate between increased destruction and decreased production of neutrophils as the cause of neutropenia.

d. **Therapy** for neutropenia is directed at underlying etiologies. The efficacy of granulocyte transfusion is controversial (except in infants); the treatment carries the risk of alloimmunization or disease [e.g., cytomegalovirus (CMV)] transmission].

2. **Neutrophilia** is an increase in peripheral blood neutrophils or precursors.

a. **Etiology** of neutrophilia is quite varied. Common causes include:
(1) Environmental factors (e.g., cold, heat)
(2) Emotional factors (e.g., anger, stress)
(3) Surgery
(4) Inflammatory conditions (e.g., rheumatoid arthritis, vasculitis, drug sensitivity, necrosis)
(5) Infections (acute, chronic)
(6) Chemicals and drugs (e.g., epinephrine, glucocorticoids, G-CSF, GM-CSF, endotoxin)
(7) Tumors
(8) Other factors (e.g., smoking, heredity, rebound after hemorrhage)

b. **Pathology.** A need for neutrophils leads to increases in the peripheral blood because of decreased margination and egress, early release from the bone marrow reserve, and, in time, increased production of new neutrophils from myeloid precursors in the bone marrow.

c. **Clinical manifestations.** Neutrophilia is generally accompanied by an **increase in total white cell count** and may be accompanied by **other reactive changes,** such as occasional atypical lymphocytes or plasma cells.
(1) **Leukopoiesis.** Neutrophilia may be accompanied by increased numbers of band neutrophils and sometimes a few metamyelocytes or earlier precursors. The presence of

less differentiated neutrophilic precursors, called a **left shift,** presumably represents an attempt by the bone marrow to provide increased numbers of granulocytes; myelocyte to blood transit time, normally 5–7 days, can be as short as 48 hours when there is demand.

(a) **Leukemoid reaction** (i.e., pronounced neutrophilia accompanied by immature myeloid precursors) is a condition that sometimes must be distinguished from myeloproliferative disorders or chronic myelogenous leukemia (CML). Leukocyte alkaline phosphatase (LAP) levels are elevated or normal in neutrophilia but low in CML; normal to elevated LAP levels with splenomegaly and a left-shifted peripheral smear suggest a myeloproliferative disorder.

(b) **Increased band neutrophils** are thought to be a useful indicator of inflammation. However, studies show that this finding generally is not specific and is by no means an invariable accompaniment of inflammation. The overall increase in white blood cell count is a more reliable clinical parameter, although clinicians occasionally may wish to evaluate carefully band levels in immunosuppressed or older patients who may be unable to mount an increased white count and in newborns.

(2) **Morphologic changes in neutrophils** that characteristically accompany neutrophilia include **Döhle bodies** (light blue cytoplasmic inclusions representing aggregates of polyribosomes), **toxic granules** (persistent strong staining of primary granules), and **cytoplasmic vacuoles.**

3. **Functional/morphologic disorders of neutrophils**

a. **Major disorders.** Disorders of neutrophil morphology and function are numerous. Important examples are listed in Table 11-5, and more common ones are described below.

(1) **Chédiak-Higashi syndrome** is an autosomal recessive disorder featuring the abnormal fusion of cytoplasmic granules to yield **giant granules** in leukocytes and cells of other organs (e.g., skin, eyes). Neutrophils are less chemotactic and adherent. The ingestion of foreign particles is normal but intracellular killing is not because of abnormal granule fusion. There is usually associated neutropenia.

(2) **Chronic granulomatous disease** (CGD) exhibits mutations that knock out the respiratory burst necessary for the generation of O_2^- and H_2O_2, in which **cytochrome b**

Table 11-5. Major Functional/Morphologic Disorders of Neutrophils

Disorder	Characteristic Abnormality	Clinical Features
Chédiak-Higashi syndrome	Large cytoplasmic granules in neutrophils, lymphocytes, and monocytes	Recurrent infections
Chronic granulomatous disease (CGD)	Impaired generation of oxygen metabolites; ingestion but no killing of catalase-positive organisms (e.g., *Staphylococcus aureus*)	Recurrent infections with catalase-positive organisms
Neutrophil adhesion defects	Decreased integrins; decreased neutrophil adherence and respiratory burst	Recurrent infections
Myeloperoxidase deficiency	Diminished lysosomal effectiveness of hydrogen peroxide	None
Other enzyme deficiencies	Lack of glutathione reductase, oxidase, or catalase	None
May-Hegglin anomaly	Döhle bodies in granulocytes and monocytes; giant platelets; autosomal dominant inheritance	Thrombocytopenia in some patients
Alder-Reilly anomaly	Prominent red–purple granules	None
Pelger-Huët anomaly	Bilobed or monolobed granulocytes; may be inherited or acquired	None; cytopenia if myelodysplastic

or **NADPH oxidase** plays a crucial role. The failure to accumulate H_2O_2 in lysosomes permits phagocytosed catalase-positive microbes to replicate intracellularly.

(a) **Mutations inactivating cytochrome b cause most X-linked forms,** which account for two-thirds of cases.

(b) **Mutations affecting NADPH oxidase activity** cause the remaining one-third of cases, which are **autosomal recessive.**

(3) **Congenital leukocyte adherence disorders** stem from deficiencies in the **integrin (CD11/CD18)** family of adhesive proteins, which compromise neutrophil adherence for purposes of chemotaxis, phagocytosis (e.g., at C3 receptor sites), and antibody-mediated cellular cytotoxicity.

(4) **Immunodeficiency syndromes,** although not an intrinsic defect of the neutrophil, compromise neutrophil function through **inability to opsonize foreign organisms with antibody or complement** (e.g., C3, C3b inactivator, other early complement components).

b. **Diagnosis.** Laboratory tests of neutrophil function are not widely available. Many are difficult to control or interpret and are suitable primarily for research. The more useful tests include the following:

(1) Nitroblue tetrazolium (NBT) dye reduction or direct measurement of O_2^- generation for respiratory burst assessment

(2) Quantitative ingestion of labeled particles to examine phagocytic capacity

c. **Therapy** for functional or morphologic disorders of granulocytes is symptomatic, although several of these conditions are without clinical effect (e.g., May-Hegglin anomaly). Since many of these disorders are inherited, bone marrow transplantation and gene therapy are areas of active investigation.

C. Disorders of eosinophils

1. **Eosinopenia** is defined as a persistently low peripheral blood eosinophil count. It is unclear whether this is due to the release of fewer cells or to increased vascular margination.

a. **Etiology.** Eosinopenia occurs in association with acute infections and with administration of adrenocorticotropic hormone (ACTH), prostaglandins, epinephrine, or glucocorticoids.

b. **Diagnosis.** Eosinophil levels derived from differential percentages multiplied by the white cell count are not accurate enough to quantitate low levels of eosinophils; an eosinophil-specific absolute count must be performed.

2. **Eosinophilia** is defined as a peripheral eosinophil count above 500/μl. It may be associated with parasitic infestation, any of several allergic states (e.g., asthma, drug reactions, inflammatory skin disorders), and neoplasms (e.g., CML).

3. **Hypereosinophilic syndrome** is defined as an unexplained sustained peripheral blood eosinophilia of more than 1500/μl.

a. **Clinical features.** Hypereosinophilic syndrome includes a complex group of entities that may be associated with **tissue damage,** presumably because of the inappropriate secretion of eosinophil granule components. Bipyramidal **Charcot-Leyden crystals** (i.e., aggregates of intracellular and perhaps membrane components) may be found with large numbers of tissue eosinophils.

b. **Therapy** generally is with antihistamines or glucocorticoids; chemotherapy may be required. Leukapheresis may be helpful for some patients.

D. Disorders of basophils and mast cells

1. **Basopenia** is not readily diagnosed nor actively investigated, because basophil levels in peripheral blood normally are low ($<$ 100/μl). Basopenia has been described in association with generalized leukocytosis owing to inflammation, thyrotoxicosis, and steroid treatment and is sometimes associated with eosinopenia.

2. **Peripheral basophilia** (basophil levels $>$ 100/μl) may be seen in reactive immunologic conditions (e.g., IgE-mediated hypersensitivity) or in chronic inflammatory disorders (e.g., rheumatoid arthritis, ulcerative colitis). Basophilia also has been noted in viral infections, following radiation, and in association with various neoplastic disorders. Basophilia is a common accompaniment to the **myeloproliferative disorders,** particularly CML.

3. **Reactive increases in mast cells** may be seen locally in tissues in association with hypersensitivity reactions, in lymph nodes draining foci of inflammation or tumors, and in lymph nodes or bone marrow affected by low-grade lymphoproliferative disorders.

4. **Mastocytosis** comprises a spectrum of disorders characterized by discrete accumulations of mast cells. Among the disorders are cutaneous mastocytosis (urticaria pigmentosa) and systemic mastocytosis.
   a. **Urticaria pigmentosa** features multiple brown papules composed of mast cells that may degranulate and cause intense itching. Older children usually are affected, with signs and symptoms abating around puberty.
   b. **Systemic mastocytosis**
      (1) **Clinical features** of systemic mastocytosis may include organomegaly and extracutaneous symptoms such as nausea, palpitations, diarrhea, and cramps in addition to itching and flushing caused by histamine release. **Dermatographism,** in which a wheal traces a pattern of cutaneous stroking, may be prominent. Most patients are adults; in some, disease is an extension of earlier urticaria pigmentosa. The course of systemic mastocytosis is highly variable but may be very aggressive.
      (2) **Diagnosis** usually is based on finding granulomas composed of mast cells, lymphocytes, and eosinophils on bone marrow biopsy, often associated with local fibrosis.

5. **Therapy for disorders of basophils and mast cells** includes local excision of symptomatic lesions or administration of antihistamines, steroids, and prostaglandin inhibitors for mild disease. Cytotoxic chemotherapy occasionally is required.

E. **Disorders of monocytes.** Normally, monocytes comprise 1%–6% of the cells in the peripheral blood; rarely does this percentage exceed 10%. In tissue, macrophages (often referred to as histiocytes) occur normally as single cells or pairs.

1. **Monocytopenia,** defined as a persistently decreased monocyte count, is unusual and most frequently occurs as part of a general decrease in white count seen in autoimmune disorders (e.g., SLE) and hairy cell leukemia and after glucocorticoid administration or chemotherapy.

2. **Monocytosis,** defined as a persistent peripheral monocyte count of more than 1000/μl, is a feature of various disorders.
   a. **Hematologic disorders.** Most commonly, monocytosis is associated with myelodysplastic syndromes, acute and chronic leukemias, and some lymphomas or myelomas. Occasionally, monocytosis occurs following splenectomy.
   b. **Generalized inflammation** may be caused by infectious diseases as well as by some autoimmune disorders. In the past, **mycobacterial infection (tuberculosis)** was the classic condition associated with monocytosis.
   c. **Neoplasms** may also be associated with significant monocytosis.

3. **Lipid storage diseases** are characterized by abnormal accumulation of lipids in monocytes and macrophages due, generally, to inherited deficiencies of lysosomal hydrolases. Several examples are described below and listed in Table 11-6.
   a. **Gaucher's disease** is a prototype lipid storage disease caused by a variety of molecular abnormalities that inactivate β-glucosidase (glucocerebrosidase), a lysosomal enzyme required for the degradation of **glucocerebroside**. The disorder is autosomal recessive, with an increased incidence in Ashkenazi Jews.
      (1) **Etiology.** Defects responsible for Gaucher's disease occur both as point mutations and as gross alterations of gene structure associated with crossovers between the functional gene and an adjacent pseudogene.
      (2) **Pathologic features.** Gaucher's disease is characterized by engorged tissue histiocytes that have a **"crumpled cigarette paper" appearance** due to extensive membrane-bound lipid inclusions. Similar histiocytes (known as pseudo-Gaucher cells) may be seen in the bone marrow and tissue in conditions with high cell turnover (e.g., CML).
      (3) **Clinical features.** Three clinical types of Gaucher's disease are recognized. Heterozygotes are normal, but carriers generally can be detected by β-glucosidase assays.
         (a) **Type I** (adult type), the most common form, features **massive splenomegaly,** often with clinical hypersplenism, hepatomegaly, skeletal lesions, and cytopenias secondary to bone marrow involvement. Serum acid phosphatase levels are increased, and white cells are deficient in β-glucosidase.
         (b) **Type II** (neuronopathic or infantile type) is a less common type that occurs early and leads to rapid neurologic compromise.
         (c) **Type III** is less well-studied, with subacute neurologic progression.
      (4) **Therapy** involves supportive transfusion and splenectomy. Replacement therapy with

recombinant glucocerebrosidase is now available. Bone marrow transplantation has been performed, and gene therapy may be a therapeutic option in the future.

b. **Other lipid storage diseases** are listed in Table 11-6, whose cumulative incidence is not insubstantial (> 1000 new cases per year in the United States). Enzyme replacement and bone marrow transplantation are increasingly being used for these diseases. Early diagnosis and transplantation are important in many patients for the best prognosis.

4. **Langerhans' cell histiocytosis.** Langerhans' cells are dendritic cells derived from bone marrow monocyte precursors. These cells can proliferate and invade various organs and tissues, producing a collection of disorders previously known as **histiocytosis X**. Individual syndromes include classically described **eosinophilic granuloma of bone** as well as **Letterer-Siwe disease, Hand-Schüller-Christian disease,** and other localized histiocytic proliferations.

a. **Pathologic features.** Langerhans' cells exhibit **grooved nuclei** and contain distinct racquet-shaped cytoplasmic bodies known as **Birbeck's granules,** which can be identified ultrastructurally. Langerhans' cells, which demonstrate positivity for the membrane marker CD1 and neural marker S-100, are believed to function in the immunologic presentation of antigen.

b. **Clinical features**

(1) Langerhans' cell infiltration may be localized, with one or more lesions in bone, or multifocal, with involvement of the skin, mucous membranes, lymph nodes, liver, spleen, lungs, and even the central nervous system (CNS).

Table 11-6. Hereditary Storage Disorders Involving Tissue Histiocytes

Disorder	Substance Accumulated	Defect	Clinical Features
Gaucher's disease	Glucocerebroside	Glucocerebrosidase	Variable; treatment available
Niemann-Pick disease	Sphingomyelin	Sphingomyelinase	Severe, foamy CNS histiocytes
Tay-Sachs disease; Sandhoff disease	GM_2 ganglioside	Hexosaminidase A (Tay-Sachs); hexosaminidase A and B (Sandhoff)	Severe CNS disease; blindness; cherry-red spots in retina; carrier screening is beneficial
GM_1 gangliosidosis	GM_1 ganglioside	β-Galactosidase	Variable onset; neurologic disease
Fabry's disease	Ceramide trihexose	α-Galactosidase A	X-linked; adult-onset renal failure; symptoms in female carriers
Metachromatic leukodystrophy	Sulfatides	Arylsulfatase A	Variable; CNS accumulation; early death; adult-onset psychosis
Mucopolysaccharidoses (MPS)*			
Hurler syndrome (MPS I)	Glycosaminoglycan	Iduronate sulfatase	Autosomal recessive; variable severity; rhinitis; hernias; dysmorphic features over time
Hunter syndrome (MPS II)	Glycosaminoglycan	Iduronate sulfatase	X-linked
Tangier disease	Cholesterol esters	HDL (α-lipoprotein)	Mild disease with risk of vascular disease in adults; organomegaly; enlarged tonsils
Wolman disease	Cholesterol esters; triglycerides	Acid lipase (esterase)	Severe, early onset; cholesterol ester deposition in bone marrow and spleen

*MPSs are a diverse group of disorders characterized by deficiency of lysosomal enzymes responsible for intracellular catabolism of mucopolysaccharides. All but Hunter syndrome are autosomal recessive conditions. MPSs vary considerably in their clinical presentation. Hurler syndrome and Hunter syndrome are prototypic MPSs.
HDL = high-density lipoprotein.

(2) Langerhans' cell histiocytosis is a disease predominantly of children and young adults. Onset in infancy, severe cytopenia, and significant hepatic or pulmonary involvement are poor prognostic features.

c. **Therapy**

(1) Excision of local lesions often is sufficient; spontaneous remissions may occur even in more widespread disease.

(2) Radiotherapy may be applied to bony lesions, and judicious restraint of activity is indicated to minimize the chance of pathologic fractures.

(3) Corticosteroids and chemotherapeutic agents are administered in more serious cases.

5. **Hemophagocytic syndromes** usually are the result of viral infection, although they may also be seen with bacterial, fungal, and parasitic infections and, rarely, with neoplasms.

a. **Clinical features and laboratory findings**

(1) Patients exhibit systemic symptoms, with significant anemia, thrombocytopenia, and leukopenia.

(2) Examination of the bone marrow or enlarged lymph nodes, liver, or spleen reveals tissue macrophages full of phagocytosed blood cells.

b. **Therapy and prognosis.** Patients may be difficult to support by transfusion. Recovery usually occurs with resolution of the infection, but immunosuppressed patients are at particularly high risk for fatal infections.

6. **Other benign histiocytic disorders** include rare and invariably fatal familial disorders (e.g., familial erythrophagocytic lymphohistiocytosis) as well as reactive lymphadenopathies (see III F 4).

F. Disorders of lymphocytes and plasma cells

1. **Lymphocytopenia** generally is defined as an absolute circulating lymphocyte count below 1000/μl, reflecting a decrease in the number of circulating T cells.

a. **Etiology and pathogenesis.** One first considers a diagnosis of cancer, infection, or collagen vascular disease when a patient presents with lymphocytopenia. Mechanisms are poorly understood in many disorders but include:

(1) **Decreased production** of lymphocytes (e.g., due to congenital immunodeficiency, aplastic anemia, or chemotherapy)

(2) **Increased destruction** of lymphocytes (e.g., due to HIV infection or an autoimmune disorder such as SLE)

(3) **Maldistribution** of lymphocytes (e.g., due to abnormal thoracic duct drainage, reticuloendothelial trapping with infection, surgery)

b. **Clinical features.** Unless associated with immunodeficiency or, possibly, infection in older patients, lymphocytopenia generally is not a helpful prognostic indicator.

c. **Therapy** is directed at the underlying condition.

2. **Lymphocytosis** is defined as an absolute circulating lymphocyte count greater than 4000/μl. In addition to the non-neoplastic causes discussed here, several neoplastic disorders often are associated with lymphocytosis, such as chronic lymphocytic leukemia (CLL), circulating lymphoma, acute lymphocytic leukemia (ALL; see Ch 12 II, III). It is essential to differentiate among these causes of lymphocytosis.

a. **Mononucleosis syndromes** are the most common cause of benign lymphocytosis.

(1) **Etiology**

(a) The most notable causes are **Epstein-Barr virus (EBV) and CMV**. EBV causes heterophile antibody-positive illness; CMV causes heterophile antibody-negative mononucleosis. General features of EBV and CMV infections are compared in Table 11-7.

(b) Hepatitis virus, adenovirus, ***Toxoplasma gondii,*** and even HIV can produce heterophile antibody-negative mononucleosis.

(2) **Epidemiology**

(a) **Age-related incidence.** EBV and CMV infections generally are inapparent in younger children. Thus, mononucleosis is rare in third world countries, where primary infection occurs in early childhood. By contrast, 60%–90% of young adults in developed countries are susceptible and develop mononucleosis during their teens (EBV) or early adulthood (CMV).

(b) **Transmission** of EBV is through saliva; CMV is spread via sexual contact or breast milk.

Table 11-7. General Features of Epstein-Barr Virus (EBV) and Cytomegalovirus (CMV) Mononucleosis Syndromes

Feature	EBV	CMV
Transmission	Oral	Venereal
Typical age at presentation	Teens	Young adults
Pharyngitis	Common	Rare
Lymphadenopathy	Present	Absent
Heterophile antibody	Present	Absent
Atypical lymphocytes	T cells	T cells

(3) **Pathophysiology**

(a) **EBV** attaches to and infects tonsillar B cells via surface receptors for complement. Infection stimulates B cell proliferation and generates an intense immune response of T cells directed against infected B cells. This leads to pharyngitis and circulating atypical lymphocytes. Occasionally, infected B cells may produce antibodies that cause autoimmune cytopenias.

(b) **CMV** infection is less well understood. The virus does not appear to infect lymphocytes but has been associated with circulating neutrophils and monocytes as well as tissue histiocytes in the liver, spleen, and other organs. Reactive T cells lead to the mononucleosis syndrome.

(4) **Clinical features and complications**

(a) After an incubation period of 4–8 weeks, patients present with fatigue, weakness, and fever. The presence of pharyngitis with lymphadenopathy distinguishes EBV from CMV.

(b) Rupture of an enlarged spleen is an uncommon complication, presumably caused by weakening of the splenic capsule by infiltrating lymphocytes.

(5) **Laboratory findings**

(a) **Circulating atypical lymphocytes.** These cells have increased, often basophilic, cytoplasm, less mature nuclear chromatin, and a tendency to show molding around adjacent red cells on peripheral blood smears.

(b) **Heterophile antibodies** are reactive against sheep, horse, and beef red cells (but not guinea pig red cells) and yield a positive **Monospot test** with EBV but not CMV infection or other causes of mononucleosis. Specific serologic tests for antibodies against EBV and CMV are useful in problem cases.

(c) **Liver function abnormalities and immune-related findings.** The latter may include Coombs'-positive anemia, cold agglutinins, thrombocytopenia, cryoglobulins, rheumatoid factor, and generalized increases in seemingly unrelated antibodies.

(d) **Inadequate T cell response.** In some immunodeficient patients [e.g., those with **X-linked lymphoproliferative disorder (Duncan's disease)],** an inadequate T cell response permits excessive B cell proliferation, leading to severe disease and, in some instances, B cell lymphomas.

(6) **Differential diagnosis.** Toxoplasmosis presents with lymphadenopathy (generally of posterior auricular nodes) but not with pharyngitis and is serologically and pathologically distinct.

(7) **Therapy.** Mononucleosis syndromes are self-limited, and specific treatment usually is unnecessary. Glucocorticoids or antiviral agents (e.g., acyclovir) may be administered in severe cases.

b. **Infections.** In infection-induced lymphocytosis, circulating lymphocytes are normal-appearing, mature, and small.

(1) ***Bordetella pertussis* infections** are associated with a significant lymphocytosis of helper T cells resulting from a bacteria-elaborated factor that inhibits lymphocyte egress from the blood.

(2) **Acute infectious lymphocytosis** is a contagious disorder of unknown etiology and pathophysiology generally seen in children and young adults. Lymphocyte counts up to 100,000/μl have been reported but usually are lower and subside in 2–7 weeks. Symptoms, if present, are usually mild.

c. **Other causes.** Lymphocytosis occasionally is reported in association with cancers, hypersensitivity reactions, thyrotoxicosis, and rheumatoid arthritis. It also may occur in association with trauma or stress, perhaps as a response to released catecholamines.

3. **Immunodeficiency disorders** can result from defects at many of the functional stages required for an intact immune response. The disorders may be hereditary or acquired but are best understood when classified as abnormalities of B cells, T cells, phagocytes, or complement. The following discussion highlights some of the major immunodeficiency disorders resulting from lymphocyte defects.
   a. **General considerations.** Depending on the cells or organs affected, a variety of immunodeficiency disorders may result from defects of B or T cell function. Deficits of T cell function may also affect B cell function, leading to combined B cell and T cell disorders. Clinical features are quite variable but often include recurrent and persistent infections and an increased incidence of malignancy, particularly B cell lymphomas.
      (1) **Patients lacking B cell function** are susceptible to bacterial infections, especially with encapsulated organisms, and have decreased or absent B cells and decreased development of B cell–dependent lymphoid organs.
      (2) **Patients lacking T cell function** are susceptible to infections by viruses, fungi, and opportunistic organisms (e.g., *Pneumocystis carinii*).
   b. **Severe combined immunodeficiency disorder (SCID)** is a heterogeneous group of disorders characterized by defects at several levels of immune development. Patients suffer recurrent bacterial, viral, fungal, and parasitic infections.
      (1) **Swiss agammaglobulinemia** is presumed to result from a lack of precursors for both B and T cells, which can be restored through allogeneic bone marrow transplants. Immunodeficiency removes the need for pretransplant cytoreduction, but donor marrow should be depleted of mature T cells to minimize graft-versus-host disease (GVHD) in the recipient.
      (2) **Adenosine deaminase (ADA) deficiency** is due to absence of mature T cells; presumably, a toxic effect of adenosine metabolites prevents T cell maturation in the thymus, where ADA levels are low. The disorder is autosomal recessive.
         (a) **Diagnosis.** The ADA gene has been cloned and localized to chromosome 20, permitting prenatal diagnosis. Several of the mutations are now known.
         (b) **Therapy.** Bone marrow transplantation is the preferred treatment. Stabilized ADA coupled to polyethylene glycol is a less desirable alternative. Restoration of normal function using molecular methods to insert a normal gene (or cDNA) into patient cells is currently being investigated.
      (3) **Other defects.** SCID patients with other defects—including expression of cytokines or their receptors, T cell antigen receptors, or HLA class II molecules—have been described and should be amenable to bone marrow transplants for reconstitution of the immune deficit.
   c. **IgA deficiency** is the most common of primary immunodeficiencies.
      (1) Often asymptomatic, IgA deficiency may be associated with respiratory infections and autoimmune or allergic disorders. Serum antibodies to IgA in many patients present the risk of severe anaphylactic reactions to transfused blood products (see Ch 17 III A 5 b).
      (2) IgA deficiency is noted in many patients with ataxia-telangiectasia, a complex disorder featuring cerebellar ataxia, telangiectasias, frequent infections, and an increased incidence of lymphomas. Many patients demonstrate decreased $CD4^+$ cell levels and variable cellular and humoral immunodeficiency.
   d. **X-linked immunodeficiencies**
      (1) **Wiskott-Aldrich syndrome** is associated with eczema, thrombocytopenia with small platelets, and decreased numbers of T cells, all due to deficits of surface membrane protein CD43. Antibody responses also are depressed, and patients have a high incidence of B cell lymphomas.
      (2) **X-linked agammaglobulinemia** (Bruton's disease) is characterized by normal T cell function but an absence of mature B cells. Causes are unknown but may reflect problems in effective immunoglobulin gene rearrangement.
      (3) **X-linked lymphoproliferative disorder** [see III F 2 a (5) (d)]. No treatment is available for this disorder.
   e. **Common variable immunodeficiency** is a mixed group of hypo- or agammaglobulinemic disorders that are not X-linked. Many cases may be due to a defect in terminal B cell maturation, although others appear to be due to primary T cell defects that result in compromised B cell function. Treatment is with immunoglobulin replacement.
   f. **DiGeorge syndrome** patients have low numbers of T cells because of variable hypoplasia of the thymus associated with maldevelopment of embryonic pharyngeal pouches. Fetal thymocyte transplants restore function in some patients.

g. Acquired immune deficiency syndrome (AIDS)

(1) Etiology. There are two distinct but related forms of HIV that cause AIDS: HIV-1 in North America, South America, Europe, and Central Africa and HIV-2 in West Africa.

(2) Epidemiology. Infected individuals come from several risk populations.

(a) High-risk groups include:

(i) Homosexual males

(ii) Intravenous drug abusers

(iii) People exposed to blood and blood products, particularly with multiple exposures, such as hemophiliacs (for more information about HIV risk and the blood supply, see Ch 17 III B 3)

(iv) Infants of HIV-infected mothers

(b) Heterosexual transmission of HIV from an infected partner may occur, although the risk is lower than that for the other groups. For this reason, the use of condoms is considered an essential safe-sex practice for sexually active individuals.

(3) Pathogenesis

(a) HIV relies on viral-encoded **reverse transcriptase** to transcribe viral RNA into DNA, from which new virions are made. Key genes unique to HIV, which are important for the expression of viral proteins are **transactivator (*tat*), regulatory (*rev*), and *nef* genes**. The function of several other genes (***vif, var, vpu,*** and ***vpx***) is under study.

(b) Infection occurs by binding of HIV through a surface glycoprotein (gp)120 to cells that express the CD4 molecule. This makes $CD4^+$ cells and monocytes the prime targets of HIV. In this process, cellular syncytia may form. After uptake, uncoating, and integration of reverse-transcribed viral DNA into host DNA, new viral proteins and virions are made.

(4) Clinical features

(a) Disease course. The Centers for Disease Control classifies HIV-induced disease as shown in Table 11-8 and described below.

(i) **Group I disease (acute infection)** presents as a mononucleosis syndrome and lasts several weeks.

(ii) **Group II disease (asymptomatic infection)** follows the acute infection and may last for many years.

(iii) **Group III disease [AIDS-related complex (ARC)]** is diagnosed when a patient develops weight loss, fever, persistent lymphadenopathy, diarrhea, or skin disorders.

(iv) **Group IV disease (AIDS)** is diagnosed when a patient develops opportunistic infections, malignancies (e.g., Kaposi's sarcoma, lymphoma), or neurologic symptoms.

(b) Opportunistic infections must be detected early to provide effective treatment. Common organisms include:

(i) **Bacteria,** such as *Mycobacterium tuberculosis* and *M. avium-intracellulare, Salmonella* species, *Shigella* species, and *Streptococcus pneumoniae*

(ii) **Fungi,** such as *P. carinii, Cryptococcus neoformans,* and *Candida albicans*

(iii) **Viruses,** such as CMV, EBV, herpes simplex virus (HSV) , and herpes zoster virus

(iv) **Protozoa,** such as *T. gondii* and *Cryptosporidium muris*

Table 11-8. Centers for Disease Control Classification of Human Immunodeficiency Virus (HIV)–Induced Disease

Classification	Disease Description
Group I	Acute infection
Group II	Asymptomatic infection
Group III	Persistent generalized lymphadenopathy
Group IV	Other disease
Subgroup A	Constitutional symptoms
Subgroup B	Neurologic disease
Subgroup C	Opportunistic infection
Subgroup D	Secondary malignancies
Subgroup E	Other conditions

(c) **Malignancies**

(i) **Kaposi's sarcoma,** a mesenchymal neoplasm of uncertain histogenesis, usually presents in homosexual males as skin plaques but may involve lymph nodes and visceral organs.

(ii) **Aggressive histology non-Hodgkin's lymphomas,** usually of B cell origin, also are a feature of AIDS (see Ch 12 III C).

(d) **CNS involvement**

(i) **Infection.** In addition to opportunistic infections of the CNS, there is evidence that HIV virus can involve the brain. AIDS patients may present with a spectrum of neurologic symptoms related to infection, **including a dementia complex unique to the disease.**

(ii) **Primary CNS lymphomas** are a complication encountered in AIDS patients.

(5) **Pathologic features**

(a) **Lymph nodes** from group III patients demonstrate a florid follicular hyperplasia, often with plasmacytosis. Lymphomas are of unfavorable large cell, immunoblastic, or undifferentiated (small noncleaved cell) histologies.

(b) **Bone marrow** generally is normocellular, with mild lymphoplasmacytosis. Granulomas associated with fungal or mycobacterial infections may be quite subtle. Some patients have a myelodysplastic picture with dyspoiesis. Viral-associated hemophagocytosis (see III E 5) can be devastating in AIDS patients.

(6) **Diagnosis** is based on the characteristic clinical features noted above and the following laboratory findings.

(a) **Immunosuppression.** The predominant effect of HIV infection is marked immunosuppression, which, in most patients, occurs after 5–10 years. This is caused by gradual but specific **loss of $CD4^+$ cells,** which are important for many immunologic functions.

(i) $CD4^+$ cell loss probably occurs through direct viral toxicity, cell-mediated immunity due to viral gp120 bound to surface CD4, and syncytia formation.

(ii) This loss results in the characteristic **flipped $CD4^+$:$CD8^+$ ratio,** which normally ranges from 2:1 to 4:1 in normal individuals.

(iii) Careful monitoring of $CD4^+$ cells is indicated when levels fall below 500/μl; the risk of an AIDS-associated illness (e.g., opportunistic infection, Kaposi's sarcoma, lymphoma) is most likely when $CD4^+$ cells fall below 200/μl.

(iv) Paradoxically, serum immunoglobulin levels are often increased in HIV-infected patients.

(b) **Serum antibodies.** Detection of serum antibodies to HIV-specific gp24, gp41, or gp120/160 is the usual test for HIV infection. For problem cases, viral culture or detection of viral DNA via polymerase chain reaction (PCR) techniques may be employed.

(c) **Peripheral cytopenia** beyond lymphocytopenia is a common feature of AIDS, including **thrombocytopenia,** which is hypothesized to be immune-mediated, along with **anemia and generalized leukopenia**. Direct infection of bone marrow precursors may also contribute to cytopenias. Concurrent infection by parvovirus B19 has been reported to cause an acute red cell aplasia.

(d) **Therapy.** No truly effective treatment is currently available for AIDS patients. Supportive measures for anemia and thrombocytopenia, if necessary, are helpful. Zidovudine (also known as AZT) provides some, occasionally short-term, benefits in the level of $CD4^+$ cells. The antiviral agent, acyclovir, has recently demonstrated promise for increased patient survival. Clinical trials treating cytopenias with recombinant cytokines (e.g., erythropoietin, G-CSF, GM-CSF) are now under way.

4. **Reactive lymphadenopathies**

a. **Etiology.** Lymph nodes react and enlarge in response to a variety of stimuli, including inflammation, infection, and cancer.

b. **Pathology**

(1) **Follicular hyperplasia** with germinal center formation reflects B cell reactivity, a common response to bacterial infections and other inflammatory stimuli.

(2) **Diffuse paracortical hyperplasia** reflects T cell reactivity, which is more a feature of reaction to viruses and cell-mediated immune responses.

(3) **Mixed patterns with follicular and diffuse components** are very common.

(4) **Sinus histiocytosis** is a generalized increase of tissue histiocytes and monocytes in lymph node sinuses seen in many benign or neoplastic disorders. Sinus histiocytosis with massive lymphadenopathy (i.e., Rosai-Dorfman disease) is a self-limited lymphadenopathy with profound lympho-erythrophagocytosis by histiocytes in children.

(5) **Granulomatous patterns** feature aggregates of histiocytes, lymphocytes, and occasional giant cells with or without necrosis. These aggregates form in response to foreign material or as a consequence of cell-mediated immunity in conditions such as toxoplasmosis, sarcoidosis, tuberculosis, and fungal infections.

(6) **Dermatopathic patterns,** seen in lymph nodes draining areas of cutaneous inflammation, exhibit prominent paracortical hyperplasia composed of reactive histiocytes and T cells.

c. **Diagnosis.** Patients with enlarged lymph nodes must be evaluated carefully. An active immune system and susceptibility to infection makes lymphadenopathy very common in children.

(1) **Localized self-limited lymphadenopathy** is likely to be benign, although the size of lymph nodes in low-grade lymphoproliferative processes can wax and wane. **Persistent lymphadenopathy** should be biopsied, taking care to sample the largest lymph node available, and evaluated by an experienced hematopathologist.

(2) **Superficial lymph nodes** of the cervical, supraclavicular, axillary, and inguinal regions are easily evaluated by physical examination. The evaluation of **nonsuperficial lymph nodes** can be performed by sophisticated imaging techniques such as magnetic resonance imaging (MRI).

5. **Amyloidosis** (see Ch 12 IV E)

STUDY QUESTIONS

Directions: Each of the numbered items or incomplete statements in this section is followed by answers or by completions of the statement. Select the **one** lettered answer or completion that is **best** in each case.

1. Phagocytosis is a primary function of

(A) neutrophils
(B) monocytes
(C) both
(D) neither

2. Basophils and mast cells, both of which contain basophilic granules on Wright's-stained preparations, are similar in that they both

(A) contain histamine
(B) derive from the same bone marrow precursor
(C) have identical granule structure
(D) may circulate in the peripheral blood normally

3. Which of the following cytokines is essential for T cell proliferation in immune responses?

(A) IL-1
(B) IL-2
(C) IL-5
(D) GM-CSF
(E) G-CSF

Directions: Each item below contains four suggested answers of which **one or more** is correct. Choose the answer

A if **1, 2, and 3** are correct
B if **1 and 3** are correct
C if **2 and 4** are correct
D if **4** is correct
E if **1, 2, 3, and 4** are correct

4. Cells that bear the CD4 surface antigen participate in

(1) HIV infection
(2) certain B cell responses
(3) phagocytosis
(4) antigen presentation for immune responses

5. Abnormalities associated with chronic granulomatous disease (CGD) include

(1) impaired generation of oxygen metabolites
(2) impaired killing of catalase-positive organisms
(3) impaired cytochrome b function
(4) abnormally large cytoplasmic granules

1-C
2-A
3-B
4-E
5-A

Directions: The group of questions below consists of lettered choices followed by several numbered items. For each numbered item select the **one** lettered choice with which it is **most** closely associated. Each lettered choice may be used once, more than once, or not at all.

Questions 6–11

Match the stages of neutrophil maturation with the appropriately lettered cell in the figure below.

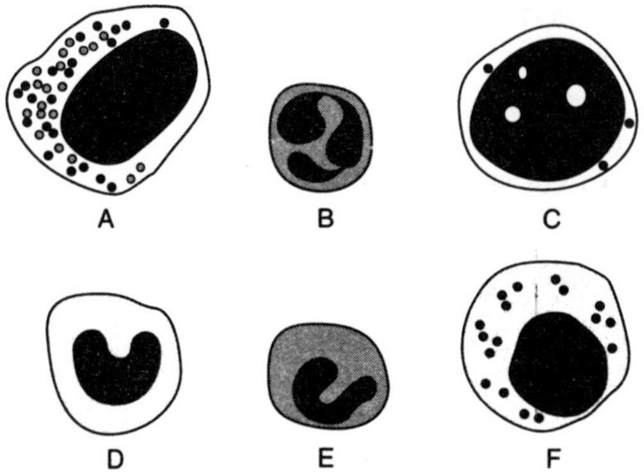

6. Myeloblast
7. Band neutrophil
8. Myelocyte
9. Mature neutrophil
10. Promyelocyte
11. Metamyelocyte

6-C 9-B
7-E 10-A
8-F 11-D

ANSWERS AND EXPLANATIONS

1. The answer is C *[I B 2 b (1), E 3 c].*
Phagocytosis is a primary physiologic function of both neutrophils and monocytes, although monocytes, particularly in tissues, may also play crucial roles in antigen presentation for immunologic responses. Actually, neutrophils are thought to be more efficient phagocytes except, perhaps, when the material to be phagocytosed is large or very abundant. One reason may be that, unlike monocytes, neutrophils contain abundant tissue glycogen stores and, therefore, are more efficient at phagocytosis in environments where oxidative metabolism is inhibited. Specialized tissue macrophages derived from circulating monocytes perform specific phagocytic functions (e.g., Kupffer's cells of the liver remove senescent erythrocytes).

2. The answer is A *[I D; Table 11-1].*
Basophils and mast cells both contain histamine in cytoplasmic granules. Although the granules of these two cell types stain similarly with polychrome stains, they are otherwise quite dissimilar. The basophil has few large granules, and the mast cell has numerous small ones. Mast cells are confined to tissue and are virtually never seen in the peripheral blood except in rare cases of severe systemic mast cell disease. Not surprisingly, these two cells, which may have some similarity in function, are not even felt to derive from a common bone marrow precursor cell.

3. The answer is B *[II E 1 b (2); Table 11-4].*
Interleukin 2 (IL-2), originally named T cell growth factor (TCGF), was first discovered as an activity in lectin-stimulated T cells, which was capable of promoting prolonged proliferation of normal T cells in vitro. IL-1 is a cofactor in many immune responses and often potentiates the action of other growth factors; it is not strictly required for T cell proliferation. IL-5 has effects primarily on the differentiation of both B and T cells as well as eosinophils. The actions of granulocyte/macrophage colony-stimulating factor (GM-CSF) and granulocyte colony-stimulating factor (G-CSF) are focused primarily on granulocyte/monocyte precursors and their progeny.

4. The answer is E (all) *[I E 1 c, 3 c; II E 2 a (1); III F 3 g (3) (b)].*
CD4 antigen is expressed on the surface of a subset of mature T cells as well as monocytes. $CD4^+$ T cells often are referred to as helper T cells, because many of these cells potentiate the effectiveness of certain B cell responses, particularly antibody production. CD4 is also the surface molecule to which human immunodeficiency virus (HIV) glycoprotein (gp)120 binds to allow the infection of cells; thus, both $CD4^+$ T cells and monocytes are targets of this virus. Two major functions of monocytes are phagocytosis and activation of lymphocytes for immune responses through the major histocompatibility complex (MHC)–restricted presentation of antigen.

5. The answer is A (1, 2, 3) *[III B 3 a (2)].*
Abnormally large cytoplasmic granules are not associated with chronic granulomatous disease; they are a feature of Chédiak-Higashi syndrome, an autosomal recessive disorder associated with recurrent infections and neutropenia. Most cases of CGD show X-linked recessive inheritance, affect males, and are due to impaired cytochrome b function, which is required for the generation of oxygen metabolites needed for the intracellular killing of microorganisms. Specifically, the inability to generate sufficient hydrogen peroxide (H_2O_2) enables catalase-positive organisms, which can degrade this compound, to replicate within neutrophil lysosomes.

6–11. The answers are: 6-C, 7-E, 8-F, 9-B, 10-A, 11-D *[I B 1 a; Figure 11-1].*
Neutrophil maturation progresses through several morphologic stages, beginning with the myeloblast. The myeloblast (*C*) is characterized by immature nuclear chromatin but no cytoplasmic differentiation; the promyelocyte (*A*) has cytoplasmic azurophilic granules; the myelocyte (*F*) demonstrates progressive chromatin condensation and emergence of secondary granules; the metamyelocyte (*D*) has additional secondary granules and nuclear indentation; the band neutrophil (*E*) demonstrates further nuclear constriction; and the mature neutrophil (*B*) exhibits nuclear segmentation.

Most peripheral blood or bone marrow cells are easily classified according to this scheme, but cells with morphologic features intermediate between different stages can always be found. Some hematologists prefer to place such cells in the more mature group. In disorders characterized by significant disturbance of myeloid maturation with asynchrony of cytoplasmic and nuclear development (e.g., myelodysplastic syndromes), classification according to normal differentiation schemes may be difficult for many cells.

12
Neoplastic Disorders of Granulocytes, Monocytes, and Lymphocytes

Jeffrey A. Kant

I. INTRODUCTION

A. Definitions

1. **Leukemia** is the neoplastic expansion of hematopoietic cells in the blood and bone marrow. The bone marrow is usually replaced by these cells; the blood generally displays an elevated white cell count but may exhibit few or even no neoplastic cells. The expansion usually occurs in the lymphoid or myeloid/monocytic lineages; it rarely affects erythroid or megakaryocytic lines. The neoplastic proliferation may be primarily of mature or immature cells.
2. **Lymphoma** is the neoplastic expansion of lymphoid cells presenting as a discrete tumor mass. Lymphoma generally, but not always, is associated with lymphoid organs such as the lymph nodes or spleen. Neoplastic lymphoid cells are generally mature.

B. Functional overlap between leukemia and lymphoma

1. **Lymphomas in blood.** Many functionally mature lymphoid cells whose role is tissue-based circulate normally via the blood among lymphoid organs. It is not surprising, therefore, that neoplastic cells may be found in the blood and bone marrow in association with lymphomas of mature lymphoid cells. Because these cancers are primarily tissue-based, patients are classified as having lymphomas, even though a leukemic peripheral blood component is present.
2. **Leukemia as tissue masses.** Similarly, circulation patterns may lead to substantial accumulations of lymphoid or myeloid cells in lymph nodes, the spleen, or other organs, even though the primary process is a leukemia. Accumulations of immature myeloid blasts are termed **granulocytic sarcomas**.

II. LEUKEMIAS

A. Introduction. Leukemias are different from other types of cancer. Since blood is the reservoir that the bone marrow supplies with leukocytes for the entire body, cells of primary hematopoietic neoplasms circulate throughout the body and, thus, are physiologically "metastatic" early in the course of the disease. Surgery has virtually no role in the treatment of leukemia; therapy must be directed at widespread disease.

1. **Classification.** The terms acute and chronic applied to leukemia are historical and refer to the course that untreated leukemias will follow. Paradoxically, with advances in therapy, "cure" can be attained in many cases of acute leukemia but rarely in chronic leukemias.
   a. **Predominant cell types** may be granulocytic/monocytic or lymphocytic in both acute and chronic leukemias.
      (1) Acute leukemias are expansions of immature cells, occasionally accompanied by cells showing some differentiation.
      (2) Chronic leukemias are expansions of more mature or differentiated cells.
   b. **Major clinical forms** observed are:
      (1) Acute myelogenous (or nonlymphocytic) leukemia (AML or ANLL)
      (2) Acute lymphocytic leukemia (ALL)
      (3) Chronic myelogenous leukemia (CML)
      (4) Chronic lymphocytic leukemia (CLL)

2. **Incidence and epidemiology.** Leukemia comprises 4%–5% of cancer among all age-groups but is the most common malignancy in children.
   a. The overall incidence is roughly 3–5/100,000 people per year in the United States, with much higher incidences associated with some predisposing causes.
   b. There is a male preponderance of roughly 1.4:1.0.
   c. All clinical forms are roughly equal in frequency overall, although the frequency is markedly variable among different age-groups.
      (1) AML is much more common in adults than in children.
      (2) ALL comprises 75%–80% of childhood acute leukemia. The incidence and type may also vary among social and ethnic groups (e.g., CLL is rare among Asians).
      (3) CLL is rarely seen in patients younger than 30 years.

3. **Etiology.** The causes of leukemia are not clearly understood, although immunosuppression or damage to bone marrow cells (and, thus, to the genetic material within cells) may be contributing factors. Other causative factors may include the following:
   a. **Radiation** in high doses (e.g., nuclear blasts, therapeutic radiation), which cause genetic damage and immunosuppression
   b. **Chemicals** (e.g., benzene, alkylating agents)
   c. **Viruses** (e.g., human T cell leukemia viruses, types I and II in adult T cell leukemia; various RNA retroviruses in animals)
   d. **Hereditary influences**
      (1) A strong genetic predisposition to leukemia is seen in certain families in association with Down syndrome (trisomy 21) and in patients with fragile chromosomes, which are present in conditions such as Bloom syndrome and Fanconi's anemia.
      (2) Certain congenital immunodeficiency disorders (ataxia telangiectasia and Wiskott-Aldrich syndrome) are also associated with an increased risk of leukemia and lymphoma, possibly due to the failure of normal host immune surveillance to eliminate transformed clones.
   e. **Nonrandom chromosome abnormalities**
      (1) The variety of consistent nonrandom chromosome abnormalities in different morphologic types of leukemia and lymphoma is a strong argument for the participation of particular genes in the cause of these neoplasms (Table 12-1).
      (2) In many cases, the translocation is in the vicinity of known oncogenes, although the role of oncogenes in the genesis of leukemia is not yet understood.

4. **Clinical course**
   a. **Infiltration of organs,** particularly the bone marrow, by leukemic cells inhibits the normal

Table 12-1. Some Consistent Chromosome Abnormalities Associated with Leukemias and Lymphomas

Chromosome Abnormality	Leukemia	Possible Oncogene
Leukemias		
t(9;22) (q34;q11)*	CML, ALL	*bcr*, c-*abl*
t(8;21) (q22;q22)	AML (M2 subtype)	?c-*mos*, ?c-*myc*
t(15;17) (q22;q12)	AML (M3 subtype)	**RAR α, PML**
t or del (11) (q23)	AML (M5, M4 subtypes)	*int*-2
inv or del(16) (p13,q22)	AML, M4 with eosinophilia	
t(4;11) (q21;q23)	ALL (children and MLL)	*int*-2
+12	CLL	
+8, −7, −7q, −5q	AML, CML (secondary change)	
Lymphomas		
t(14;18) (q32;q21)	NSCC	*bcl*-2
t(8 or 2 or 22;14) (q32)	Burkitt's lymphoma	c-*myc*
t(11;14) (q13;q32)	SLL, CLL, DLCL	*bcl*-1
t(7;14 or 11 or 9)	T cell lymphomas	*tcl*-1, *tcl*-2, *tcl*-3

t = translocation; inv = inversion; del = deletion; + = trisomy; − = monosomy; q = long arm; p = short arm; AML = acute myelogenous leukemia; ALL = acute lymphocytic leukemia; CML = chronic myelogenous leukemia; CLL = chronic lymphocytic leukemia; NSCC = nodular small cleaved lymphoma; SLL = small lymphocytic lymphoma; DLCL = diffuse large cell lymphoma; MLL = mixed lineage acute leukemia.

*Philadelphia chromosome.

production of erythrocytes, platelets, and granulocytes via direct suppression of hematopoiesis by poorly understood mechanisms.

b. Granulocytopenia predisposes to infection, and **thrombocytopenia** often leads to easy bruising or frank bleeding in the skin, gums, gastrointestinal tract, or genitourinary tract. Local infiltration can cause hepatosplenomegaly, lymphadenopathy, or bone pain. Central nervous system (CNS) symptoms may portend the ominous presence of leukemic cells in this area, which is difficult to treat.

c. Nonspecific symptoms of fatigue, weakness, and weight loss probably reflect the effects of **anemia,** increased catabolism by leukemic cells, and loss of appetite due to hepatosplenomegaly or other metabolic consequences of leukemia.

d. Aggressive cytotoxic chemotherapy used to treat some leukemias further compromises bone marrow function since it kills normal cells along with the leukemic cells. **Most patients who succumb to leukemia die of complications of bone marrow failure,** usually infection or hemorrhage, caused by the leukemia and its treatment.

e. Increased blood viscosity, stasis of cerebral blood flow, hemorrhage, brain damage, and death may result from high numbers of leukemic cells in the circulation ($> 200,000/\mu l$).

B. Acute leukemias

1. Classification. Acute leukemias are generally classified by their **origin from lymphoid or myeloid (including other nonlymphoid) progenitors**. The determination of lymphoid or myeloid is based on the results of morphologic, cytochemical, immunologic, and molecular studies (see II B 2) and has important implications for the therapy given and the overall prognosis, particularly in children. The FAB (French, American, and British) classification in use today (Table 12-2) attempts to standardize diagnostic criteria throughout the world.

a. Acute myelogenous leukemia (AML)

(1) Clinical subtypes

(a) Most AML is of the M1, M2, and M4 types. M2 and M4 are easily diagnosed from their characteristic morphology and cytochemistry. M1 must be distinguished from ALL.

Table 12-2. FAB Classification of Acute Leukemia

Acute myelogenous (or nonlymphocytic) leukemia (AML or ANLL)	
M0	Acute myelogenous leukemia without differentiation*
M1	Acute myelogenous leukemia without differentiation
M2	Acute myelogenous leukemia with differentiation
M3	Acute promyelocytic leukemia
M4	Acute myelomonocytic leukemia
M5	Acute monocytic leukemia
M6	Erythroleukemia
M7	Acute megakaryocytic leukemia
Acute lymphocytic leukemia (ALL)	
L1	Acute lymphocytic leukemia (relatively homogeneous morphologically)
L2	Acute lymphocytic leukemia (more heterogeneous morphologically)
L3	Acute lymphocytic leukemia (Burkitt-like)
Acute undifferentiated leukemia (AUL)	
This designation is applied to leukemias that cannot be identified as myeloid or lymphocytic in origin after cytochemical or immunologic (or both) marker studies.	

FAB = French, American, and British.
*M1 cases show myelogenous differentiation by cytochemical and immunologic analysis; M0 cases by immunologic analysis only.

(b) **M3 (acute promyelocytic leukemia)** is a proliferation almost entirely of **promyelocytes with numerous primary granules,** which frequently coalesce into eosinophilic needle-like aggregates (Auer rods). Because of procoagulant activity associated with substances in the heavily granulated leukemic cells, many patients present with **disseminated intravascular coagulation (DIC)** or are at risk for DIC because of cell destruction when therapy is initiated. A variant microgranular form of M3 has been viewed by electron microscopy.

(c) **M5 (acute monocytic leukemia)** actually comprises two subtypes: **M5a (monoblastic leukemia),** which is more common in children and has circulating cells that are blastic in appearance, and **M5b (monocytic leukemia),** in which circulating cells are mature or maturing monocytes. Prominent tissue infiltration (e.g., of the gums) may be a feature of acute leukemia with numerous monocytes (M4 and M5 types).

(d) **M6 (erythroleukemia)** derives its name from prominent and disordered proliferation of erythroid precursors associated with an increase in myeloblasts greater than 30% of bone marrow nonerythroid cells. With time, most patients develop a more classic form of AML (usually M1, M2, or M4). It is hypothesized that leukemic precursors retain a capability to differentiate into erythroid cells that is used less as the disease progresses.

(e) **M7 (megakaryocytic or megakaryoblastic leukemia)** is a rare form of AML associated with prominent bone marrow fibrosis, perhaps because of elaboration of growth-promoting factors for stromal cells. Early cases were termed acute myelofibrosis or malignant myelosclerosis. Megakaryoblasts are most easily distinguished by immunostaining with antiplatelet glycoprotein antibodies. They can be seen as a subpopulation in other types of AML or in the blast crisis of CML. Abnormal platelets may be seen; platelet counts are normal or increased.

(f) **Mixed lineage leukemias (MLL),** sometimes called **biphenotypic leukemias,** show expression of myeloid and lymphoid markers on the same blasts. This may indicate the potential for differentiation along myeloid and lymphoid lines or aberrant expression as documented in a number of neoplasms. Some studies suggest that MLL portends a poor prognosis.

(2) **Prognosis.** The FAB morphologic subtype does not correlate strongly with prognosis. Older age, high white cell count, and low platelet count at diagnosis are indicators of a poor prognosis. Chromosome abnormalities can negatively (monosomy 5 or 7, −5q, −7q, hyperdiploid) or positively [t(8;21), inv(16), trisomy 21] affect prognosis.

(3) **Preleukemic (myelodysplastic) syndromes**

(a) **Refractory cytopenia of red cells, white cells, or platelets** is present for a time in a number of patients who develop AML. Many patients die as a result of defective hematopoiesis; most are elderly. Peripheral blood and bone marrow studies demonstrate abnormalities of maturation known as **dyspoiesis**.

(b) An **increase in bone marrow blasts** to between 5% and 30% is seen in most patients who endure a preleukemic phase of cytopenia and subsequently develop AML. This increase is less than the 30% required for a diagnosis of AML. There are fewer than 5% blasts in the bone marrow of normal patients.

(c) Studies indicate that myelodysplastic syndromes are clonal proliferations that share many of the same **chromosome abnormalities** described in patients with AML.

(d) The cause of the myelodysplastic syndrome cannot be defined in many patients, which is also true in AML. Some studies suggest patients are likely to have a history of **toxic exposure**. Myelodysplasia—often with progression to AML—is a well-known complication of aggressive chemotherapy with alkylating agents for breast and ovarian cancer, multiple myeloma, and Hodgkin's and non-Hodgkin's lymphomas.

b. Acute lymphocytic leukemia (ALL)

(1) **Clinical subtypes**

(a) **L1 and L2.** Subtle morphologic criteria are employed to subclassify acute leukemias as L1 or L2; reproducibility may be problematic, and there may be disagreement even among experienced observers.

(i) L1 ALL is more common in young children, who tend to have a better prognosis than children with L2 (Table 12-3). Children with L2 ALL tend to be older, have higher peripheral white cell counts, and experience a more aggressive disease course.

Table 12-3. Prognostic Factors in Childhood Acute Lymphocytic Leukemia (ALL)

	Prognostic Factors	
Parameters	**Good**	**Poor**
White cell count*	Low (< 50,000)	High
Age*	Young (1–10 years)	Older (> 10 years), infants
CALLA (common ALL antigen, CD10)	Present	Absent
Lymphoid cell type	Early B cell	T cell
Cytogenetics	Normal	Abnormal
FAB classification	L1	L2

FAB = French, American, and British.
*Dominant factors.

(ii) The L2 subtype occurs more frequently than the L1 subtype in adults. It is unclear whether either subtype behaves different clinically.

(b) L3. The rare L3 type reflects the leukemic phase of an aggressive B cell lymphoma (Burkitt's or undifferentiated lymphoma) usually found in children and young adults.

(2) Pathology

(a) ALL occurs in both the T and B cell lineages. Among children, 15%–25% of cases involve T cells. The disease often presents in adolescence with a mediastinal mass and a propensity for CNS involvement.

(b) Immunologic subtypes of non–T cell ALL

(i) Common ALL ($CD10^+$ antigen*, B cell antigens, immunoglobulin gene rearrangement)

(ii) Null ALL (lacks CD10 antigen or B cell markers)

(iii) Pre-B ALL (similar to common ALL but expresses cytoplasmic immunoglobulin)

(iv) B ALL (rare, expresses monoclonal surface membrane immunoglobulin)

(3) Prognosis

(a) Childhood ALL. Patients with common ALL and pre-B ALL do best; those with null ALL [without common ALL antigen (CALLA)] and T cell ALL do less well; patients with rare B cell ALL do very poorly. There is evidence that pre-B ALL has a poorer prognosis than common ALL.

(b) Adult ALL. Patients with prolonged time to complete remission, older age, higher white cell counts, hepatosplenomegaly, a bleeding diathesis at diagnosis, and null or common immunologic subtypes have a poor prognosis.

2. Diagnosis of acute leukemia is made from peripheral blood and bone marrow studies; more than 30% of nucleated cells in the bone marrow must be immature blasts. Classification as lymphoid or myeloid is made on the basis of morphologic appearance supplemented by cytochemical, immunologic, and molecular studies (Table 12-4). Certain FAB subtypes such as M3 and M5 exhibit predominantly maturing cells with fewer than 30% blasts but behave clinically as acute leukemia.

3. Treatment. AML and ALL are treated with somewhat different chemotherapeutic agents. Since treatments usually potentiate already significant cytopenias, supportive therapy with blood components (red cells, platelets, and, less frequently, white cells) is often required.

a. Standard therapy

(1) AML. Using combination chemotherapy (e.g., daunorubicin, cytosine arabinoside, 6-thioguanine, or daunorubicin-idarubicin), it is possible to induce, but difficult to maintain, remission in 30%–90% of patients with AML. (The highest percentage of remissions is in children, the lowest is in older adults.) Continuous complete remissions of 5 years are seen in fewer than 25% of all patients, some of whom may be cured. Children with AML demonstrate 5-year continuous complete remission rates of up to 40%.

---

*Because antibodies from different sources often recognize identical antigens, **cluster designations (CD)** have been defined for most surface antigens (see Ch 11 II A 2; Table 11-2).

Table 12-4. Laboratory Tests Used to Distinguish Acute Myelogenous Leukemia (AML) and Acute Lymphocytic Leukemia (ALL)

Test	AML	ALL
Cytochemistry		
Sudan black, myeloperoxidase (granulocytes)	+ +	−
Periodic acid-Schiff (PAS)	−	+ (blocks)
Nonspecific esterases (monocytes)	+ + (M4 and M5)	−
Immunologic studies		
Terminal deoxynucleotidyl transferase (TdT)	− (small % +)	+ +
CALLA (common ALL antigen, CD10)	−	+ + (ALL)
B and T lymphocyte antigens	−	+ +
Myeloid/monocyte antigens	+ +	−
Cytoplasmic immunoglobulin	−	+ (pre-B)
Molecular tests		
Immunoglobulin gene rearrangements or T cell receptor gene rearrangements	− (some +)	+ +

(2) **ALL**

(a) Most childhood ALL is the common immature B cell type, which has a good prognosis and can be treated with mild therapies, including agents such as vincristine and prednisone. Treatment of ALL among children represents a major triumph; more than 90% of such patients attain remission, and continuous remission after therapy suggests that 50%–75% can be cured!

(b) Poor prognosis ALL in children is treated with more aggressive regimens with less favorable, but still excellent, results.

(c) The therapeutic outcome for adult ALL is poor, with results resembling those of AML.

b. **Bone marrow transplantation** is being used increasingly to treat poor-risk patients such as adults with ALL in first remission, children with ALL who have relapsed, and patients with all varieties of AML. Although survival figures associated with autologous transplantation approach those of allogeneic bone marrow transplantation, significant differences exist.

(1) **Allogeneic transplantation,** in which the donor is a human leukocyte antigen (HLA) –compatible relative, provides normal bone marrow and carries a high risk of disabling graft-versus-host disease (GVHD). For this reason, allogeneic transplantation is **restricted to patients younger than 40 years** of age. The use of antibodies to purge the bone marrow of cytotoxic T lymphocytes before infusion is under investigation.

(2) **Autologous transplantation,** in which the patient's own bone marrow, harvested after attaining clinical remission, is used for rescue after lethal ablation therapy, poses no risk of GVHD; however, the marrow may contain microscopic leukemia. Protocols to destroy residual leukemic cells with antibodies and chemotherapeutic agents in vitro are under study.

C. **Chronic leukemias.** In contrast to acute leukemias, chronic leukemias exhibit an accumulation of morphologically mature rather than immature cells in the lymphoid or myeloid lines (see II A 1 a). The basic defect in growth control presumably affects progenitor cells, but in these disorders most neoplastic cells differentiate. Since maturing cells generally have less capacity for division, lower growth fractions are presumed to be a reason for resistance to cure by chemotherapy aimed at dividing cells.

1. **Chronic myelogenous leukemia (CML)** is often considered a myeloproliferative disorder (see Ch 3 III C), although it has a distinct clinicopathologic picture.

a. **Clinical presentation.** CML is generally seen in young or middle-aged adults who present with high white cell counts (often > 100,000/μl) and marked splenomegaly, owing to leukemic infiltration and extramedullary hematopoiesis.

b. **Diagnosis**

(1) A spectrum of **granulocytes at all stages of maturation** are seen in the peripheral blood and bone marrow. **Basophilia** and **eosinophilia** are often present. Isoenzyme studies of glucose-6-phosphate dehydrogenase (G6PD) indicate that the defect in many cases

of CML occurs in an early stem cell capable of also giving rise to erythrocytes, megakaryocytes, and sometimes B lymphocytes.

(2) **Serum vitamin B_{12} levels** are often markedly **elevated,** and the granulocytes have an acquired **deficiency** of the enzyme **leukocyte alkaline phosphatase (LAP)**.

(3) The **Philadelphia (Ph) chromosome** is exhibited in more than 95% of patients. In the Ph chromosome, much of the long arm of chromosome 22 is translocated to other chromosomes, usually chromosome 9. It appears that there are rare true cases of CML in which the Ph chromosome is not present, and in these patients the disease may behave in a more indolent manner. However, most prior diagnoses of Ph-negative CML were other disorders, including myelodysplasia, other myeloproliferative disorders, and reactive conditions.

(4) CML must be differentiated from granulocytic hyperplasias and leukemoid reactions. White cell counts are generally lower in these conditions, with fewer immature cells in reactive conditions, and LAP levels are normal or elevated.

c. **Clinical course and treatment**

(1) **Stable phase.** The characteristic proliferation of maturing granulocytes is usually not eradicated but can be controlled by therapy for a number of years. Bone marrow transplantation is increasingly used in the treatment of CML. Preliminary data suggest that transplantation is best performed early in the stable phase. In autologous transplantation, it is hoped that the stable phase can be prolonged or restored.

(2) **Blast crisis and accelerated phases.** Most patients progress in 3–5 years to an accelerated phase heralded by increased numbers of immature blasts and frank blast crisis, which is indistinguishable from acute leukemia but is difficult to treat effectively. Despite the myeloid nature of cells in the stable phase, a lymphoid blast crisis is seen in some patients and treated with therapies directed at ALL.

2. **Chronic lymphocytic leukemia (CLL)**

a. **Clinical presentation.** CLL usually presents in an indolent fashion in older patients; it is virtually never seen in children.

b. **Diagnosis**

(1) The diagnosis is often made incidentally from a **persistent lymphocytosis**.

(2) CLL cells are generally clonal populations of **mature B lymphocytes,** exhibiting monoclonal surface immunoglobulin. An unusual feature is expression of the **CD5 membrane antigen** seen on mature T lymphocytes.

c. **Clinical course**

(1) Cells accumulate slowly in the bone marrow, spleen, liver, and lymph nodes. Roughly half of CLL patients exhibit decreased immunoglobulin production and show an increased susceptibility to infection. Immune-mediated anemias or thrombocytopenias are also seen.

(2) The course of disease is dependent on the leukemia burden, which can be assessed by clinical staging systems, such as the proposal by Rai, which take into account blood counts and organ involvement by CLL (Table 12-5).

(3) CLL of T lymphocytes is rare but seems to behave similarly to B cell CLL, with the exception of more aggressive entities such as human T cell lymphotropic virus (HTLV)–associated proliferations.

Table 12-5. Clinical Staging in Chronic Lymphocytic Leukemia (CLL) [Modified Rai Classification]

	Risk		
Clinical Features	**Low (Stage 0)**	**Intermediate (Stages I, II)**	**High (Stages III, IV)**
Lymphocytosis*	Present	Present	Present
Lymphadenopathy/splenomegaly	Absent	Present	May be present
Thrombocytopenia†	Absent	Absent	Present
Anemia‡	Absent	Absent	Present
Median survival (years)	> 10	6–8	1–2

*$> 15,000$ lymphocytes/μl.
†$< 100,000$ platelets/μl.
‡Hemoglobin concentration < 11 g/dl.

(4) Occasionally CLL transforms into a clinically and morphologically more aggressive phase resembling prolymphocytic leukemia [PLL; see II C 2 e (1)]. Five percent of CLL patients subsequently develop a large cell lymphoma (Richter's syndrome), which studies indicate may or may not arise from the original neoplastic CLL clone.

d. Treatment

(1) Since survival is similar to that of age-matched controls, treatment is recommended only for progressive disease in low-risk patients.

(2) Symptomatic intermediate-risk patients may benefit from the administration of chlorambucil, prednisone, or both.

(3) High-risk patients generally require chemotherapy with combination regimens or chlorambucil–prednisone.

(4) Novel approaches such as anti-idiotypic antibodies and biologic-response modifiers (e.g., lymphokines), which attempt to circumvent the limitations of chemotherapy associated with the low-growth fraction of neoplastic CLL cells, may have a role in treatment but require further evaluation.

e. Related disorders

(1) **PLL** is a related but more aggressive leukemia of prolymphocytes. A prolymphocyte looks like an activated lymphocyte, exhibiting a larger nucleus and usually a prominent nucleolus, much like the immunoblast in Figure 12-1. It presents explosively with a very high white cell count and massive splenomegaly. Rare T cell forms also involve lymph nodes and the skin.

(2) **T_γ lymphocytosis syndrome.** T_γ lymphocytosis is also called large granular lymphocytic leukemia and T suppressor chronic lymphocytic leukemia. Patients are usually older adults with significant neutropenia and splenomegaly. The peripheral blood generally shows a modest proliferation of medium-sized lymphocytes with granules that usually have a T suppressor cell phenotype (CD2, CD3, CD8) but lack the pan–T cell marker CD5. Most cases appear to be clonal proliferations of T cells by molecular analysis, although cases have been reported that are polyclonal. The clinical course is generally indolent. Death is due to neutropenia-related sepsis or progressive disease. Splenectomy is not helpful, and chemotherapy is of limited use.

3. Hairy cell leukemia

a. Clinical presentation. Hairy cell leukemia is a low-grade leukemia of B lymphocytes occurring primarily in middle-aged and older men. Because of extensive bone marrow infiltration and hypersplenism owing to splenic involvement and enlargement, patients usually present with pancytopenia, including monocytopenia.

b. Diagnosis. The characteristic leukemic lymphocytes have ruffled borders (hence the name) and moderate cytoplasms but may be difficult to identify. The **lymphocytes** in approximately 90% of cases contain **tartrate-resistant acid phosphatase (TRAP)**. Hairy cell leukemia has a characteristic morphologic involvement in the bone marrow and spleen where, unlike lymphomas, it primarily involves the red pulp. Specific immunophenotypic markers of hairy cells have been described, including expression of the interleukin-2 (IL-2) receptor (CD25).

c. Clinical course and treatment. The clinical course is usually indolent, although problems arise more quickly than in CLL because of pancytopenia. For this reason, splenectomy may be done first in an attempt to improve blood counts, with chemotherapy used judiciously when necessary. Many patients benefit from **interferon-α** treatment, and **pentostatin** (2′-deoxycoformycin) has shown significant effects in trials to date. **2-Chlorodeoxyadenosine** has shown extremely promising results in limited trials.

4. Adult T cell leukemia/lymphoma (ATLL) is found primarily in endemic regions (southwest Japan, the Caribbean basin, and southeastern United States). All patients have **antibodies to HTLV type I** (HTLV-I). Patients present with skin lesions, lymphadenopathy, and often circulating mature $CD4^+$ T lymphocytes with lobulated "cloverleaf" nuclei. Many patients display lytic bone lesions and hypercalcemia. ATLL behaves aggressively in most patients, although occasional chronic cases are seen. Its description is included with chronic leukemias because it was and is confused with CLL.

5. Sézary syndrome. In the Sézary syndrome of mycosis fungoides or cutaneous T cell lymphoma, neoplastic atypical lymphoid cells with characteristic convoluted nuclei frequently circulate in the blood. These cells are usually mature $CD4^+$ T lymphocytes.

III. MALIGNANT LYMPHOMAS.

Two major classes of malignant lymphomas exist that behave clinically as distinct entities: **Hodgkin's** and **non-Hodgkin's lymphomas**. Most present as tumors involving lymph nodes or other lymphoid organs such as the spleen, but extranodal presentations are seen. Important clinical features of Hodgkin's and non-Hodgkin's lymphomas are compared in Table 12-6.

A. Introduction

1. **Incidence.** The overall incidence of malignant lymphomas is 5–10 cases per 100,000 population each year. There are approximately 2 cases of non-Hodgkin's lymphoma for each case of Hodgkin's disease. Lymphoma as a class shows a 3:2 predilection for males.

2. **Etiology**
   a. **Infectious agents and viruses.** Simultaneous clustered cases of Hodgkin's disease have suggested the possibility of an infectious agent, although this has yet to be confirmed. As mentioned in II C 4, HTLV-I is clearly associated with acute T cell lymphoma/leukemia in Japan. Epstein-Barr virus (EBV) is associated with Burkitt's lymphoma of African origin.
   b. **Immunologic dysfunction.** A variety of immunologic dysfunctions are associated with increased rates of non-Hodgkin's and Hodgkin's lymphomas. Immunologically deficient patients, including those with inherited immunodeficiencies, acquired immune deficiency syndrome (AIDS), immunosuppression after renal, cardiac, or other types of transplantation, and autoimmune disorders such as Sjögren's syndrome, systemic lupus erythematosus, and others, are at increased risk for the development of non-Hodgkin's lymphomas, usually the more aggressive types.
   c. **Heredity.** Apart from those associated with inherited immunodeficiencies, genetic associations with lymphoma have occasionally been noted, including identical Hodgkin's lymphomas in twins. Many such lymphomas are likely related to poorly characterized underlying immunodeficiencies or infectious agents.
   d. **Chemicals.** Farmers with significant exposure to herbicides carry a higher risk of non-Hodgkin's lymphomas. Increased risk has also been reported with exposure to benzene and dioxins.

3. **Diagnosis.** Pathologic distinction of lymphomas from reactive conditions may be difficult; it is important that Hodgkin's and non-Hodgkin's lymphomas be accurately distinguished for the purposes of staging, treatment, and prognosis. Diagnostic tissue should be examined by an experienced pathologist.

4. **Diagnosis and treatment**
   a. Accurate clinical and pathologic staging is important as a prognostic indicator and for the choice of proper therapy. The **Ann Arbor system** is widely used for lymphomas, particularly for Hodgkin's disease (Table 12-7). Staging data are obtained by comprehensive studies, including physical examination, chest x-rays, liver and spleen scans, magnetic resonance imaging (MRI) and computed tomography (CT) scans, bone marrow biopsy, and laparotomy, if indicated.
   b. Lymphoma treatment with radiation and combination chemotherapy is generally best done at a center that sees many patients with these disorders.

Table 12-6. Comparison of Hodgkin's and Non-Hodgkin's Lymphomas

Hodgkin's Disease	Non-Hodgkin's Lymphomas
Orderly spread by contiguity	More random spread, probably via blood
Extranodal presentation rare	Extranodal sites in unfavorable lesions
Systemic symptoms, prognostic importance	Systemic symptoms less common
Involves central and axial lymph nodes, but rarely mesenteric lymph nodes, blood, or lymphoid tissue of Waldeyer's ring (oronasopharynx)	More frequent involvement of peripheral and mesenteric lymph nodes, blood, Waldeyer's ring
Single disease in terms of clinical treatment; cure possible for all types and stages	Multiple diseases (at least two) clinically; cure rare in low-grade tumors

Table 12-7. Ann Arbor Staging Classification

Stage	Extent of Disease
I	One lymph node region or one extralymphatic site (I_E)
II	Two or more lymph node regions on the same side of the diaphragm One or more lymph node regions plus one extralymphatic site, same side of diaphragm (II_E)
III	Lymph node regions on both sides of the diaphragm possibly with involvement of spleen (III_S), an extralymphatic site (III_E), or both (III_{SE})
IV	Disseminated disease involving one or more extralymphatic sites (e.g., bone marrow, liver, noncontiguous lung involvement) usually with lymph node involvement
Systemic symptoms	
A	Asymptomatic
B	Temperature ≥ 38° C, night sweats, or unexplained weight loss of more than 10% body weight in the prior 6 months

B. Hodgkin's disease

1. Clinical presentation (see Table 12-8)

a. Disease occurs in a bimodal age distribution—late adolescence/early adulthood (nodular sclerosis), with subsequent second peak in older adults.

b. A characteristic feature of Hodgkin's disease is its **pattern of spread in a contiguous fashion** from one lymphoid region to the next, presumably by efferent lymphatics. Hematogenous dissemination to distant sites (bone marrow, liver) may occur in aggressive disease.

c. Defects in cellular immunity are frequently reflected in anergy and increased susceptibility to infections in these patients and are generally correlated with the stage of the disease. This may persist even during remission or following cure.

2. Diagnosis

a. Reed-Sternberg (RS) cells

(1) RS cells are the diagnostic hallmark of Hodgkin's disease. They are large cells with two or more nuclei demonstrating prominent central nucleoli. Characteristic variant RS cells are useful in pathologic diagnosis.

(2) Recent studies indicate that RS cells are derived from B lymphocytes in lymphocyte-predominant Hodgkin's disease and T lymphocytes or tissue monocytes in the other major subtypes. Some investigators have proposed that the RS cell is a neoplastic derivative of interdigitating reticulum cells found in the paracortex of lymph nodes that may play a role in antigen presentation to T lymphocytes in the normal immune response.

(3) Hodgkin's disease is an unusual "tumor": Clonal neoplastic RS cells form a small percentage (usually < 1%) of the lesion. The remainder consists of polyclonal lymphocytes, monocytes, plasma cells, eosinophils, neutrophils, and connective tissue. Four major pathologic subtypes based on the architecture of the lymphoma and the relative number of lymphocytes and RS cells or characteristic RS variants are defined in Table 12-8.

b. Special studies, including immunohistochemistry and immunoglobulin or T cell receptor gene rearrangement studies help **distinguish Hodgkin's from non-Hodgkin's lymphoma,** a common diagnostic problem with important therapeutic implications.

3. Prognosis

a. The clinical and pathologic stage is the major prognostic indicator. Patients with high-stage disease do poorly. In this context, older age, massive mediastinal disease, B symptoms (see Table 12-7) in low-stage disease, multiple (five or more) splenic nodules, and stage III disease beyond the upper abdomen are adverse signs.

b. The **likelihood of cure in early stage disease is 90% or better,** with better than 60+% 10-year survival for all patients. Even without cure, many patients live for extended periods.

c. Extended survival after therapy unfortunately has as a consequence secondary aggressive non-Hodgkin's lymphoma or AML in up to 10% of patients. Secondary hypothyroidism and sterility may occur.

Table 12-8. Histopathologic/Clinical Features of Hodgkin's Disease

Subtype	Frequency	Features
Nodular sclerosis	50+%	Young adults, only type more common in women, lacunar RS variants, fibrosis, nodules
Lymphocyte predominant	< 10%	Younger patients, rare RS cells, many lymphocytes, evidence of B lymphoid origin fairly strong, usually stage I/II
Mixed cellularity	30+%	More abundant RS cells, rich infiltrate of inflammatory cells, broad diagnostic group
Lymphocyte depleted	Uncommon	Numerous RS and other atypical cells, easily confused with large cell non-Hodgkin's lymphoma

RS = Reed-Sternberg (cells).

4. Treatment

a. Radiation therapy is very effective for early stage (I and II) disease and is usually given to treat supradiaphragmatic disease (mantle), subdiaphragmatic disease (inverted Y), or both.

b. Multiagent chemotherapy regimens such as MOPP–ABVD [mechlorethamine, Oncovin (vincristine), procarbazine, and prednisone–Adriamycin (doxorubicin), bleomycin, vinblastine, and dacarbazine] give excellent results in higher stage (II–IV) disease.

c. Patients who relapse after radiation therapy can be treated with chemotherapy; those who relapse after chemotherapy are considered for bone marrow transplantation.

C. Non-Hodgkin's lymphomas

1. Pathology. Non-Hodgkin's lymphomas are neoplastic clones of lymphocytes arrested at or arising from discrete stages of normal lymphoid differentiation (Figure 12-1).

a. Anatomic, phenotypic, proliferative, and functional characteristics

(1) Lymphomas of morphologically mature cells share the migratory habits and low proliferative potential of their normal counterparts. They generally show distant dissemination, usually in the bone marrow, at diagnosis, but patient survival is prolonged since cell proliferation is slow and probably subject to some of the body's normal growth controls.

(2) Non-Hodgkin's lymphomas of larger and less mature cells usually obliterate normal lymph nodes, presumably because of their higher growth potential, analogous to the proliferative responses of lymphocytes that have "transformed" in response to antigenic stimuli. Transformed cells circulate less extensively, and it is more likely that large cell lymphomas, the tumors of transformed-appearing lymphocytes, are found to be localized at diagnosis.

(3) From 65% to 75% of lymphomas are of B lymphoid origin, and 25% to 35% are of T lymphoid origin. B cell tumors localize in and spread to B cell regions of lymphoid tissues (e.g., follicular lymphomas), whereas T cell tumors often preferentially involve T cell regions of the lymph node (paracortex).

(4) Lymphomas of mature B cells may produce immunoglobulin paraproteins (e.g., Waldenström's macroglobulinemia), whereas **tumors of mature T cells may be associated with hypergammaglobulinemia,** suggesting that neoplastic T cells can participate as "helpers" for immunoglobulin production by the immune network.

b. Pattern (follicular/nodular versus diffuse) **and cell type** (small mature cells with or without cleaved nuclei or large cells with "transformed" nuclei) are important clinicopathologic features in classification (Table 12-9). The National Cancer Institute's (NCI) working formulation classifies lymphomas as low-, intermediate-, and high-grade types in terms of untreated clinical behavior.

(1) Indolent tumors have small, morphologically mature cells and often a follicular pattern. Mature cells have relatively small nuclei with evenly dispersed but clumped nuclear chromatin and small to modest amounts of cytoplasm.

(2) Aggressive tumors have a diffuse pattern and large or less-differentiated lymphoid cells. All high-grade tumors have a diffuse pattern.

c. Histologic progression

(1) Some patients with low-grade non-Hodgkin's lymphomas subsequently develop an

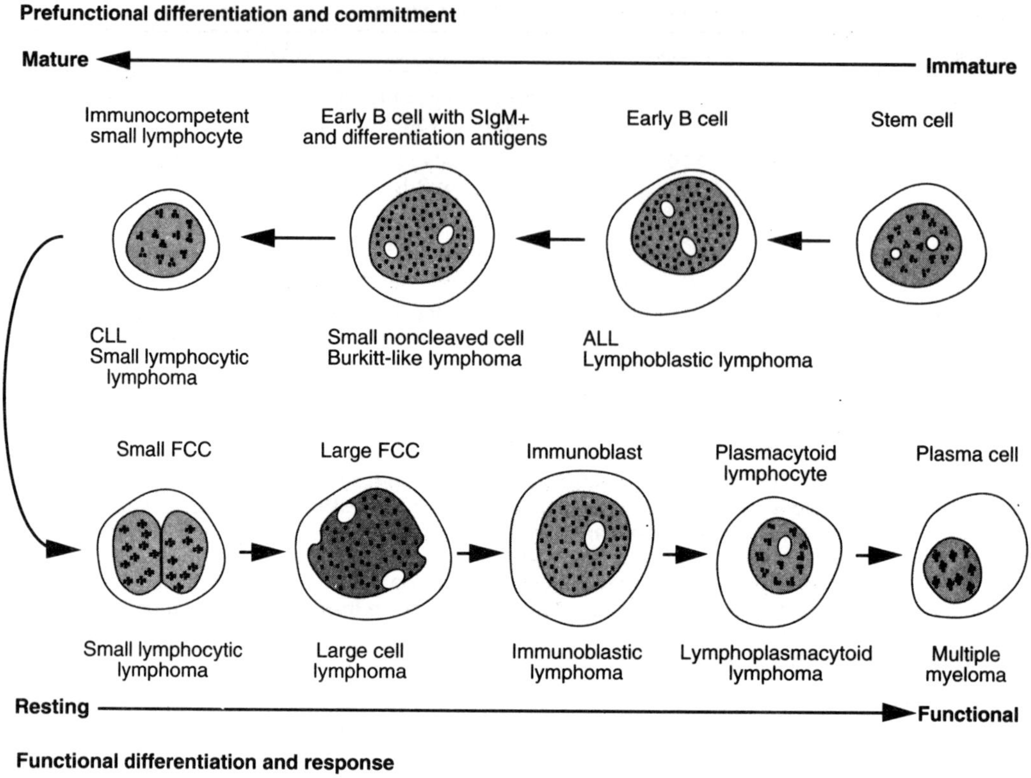

Figure 12-1. Non-Hodgkin's lymphomas as neoplasias that mirror normal B lymphoid development and function. The stages of B lymphoid development and functional differentiation are illustrated, with corresponding lymphomas listed below each stage. *SIgM+* = surface membrane immunoglobulin M–positive; *CLL* = chronic lymphocytic leukemia; *ALL* = acute lymphocytic leukemia; *FCC* = follicular center cell.

intermediate- or high-grade lymphoma that, in most cases, demonstrates the same clonal markers as the low-grade lymphoma.

(2) Occasionally, there are patients who present with a high-grade tumor who then later recur with a low-grade lymphoma. This probably reflects "cure" of the large-cell component of what initially was a high-grade lesion that also contained mature neoplastic lymphocytes that were not susceptible to therapy and that continued to proliferate at a low rate to manifest again at a later time.

2. Cytogenetics. Major cytogenetic abnormalities are listed in Table 12-1. Several translocations into the immunoglobulin heavy chain locus occur on chromosome 14 and are associated with increased gene expression, leading investigators to hypothesize overexpression of normally quiescent genes via the immunoglobulin gene promoter. Most (14;18) translocations occur within a 250–300 base-pair region on chromosome 18 in follicular and in some diffuse lymphomas. This unique junction fragment can be monitored by the polymerase chain reaction to detect small numbers (1 in 100,000 or more) of neoplastic cells.

3. Clinical presentation

a. Most patients present with one or several **enlarged painless lymph nodes**. Cervical, inguinal, and axillary nodes are most frequently involved.

b. One-fifth to one-third of patients with intermediate- and high-grade lymphomas present in **extranodal sites** such as Waldeyer's ring, the gastrointestinal tract, skin, salivary glands, and bone.

c. Most patients have clinical **stage III or IV disease at diagnosis,** as determined by chest x-rays, bone marrow and liver biopsies, and various imaging procedures. Laparotomies,

Table 12-9. National Cancer Institute (NCI) Working Formulation for Lymphoma Classification

Low-grade
Diffuse small lymphocytic (old DWDL)
Follicular small cleaved cell (old NPDL)
Follicular mixed small and large cell
Intermediate-grade
Diffuse small cleaved cell
Diffuse mixed small and large cell
Diffuse large cell lymphoma*
Follicular large cell lymphoma†
High-grade
Immunoblastic lymphoma*
Small noncleaved cell, Burkitt-type (old undifferentiated)
Lymphoblastic lymphoma

DWDL = diffuse well-differentiated lymphocytic leukemia.

NPDL = nodular poorly differentiated lymphocytic lymphoma.4z

*Both groups previously termed diffuse "histiocytic" lymphomas (DHL).

†Recent evidence suggests this class may best be placed in the low-grade group; this subtype is uncommon.

which are used much less frequently than in Hodgkin's disease, primarily help assess potentially low-stage intermediate-grade lymphomas, which are candidates for radiation therapy.

4. **Subtypes**
   a. **Lymphoblastic lymphoma is the tissue equivalent of ALL.** It is usually of T lymphocyte origin and often presents in adolescents as a mediastinal mass. Lymphoblastic lymphomas quickly disseminate into the peripheral blood and CNS and must be treated aggressively.
   b. **Small noncleaved (Burkitt's) lymphoma** is a rapidly growing tumor that characteristically presents in the jaw in children from Third World countries and in the bowel or abdominal lymph nodes in children from developed countries. A strong association with Epstein-Barr virus has been noted in African patients. These tumors are always of B cell origin.
   c. **Intermediate differentiation** (mantle zone) **lymphomas,** which are not listed in the NCI working formulation, may show modest nuclear irregularity and B cell antigens (e.g., CD20); surface immunoglobulin levels are intermediate between those of small lymphocytic and small cleaved lymphomas.
   d. In a number of T cell lymphomas, neoplastic cells exhibit an affinity for, and are usually first diagnosed, in the skin. These are generally referred to as **cutaneous T cell lymphomas** and include distinct clinicopathologic entities such as mycosis fungoides. The **Sézary syndrome** is characterized by diffuse erythroderma, skin involvement by mycosis fungoides, and circulating lymphoma cells with hyperconvoluted nuclei.

5. **Treatment**
   a. Patients with **favorable low-grade lesions** may not require immediate treatment. For a very few patients with early-stage (I or II) disease, radiation therapy may produce durable remission. It is difficult to maintain remission in patients with high-stage disease, and clinicians may watch and wait until patients are symptomatic before employing total lymphoid radiotherapy or low-toxicity single-agent chemotherapy for palliation. Paradoxically, few patients with low-grade lesions achieve cures; however, median survival is 5–10 years.
   b. Patients with **unfavorable intermediate- and high-grade lesions,** who require immediate and aggressive treatment, receive high-dose radiation for stage I disease and combination chemotherapy for high-stage disease. A response is seen in 70%–80% of patients; attainment of complete clinical remission is a crucial determinant for cure. Overall long-term survival is 50% or more, despite unfavorable histology. Bone marrow transplantation is being investigated now for patients who relapse.
   c. Patients (usually children) with **Burkitt's and lymphoblastic lymphomas** receive specific multiagent chemotherapy and CNS prophylaxis; long-term survival is 50%–70%.

IV. PLASMA CELL AND LYMPHOPLASMACYTIC NEOPLASMS represent expansions of fully differentiated functional B cells that produce and usually secrete homogeneous clonal immunoglobulins often referred to as **paraproteins**. Three major groups are recognized: monoclonal gammopathy of uncertain significance (MGUS), multiple myeloma, and macroglobulinemía.

A. Introduction

1. **Incidence.** Plasma cell and lymphoplasmacytic disorders are seen with increasing incidence in older patients (e.g., MGUS is seen in 1% of all individuals older than 25 years, in 3% of all individuals older than 70 years, and in 10% of all individuals older than 80 years).

2. **Diagnosis** relies on laboratory (immunoelectrophoresis or immunofixation) detection of **monoclonal immunoglobulins,** often termed **M proteins** or paraproteins, in serum and urine. The **class of immunoglobulin** produced in plasmacytic disorders corresponds to the morphology of neoplastic cells. MGUS and myeloma generally produce IgG, IgA, IgD, and IgE or light chains. IgM is generally produced by lymphoplasmacytoid lymphomas with or without lymphocytosis. The overall distribution of paraproteins is about 50% IgG, 20%–25% IgA, 15% IgM, and 10% light chain only.
   a. Overproduction of clonal immunoglobulin is usually associated with decreased levels of other immunoglobulins through suppressive mechanisms that are not well understood.
   b. The relative frequency of paraproteins MGUS, multiple myeloma, and macroglobulinemia closely parallels the percentage of isotypes in lymphoid cells in normal individuals producing IgA, IgE, IgD, IgG, and IgM, suggesting neoplastic transformation is not restricted to certain classes of lymphocytes.
   c. **Rouleaux** are commonly observed in peripheral blood smears of patients with paraproteins, and the erythrocyte sedimentation rate is elevated.

3. **Clinical course.** The disease course of MGUS, myeloma, and Waldenström's macroglobulinemia is generally indolent if patients do not present with symptoms, signs, or laboratory evidence of rapid tumor expansion. Both in this respect and as neoplastic expansions of mature cells, they mimic low-grade non-Hodgkin's lymphomas.

B. Monoclonal gammopathy of uncertain significance is often termed benign or essential monoclonal gammopathy.

1. **Incidence and immunoglobulin classes** produced are discussed in IV A.

2. **Diagnosis** results from incidental laboratory detection of a paraprotein, sometimes referred to as an **M** (**m**yeloma or **m**acroglobulinemia) **component,** in the serum or urine. MGUS shares many of the features of indolent myeloma (Table 12-10), although bone marrow plasmacytosis is uncommon and serum levels of M components are generally below 3 g/dl. Some patients with other lymphoproliferative processes also have low-level M components.

3. **Clinical presentation.** Most patients are asymptomatic. A number of patients with peripheral neuropathy present with benign monoclonal gammopathy, apparently because of immunoglobulin directed against peripheral nerve components such as myelin and glycolipids.

4. **Clinical course.** Much like myelodysplastic syndromes, MGUS appears to behave in some patients as a preneoplastic plasma cell disorder with a variable likelihood of developing into multiple myeloma. A minority of patients (approximately 20%) develop myeloma; no clinical change is observed in others, although 50% show an increase in the serum M component level.

Table 12-10. Features of Indolent and Active Myeloma

	Myeloma	
Features	**Indolent**	**Active**
Clinical symptoms	Asymptomatic	Symptomatic
Radiographs	Normal	Lytic lesions
Blood values	More or less normal	Elevated β_2 microglobulin Hypercalcemia Increasing M component concentration Anemia
Labeling index	Low	Elevated
Morphology	Differentiated	More likely to be less differentiated

5. **Treatment** is not required. Patients are followed to evaluate a change in symptoms or a change in their M component.

C. Multiple myeloma (plasma cell myeloma)

1. **Incidence** of multiple myeloma is 1–2 cases per 100,000 population in whites each year and is almost 2–4 per 100,000 in blacks. Incidence rises dramatically in the elderly, and there is a modest male predominance. An increased incidence in some geographic regions probably reflects better and earlier detection.

2. **Pathology**
   a. Mouse plasmacytomas, unlike human myeloma, frequently show overexpression of and chromosome translocations of the c-*myc* oncogene into the immunoglobulin heavy chain gene, as in Burkitt's lymphoma. Translocations into the heavy chain locus on chromosome 14 as well as trisomy (3, 5, 7, 9, 11) and monosomy (8, 13) are seen in myeloma.
   b. Circulating monoclonal lymphoid or lymphoplasmacytic cells that share the myeloma idiotype indicate that myelomas arise because of disordered maturation processes in precursors, probably at the stem cell or pre-B stage.
   c. **Clinical presentation.** Hypercalcemia and lytic bone lesions **are due to elaboration of osteoclast-activating factors,** probably cytokines, by myeloma cells.

3. **Diagnosis** requires the presence of a monoclonal immunoglobulin, usually at levels greater than 3 g/dl, and at least 10% plasma cells in the bone marrow in a patient with the clinical stigmata of multiple myeloma. Since 10% plasma cells may occur in MGUS or reactive conditions, many authorities insist plasma cells also must form large aggregates of "sheets" for diagnosis. Plasma cell distribution may be spotty in the marrow, and diagnosis may require the directed biopsy of a lytic bone lesion. Rare patients elaborate little or no immunoglobulin but have diagnostic morphology and clinical features; this is termed **nonsecretory myeloma**.

4. **Clinical presentation**
   a. **Multiple osteolytic bone lesions** in the skull and other bones occur in 85% of patients. Fractures and bone resorption resulting from inactivity and **hypercalcemia** are a major problem and may contribute to the common complaint of **back pain** with which many patients present.
   b. **Weakness** and **fatigue** are associated with bone marrow suppression and anemia.
   c. **Renal impairment** is due to toxic effects of filtered light chains, hypercalcemia, and amyloid deposits. Lambda (λ) light chains seem more likely to produce tubular disease, whereas kappa (κ) light chains may give rise to a nephrotic syndrome because of glomerular dysfunction.
   d. **Serious infections** may occur, particularly with gram-positive *Streptococcus* or *Staphylococcus* species secondary to hypogammaglobulinemia and neutropenia.
   e. **Elevated levels of serum β_2 microglobulin** correlate with the myeloma tumor burden.

5. **Clinical staging.** Several staging systems are based on the assumption that the myeloma burden correlates with easily measured laboratory parameters, in particular the M component. Stage I patients have little radiologic disease and normal serum calcium; stage III patients have extensive bone disease and hypercalcemia. β_2 Microglobulin and albumin levels also correlate (Table 12-11).
   a. Multiple myeloma can be clinically indolent (sometimes called smoldering) or active (see Table 12-10).
   b. Median survival is 5–6 years for stage I, indolent disease and 1–3 years for active stage III disease.

6. **Treatment**
   a. Treatment is useful only if the patient is symptomatic or the myeloma shows signs of progression, such as increasing serum or urine levels of the M component, renal insufficiency, or anemia.

Table 12-11. Comparison of Clinical Stages of Multiple Myeloma

Stage	M Component (g/dl)	Hemoglobin (g/dl)	β_2 Microglobulin (mg/L)	Albumin (g/L)
I	IgG < 5; IgA < 3	> 10	< 6	> 30
II	IgG 5–7; IgA 3–5	8.5–10	> 6	> 30
III	IgG > 7; IgA > 5	< 8.5	> 6	< 30

(1) **Chemotherapy** benefits symptomatic patients and improves survival. Cure is probably not attainable now in myeloma, although there are rare reports of prolonged remissions. Therapy is usually continued for several months after the M component concentration has stabilized. Patients are then followed carefully for signs of relapse.

(a) **Alkylating agents** such as melphalan or cyclophosphamide (Cytoxan) are generally used. Toxicity is assessed by blood counts.

(b) **Steroids,** such as prednisone and dexamethasone, reduce serum calcium, have some effect on M component levels, and can be useful for patients with low white cell counts.

(2) **Radiation therapy** is frequently used for local treatment of pathologic fractures, for nerve root compression, and for large bone or solitary extramedullary plasmacytomas. Wide-field radiation has more limited use for generalized bone pain in selected patients.

(3) Bone marrow transplantation, is used to sustain a stable type of disease. **Autologous grafts** are used following melphalan and total body irradiation to reduce the tumor cell burden.

b. Response to treatment is monitored by serum levels of the M component and β_2 microglobulin levels. Patients whose M component levels are reduced significantly (> 50%) are responders. Patients whose M component or calcium levels are not reduced, who continue to exhibit symptoms, or who have plasma cell masses have a median survival of 2–3 years or less.

c. Ambulation and adequate fluid intake are extremely important adjuncts to treatment to minimize hypercalcemia.

D. Macroglobulinemia. There is a spectrum of clinical entities with which monoclonal macroglobulinemia is associated. These include **essential (benign) macroglobulinemia, plasmacytoid B cell lymphomas,** and classic **Waldenström's macroglobulinemia**.

1. **Diagnosis.** Patients with essential macroglobulinemia are generally asymptomatic with low levels of IgM paraprotein. In Waldenström's macroglobulinemia, the level of the M component is above 3 g/dl and the patient exhibits organomegaly, hyperviscosity syndrome, and anemia.

2. **Clinical presentation**

a. Presentation is indolent and similar to that of other neoplasms of mature lymphocytes, involving weight loss, fatigue, and mild bleeding (usually epistaxis).

b. Bone marrow contains lymphoplasmacytic and plasma cells, which are also present in peripheral blood in varying degrees. Lymphadenopathy and splenomegaly are common.

c. Monoclonal IgM that is present is usually associated with κ light chain.

(1) Cold agglutinins are usually monoclonal IgM molecules with autoimmune specificity to the I, i, or Pr blood-group antigen. These agglutinate red cells in the cold (which may be 25° C or higher) and cause severe hemolysis in some patients. Cryoglobulins associated with cold urticaria or Raynaud's phenomenon are seen in some patients.

(2) **Hyperviscosity syndrome** caused by IgM manifests as:

(a) Generalized neurologic dysfunction, progressing in some cases to coma

(b) A bleeding diathesis, owing to impaired platelet function

(c) Generalized hypervolemia, which may progress to congestive heart failure

(d) Retinal changes, particularly dilated tortuous vessels, often associated with hemorrhages and papilledema

(3) Striking sensorimotor peripheral neuropathy has been demonstrated in some patients, caused by monoclonal IgM with specificity for myelin-associated glycoproteins.

(4) Other features commonly seen in multiple myeloma such as renal impairment and bone disease are rare in macroglobulinemia.

3. **Clinical course.** Essential macroglobulinemia behaves in a manner similar to MGUS. Lymphomas associated with the IgM M component generally have favorable low-grade histologies; Waldenström's macroglobulinemia behaves variably, with a median survival rate of about 3 years.

4. **Treatment** is directed at patients with Waldenström's macroglobulinemia who have clinical or laboratory evidence of active disease.

a. Chemotherapy utilizing chlorambucil or regimens used in the treatment of myeloma [see

IV C 6 a (1)] significantly reduces IgM levels, tumor burden, and clinical symptomatology in many patients, although cure is not attainable. Early trials with interferon-α show beneficial effects in some individuals.

b. Plasmapheresis is particularly important for the rapid treatment of hyperviscosity syndrome.

E. Amyloidosis is associated with both neoplastic and nonneoplastic conditions, and it encompasses several syndromes that differ in pathogenesis and biochemistry. Tissue compromise is common to these syndromes because of **extravascular deposition of proteinaceous material**. Diagnosis requires aspiration of the abdominal fat pad or biopsy (gingiva or rectum) to demonstrate characteristic birefringence following staining of amyloid with Congo red. Treatment is directed at underlying diseases, although colchicine may inhibit deposition in primary as well as secondary amyloidosis.

1. **Primary amyloidosis** is due to the deposition of monoclonal immunoglobulin light chains, usually in the heart, tongue, gastrointestinal tract, liver, and connective tissue (e.g., carpal tunnel syndrome). Primary amyloidosis may occur with multiple myeloma.
2. **Secondary amyloidosis** is due to the deposition of amyloid A protein, generally in the liver, spleen, adrenals, and kidney, and is associated with chronic inflammatory diseases such as rheumatoid arthritis, osteomyelitis, tuberculosis, and carcinoma.
3. **Familial amyloidoses** are caused by specific genetic mutations in a variant prealbumin protein called transthyretin, with various target organs depending on the mutation.

F. Heavy-chain diseases are rare and are characterized by the presence of immunoglobulin heavy chains in the serum.

1. **α-Chain disease** occurs most commonly in underdeveloped countries. Initially an extensive plasmacytic infiltrate (usually in the gastrointestinal tract), it may progress to aggressive large cell lymphoma. Chronic antigen stimulation due to bacteria or parasites may play a role in etiology, since some patients recover on antibiotics alone.
2. **γ (IgG) and μ (IgM) forms** present in association with low-grade lymphoproliferative disorders or CLL, respectively.

V. NEOPLASTIC DISORDERS OF MONOCYTES AND HISTIOCYTES most often occur as expansions from hematopoietic precursors, with varying degrees of overproduction of granulocytic cells, as occurs in acute myelomonocytic leukemia, acute monocytic leukemia, and chronic myelomonocytic leukemia.

A. There is a debate among hematopathologists as to whether **malignant histiocytosis** is a discrete clinicopathologic entity. Many cases so diagnosed may be large cell lymphomas associated with erythrophagocytosis by normal macrophages secondary to cytokines secreted by lymphoma cells. Chemotherapy in the treatment of malignant histiocytosis has been successful utilizing the regimens used for unfavorable-prognosis non-Hodgkin's lymphomas.

B. A few large cell non-Hodgkin's lymphomas show only cytochemical and immunologic markers of monocytic origin and are called **"true" histiocytic lymphomas**.

STUDY QUESTIONS

Directions: Each of the numbered items or incomplete statements in this section is followed by answers or by completions of the statement. Select the **one** lettered answer or completion that is **best** in each case.

1. Each of the following laboratory procedures is likely to be useful in distinguishing acute myelogenous leukemia (AML) from acute lymphocytic leukemia (ALL) EXCEPT

(A) immunoglobulin and T cell receptor gene rearrangement studies
(B) periodic acid-Schiff (PAS) cytochemistries
(C) terminal deoxynucleotidyl transferase (TdT) studies
(D) cytochemical stains for peroxidase
(E) serum vitamin B_{12} level measurement

2. A lymph node removed from a 32-year-old man shows diffuse large cell lymphoma. Which of the following clinical characteristics of the lymphoma in this type of patient are most likely?

(A) Disseminated disease at presentation, prolonged survival, but an eventual succumbing to the lymphoma or its complications
(B) Rapid development of circulating immature blasts requiring aggressive cytotoxic therapy
(C) Survival of more than 90% of patients with this type of lymphoma at 10 years after diagnosis
(D) Rapid death if therapy is unsuccessful; a good chance for long-term survival if therapy achieves complete response
(E) Spontaneous remission in 20% of patients

3. A 28-year-old man notices a swelling in his neck while shaving. He has no other symptoms. The swelling is one of several enlarged lymph nodes; these are biopsied and sent for pathologic examination. A diagnosis of nodular sclerosing Hodgkin's disease is made, and an extensive investigation for additional disease is carried out, including staging laparotomy. Involved lymph nodes are found in the mediastinum, but abdominal nodes and the spleen are not involved. Liver and bone marrow biopsies are negative. What is the patient's disease stage?

(A) I
(B) II
(C) III
(D) IV

4. Myeloblasts are commonly observed in which of the following leukemias?

(A) Chronic myelogenous leukemia (CML)
(B) Erythroleukemia
(C) Both
(D) Neither

5. The Philadelphia (Ph) chromosome is observed in which of the following leukemias?

(A) Chronic myelogenous leukemia (CML)
(B) Acute lymphocytic leukemia (ALL)
(C) Both
(D) Neither

6. More aggressive non-Hodgkin's lymphomas are associated with which of the following pathologic patterns?

(A) Diffuse pattern
(B) Smaller, more mature cells
(C) Both
(D) Neither

1-E 4-C
2-D 5-C
3-B 6-A

Directions: Each item below contains four suggested answers of which **one or more** is correct. Choose the answer

A if **1, 2, and 3** are correct
B if **1 and 3** are correct
C if **2 and 4** are correct
D if **4** is correct
E if **1, 2, 3, and 4** are correct

7. Which of the following clinical manifestations would point to a diagnosis of hairy cell leukemia?

(1) Clonal proliferation of B lymphoid cells
(2) Pancytopenia
(3) Splenomegaly
(4) Prominent generalized lymphadenopathy

8. The poorest prognosis for patients with chronic lymphocytic leukemia (CLL) is associated with which of the following features?

(1) Anemia
(2) Splenomegaly
(3) Thrombocytopenia
(4) White cell count > 15,000/μl

7-A
8-B

ANSWERS AND EXPLANATIONS

1. The answer is E *[Table 12-4].*
Vitamin B_{12} levels are useful, when low, in confirming megaloblastic anemia resulting from vitamin B_{12} deficiency and are useful, when high, in supporting a diagnosis of chronic myelogenous leukemia (AML) or myeloproliferative disorder. Table 12-4 illustrates useful features in the distinction of AML and acute lymphocytic leukemia (ALL), utilizing morphology, cytochemistry, immunophenotypic markers, and molecular studies.

2. The answer is D *[III C 5; Table 12-9].*
Paradoxically, patients with histologically "unfavorable" high-grade lymphomas show long-term survival if a complete clinical remission can be attained, whereas it is rare to attain cure in histologically low-grade, "favorable" non-Hodgkin's lymphomas, from which patients die gradually from bone marrow compromise or lymphoma over many years. Long-term survival after 5 years for diffuse large cell lymphomas is roughly 50%. Those who do not attain complete remission usually die within several years. Spontaneous remissions are rarely seen in aggressive lymphomas.

3. The answer is B *[Table 12-7].*
Stage II disease is defined as involvement of two or more separate lymph node groups on the same side of the diaphragm. The patient's lack of symptoms would place him in the IIA group, for which total nodal radiotherapy might be given. Chemotherapy is also an option, particularly if he were to have B symptoms or bulky mediastinal disease. Disease on both sides of the diaphragm is defined as stage III, with "disseminated" involvement, such as liver, bone marrow, or other distant organs, defined as stage IV.

4. The answer is C *[II B 1 a (1) (d), C 1].*
Myeloblasts are seen in chronic myelogenous leukemia (CML) both in the stable or chronic phase, where they are relatively infrequent members of what is basically a proliferation of myeloid cells at all stages of maturation and during blast crisis or transformation. Myeloid blast crisis is seen in 75% of CML patients, and lymphoid blast crisis is seen in 25% of CML patients. Myeloblasts are required for the diagnosis of erythroleukemia FAB classification M6 [French, American, and British (FAB) classification M6], even though the dominant histologic feature is erythroid hyperplasia associated with disordered maturation (dyspoiesis). Stage M6 patients often die in a clinical state resembling that of stage M1, with immature blasts replacing the entire bone marrow with a reduced erythroid component at that time.

5. The answer is C *[II C 1 b (3); Table 12-1].*
The Philadelphia (Ph) chromosome is classically associated with chronic myelogenous leukemia (CML); it was the first chromosome abnormality consistently linked to a specific neoplasm. The Ph chromosome is also seen with regularity in acute lymphocytic leukemia (ALL), where it is associated with poorer prognosis. Although classically detected by cytogenic karyotyping as an identical-appearing 9;22 translocation in both CML and ALL, sensitive molecular assays have demonstrated different breakpoints in the *bcr* gene on chromosome 22 for CML and most AML translocations.

6. The answer is A *[III C 1 b].*
A diffuse pattern and larger transformed or less-differentiated lymphoid cells are associated with more aggressive behavior in non-Hodgkin's lymphomas, although, paradoxically, roughly 50% of patients achieve long-term disease survival with intensive chemotherapy. Smaller, more mature cells are invariably associated with less aggressive types of lymphoma, which often have a follicular pattern. Interestingly, small lymphocytic lymphoma may occur with a diffuse pattern, but it still behaves indolently.

7. The answer is A (1, 2, 3) *[II C 3].*
Pancytopenia with splenomegaly is the classic clinical presentation of patients with hairy cell leukemia. Clonal proliferation of B lymphoid cells with monoclonal surface immunoglobulin is demonstrated in virtually all cases. About 85% to 90% of cases show a tartrate-resistant acid phosphatase (TRAP) isoenzyme. Although this reaction is characteristic of hairy cell leukemia, it is occasionally seen in non-Hodgkin's lymphomas. Prominent lymphadenopathy is not generally seen in any type of leukemia and would be more suggestive of a non-Hodgkin's or Hodgkin's lymphoma.

8. The answer is B (1, 3) *[Table 12-5].*
Patients who have chronic lymphocytic leukemia (CLL) with anemia (hemoglobin concentration < 11 g/dl) or thrombocytopenia (< 100,000 platelets/μl) have the poorest survival rates, with a survival mean of only several years. Presumably, this reflects extensive infiltration of the bone marrow, with compromised normal hematopoiesis and a large total body tumor burden. Patients with isolated leukocytosis/lymphocytosis with or without lymph node, spleen, or liver involvement show overall better survival, with means ranging from at least 5 to more than 10 years. Observations of this type have been codified into clinical staging systems such as that developed by Rai to predict patient prognosis in CLL.

13
Platelets

Patricia M. Catalano

I. PLATELET STRUCTURE (Figure 13-1). Platelets are disk-shaped cells, 3–4 μm in diameter, that normally exist in whole blood in a concentration of 200,000–400,000/μl. The major structural features of the platelet include a typical cell membrane, a circumferential microtubular system, a dense tubular system, various granules, and an externally communicating open canalicular system.

A. Bilipid membrane and membrane proteins. The bilipid membrane around the platelet contains several important **glycoproteins** that function as **surface receptors**. The bilipid membrane is also the site of some of the complex coagulation activities of the platelet (Figure 13-2).

1. **Glycoprotein Ib (GP Ib)** is an intrinsic transmembrane protein with a molecular weight of about 140 kilodaltons. It serves as the binding site for **von Willebrand factor (vWF)**. Binding of vWF is necessary for platelet adhesion, an important first step in platelet function.

2. **Glycoprotein IIb-IIIa (GP IIb-IIIa)** is a prominent calcium-dependent membrane protein complex that functions as a **fibrinogen** receptor. Fibrinogen binding is necessary for platelet aggregation to occur.

B. Microtubules and microfilaments

1. **Microtubules** lying just beneath the platelet membrane form a band in the plane of greatest circumference. The microtubules are composed of tubulin and participate in cytoskeletal support of the platelet and in contraction of the stimulated cell.

2. Closely associated **microfilaments** contain actin and participate in platelet pseudopod formation.

C. Dense tubular system. The dense tubular system is so-named because of the presence of an amorphous, electron-dense material. The system selectively binds divalent cations and serves as the platelet **calcium** reservoir (calcium flux is critical to platelet function). The dense tubular system also is the site of platelet **cyclooxygenase** and of prostaglandin synthesis.

D. Granules store various substances that are secreted during platelet aggregation or are instrumental to aggregation.

1. **Dense granules** are electron-dense particles that contain high concentrations of **adenosine diphosphate (ADP)** and **calcium** as well as **serotonin** and other nucleotides. These substances, released upon platelet stimulation, enhance platelet aggregation.

2. α **Granules** store a variety of proteins that are secreted by stimulated platelets. These include **platelet factor 4, β-thromboglobulin, platelet-derived growth factor, fibrinogen, factor V, vWF,** and various glycoproteins important to adhesion, most notably **thrombospondin** and **fibronectin**.

E. Canaliculi. The open canalicular system is a complex network of surface membrane invaginations that look like vacuoles in the platelet and greatly increase the platelet's surface area. The contents of platelet granules are released through this system.

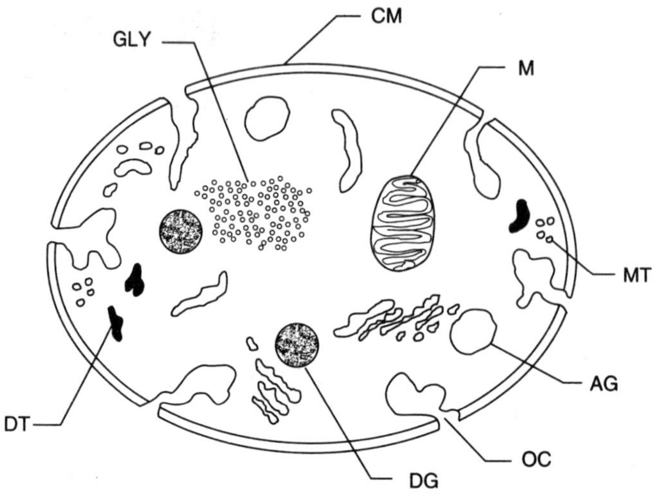

Figure 13-1. Schematic diagram of a platelet in cross section, illustrating the major morphologic features of the cell. *AG* = α granule; *CM* = cellular membrane; *DG* = dense granule; *DT* = dense tubule; *GLY* = glycogen; *M* = mitochondrion; *MT* = microtubule; *OC* = open canaliculus.

II. PLATELET KINETICS. As with other cellular elements, the balance between production and destruction determines whether adequate numbers of platelets are maintained in the peripheral blood for normal hemostasis.

A. Platelet production

1. **Proliferation and maturation** (Figure 13-3). Platelets are shed from the cytoplasm of **megakaryocytes.**
   a. **Stem cells and precursors.** Megakaryocytes develop in the bone marrow from **megakaryocyte colony-forming units (CFU-Meg)** derived from the pluripotential stem cells.
   b. **Megakaryocyte maturation.** The maturing cell becomes larger, with an increasingly lobulated nucleus.
      (1) Megakaryocytes are the largest hematopoietic cells in the bone marrow. The mature megakaryocyte is 20–50 μm in diameter and is easily recognized with a light microscope by its **multilobular, polyploid nucleus** and irregular, granular cytoplasm.
      (2) Megakaryocyte maturation is characterized not only by morphologic changes, but also by an **increase in DNA content,** which occurs because cell division does not accompany mitosis after a certain point in this cell line.
      (3) Megakaryocytes are the only normally polyploid hematopoietic cells. Although the most immature definable megakaryocytes may be diploid, many already have 4N or 8N chromosomes.
   c. **Platelet formation and release**
      (1) As megakaryocytes mature, the cytoplasm begins to acquire **morphologic features,** such as granules, which are characteristic of platelets. Platelet-associated **proteins** such as vWF also become identifiable. As maturation progresses, **demarcation membranes** form, defining future platelets.
      (2) Finally, **platelets are shed** from the most mature cells into the marrow sinuses and from there are released into the peripheral blood.
2. **Humoral regulation of platelet production.** One or more plasma factors are believed to control the peripheral platelet count in a manner similar to the humoral controls for other blood cells. Some investigators believe that there is a single humoral regulator of platelet production.
   a. Thrombopoietin or possibly another factor may act to **stimulate CFU-Meg.**
   b. **Megakaryocyte maturation** is thought to be supported or stimulated by thrombopoietin.
   c. **Platelet production** has been shown to be stimulated by thrombopoietin.

B. Platelet distribution

1. **Peripheral blood and spleen**
   a. Normally, about two-thirds of the body's platelets are in the peripheral blood, with the remainder almost entirely in a splenic pool of platelets.

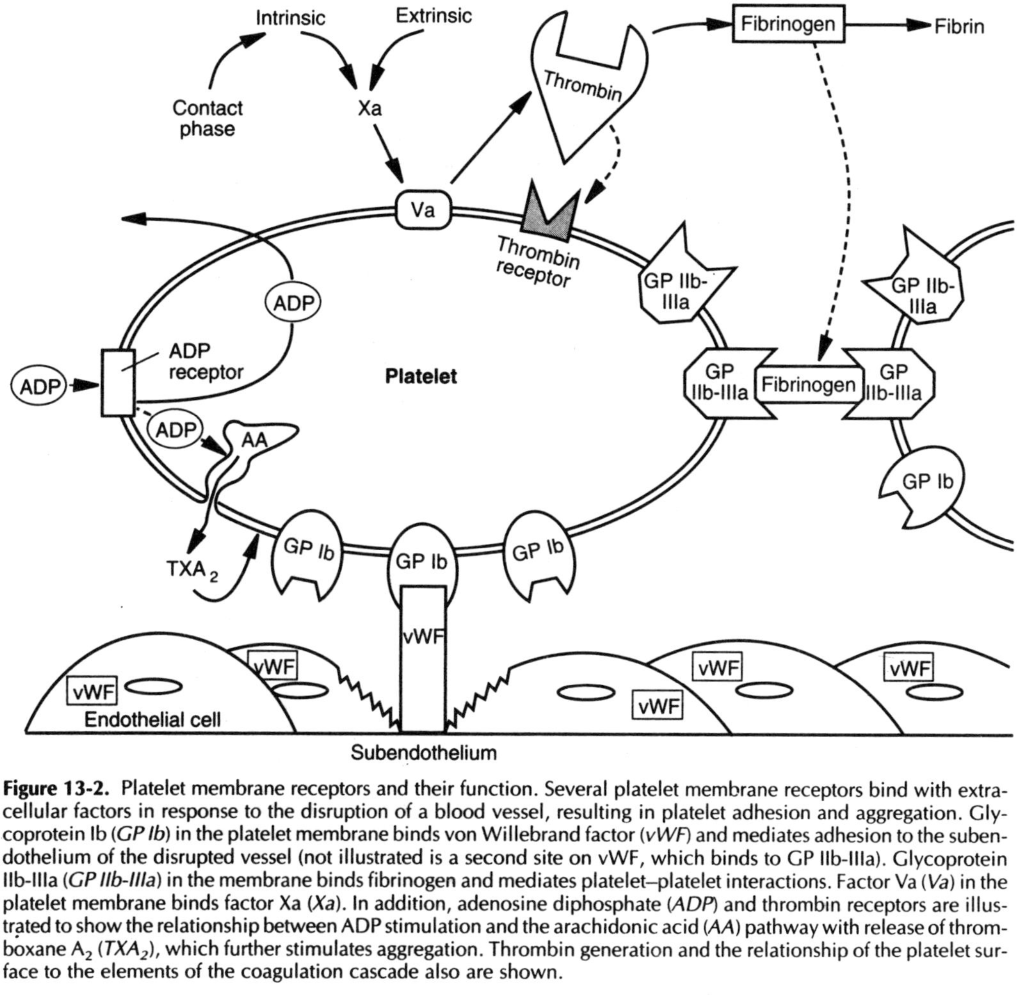

Figure 13-2. Platelet membrane receptors and their function. Several platelet membrane receptors bind with extracellular factors in response to the disruption of a blood vessel, resulting in platelet adhesion and aggregation. Glycoprotein Ib (*GP Ib*) in the platelet membrane binds von Willebrand factor (*vWF*) and mediates adhesion to the subendothelium of the disrupted vessel (not illustrated is a second site on vWF, which binds to GP IIb-IIIa). Glycoprotein IIb-IIIa (*GP IIb-IIIa*) in the membrane binds fibrinogen and mediates platelet–platelet interactions. Factor Va (*Va*) in the platelet membrane binds factor Xa (*Xa*). In addition, adenosine diphosphate (*ADP*) and thrombin receptors are illustrated to show the relationship between ADP stimulation and the arachidonic acid (*AA*) pathway with release of thromboxane A_2 (*TXA_2*), which further stimulates aggregation. Thrombin generation and the relationship of the platelet surface to the elements of the coagulation cascade also are shown.

b. In asplenic patients, the peripheral blood accounts for about 90% of platelets. Conversely, increased splenic pooling can be demonstrated in patients with splenomegaly or hypersplenism.

2. Bone marrow also is a site of platelet pooling, but to a much lesser extent.

C. Platelet life span

1. General considerations

a. Platelet survival curves (Figure 13-4) obtained by most techniques appear linear in normal persons, although evidence suggests that the curves result from both linear and exponential decay, reflecting age-dependent and random destruction of platelets.

b. Clinical applications. Determinations of platelet life span are useful for evaluating thrombocytopenic mechanisms in various diseases. However, most clinical decisions are based on circumstantial evidence for a shortened or normal life span, because techniques for determining platelet life span are not widely available.

2. Techniques for determining platelet life span

a. Platelet transfusion monitoring

(1) Technique. The platelet count is simply monitored after platelet transfusions in a thrombocytopenic patient. This can provide useful information about the cause of the disorder.

(a) If marrow failure is the cause (e.g., in aplasia or acute leukemia), transfused platelets can result in measurably increased platelet counts for several (3–5) days.

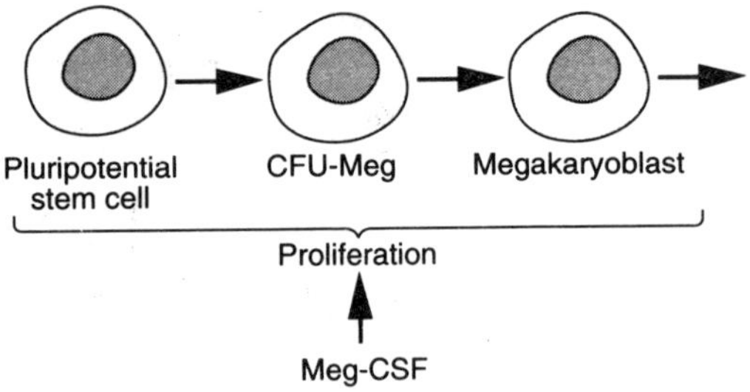

Figure 13-3. Megakaryocyte proliferation and maturation. The megakaryocyte colony-forming unit (*CFU-Meg*) arises from the pluripotential stem cell and gives rise to megakaryoblasts, which differentiate into megakaryocytes. Megakaryocytes are morphologically identified by their multilobed, polyploid (often 16N or 32N) nuclei. Cytoplasmic maturation proceeds, with the formation of demarcation membranes and, ultimately, shedding of platelets. Presumed sites of action of megakaryocyte colony-stimulating factor (*Meg-CSF*) and thrombopoietin (*TP*) are shown.

(b) If platelet destruction is the cause, transfused platelets may have such a short survival that the platelet count shows no measurable change or only a small, very brief increase.

(2) Advantages. Platelet transfusion is a simple technique that is readily available and may even be necessary to support a patient with severe thrombocytopenia. Further, it carries no additional risk beyond that of the transfusion.

(3) Disadvantages

(a) This technique has limited utility, being most accurate only in severely thrombocytopenic patients.

(b) The results of the method may be affected by prior sensitization to blood products, since the patient is given platelets from another person. Thus, the basic mechanism of the thrombocytopenia may be decreased production, but repeated transfusions may stimulate production of antiplatelet antibodies, causing destruction of the transfused platelets.

b. Radiolabeling

(1) Technique. Platelet survival is determined by serial measurement of radioactivity in blood samples after the infusion of platelets labeled in vitro with a radioisotope.

(a) Chromium 51 (^{51}Cr) has traditionally been used for the study of platelet kinetics (see Figure 13-4).

(b) However, **indium 111 (^{111}In)** has become the isotope of choice in many laboratories because it offers greater labeling and counting efficiency than ^{51}Cr. These properties allow autologous studies even in thrombocytopenic patients as well as lower radiation doses in all patients.

(2) Advantages. Radiolabeling is much more sensitive than measuring platelet counts. Radiolabeling is also well standardized, and autologous studies can be performed in many patients.

(3) Disadvantages

(a) Radiolabeling exposes the patient to radiation.

(b) Radiolabeling of platelets is not widely available, and it requires a specialized laboratory.

(c) In severely thrombocytopenic patients (especially when ^{51}Cr is used), it may be necessary to use platelets that may be subject to increased destruction as a result of prior sensitization.

c. Pharmacologic labeling

(1) Technique. The rate of new platelet formation is estimated by measuring the return of platelet cyclooxygenase activity after a single dose of **aspirin**.

(a) Aspirin prevents arachidonic acid metabolism via the cyclooxygenase pathway by irreversibly acetylating platelet cyclooxygenase.

(b) In the steady state, platelet production equals platelet destruction, and therefore the return of cyclooxygenase activity is also a reflection of platelet life span.

(2) Advantages. Pharmacologic labeling always is autologous, requires minimal specialized laboratory facilities, and does not expose patients to radiation.

(3) Disadvantages

(a) This technique has been used only as a research tool in very few laboratories and is not widely available.

(b) The technique involves transient inhibition of platelet function in thrombocytopenic patients. Also, there are technical impediments to applying this technique in severely thrombocytopenic patients as well as possible discrepancies between platelet production and survival.

Figure 13-3. Continued

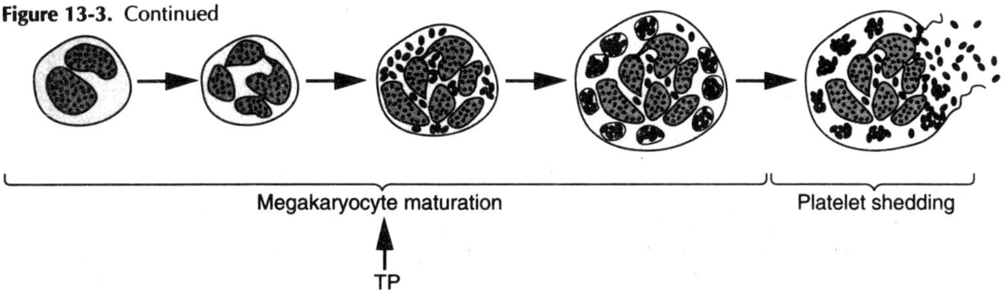

(c) Aspirin may also inhibit megakaryocyte cyclooxygenase, which could confound the interpretation of platelet survival curves and may explain the discrepancies noted among results of various assays.

III. PLATELET FUNCTION (Figure 13-5). Platelets participate in a sequence of events that lead to the formation of a **platelet plug** and ultimately to the formation of a stable **fibrin clot** at the site of vessel interruption.

A. Adhesion

1. **General considerations**
   - **a.** Normally, platelets do not adhere to intact vascular endothelium. This is at least in part due to the action of **prostacyclin [prostaglandin I_2 (PGI_2)],** which is produced by the endothelial cell and is a potent inhibitor of platelet function.
   - **b.** However, within seconds after a vessel is broken, platelets can be seen by light microscopy to adhere to the site, the first step in hemostasis.
2. **Constituents required for platelet adhesion**
   - **a. Collagen** is an important substrate for platelet adhesion. Collagen also stimulates platelet aggregation. Collagen is present in blood vessel interstitium and in basement membrane.
   - **b. GP Ib.** Laboratory models using isolated vessel segments show that adhesion does not occur when GP Ib–deficient platelets are used or when anti–GP Ib antibodies are present.
   - **c. vWF** is a complex multimeric protein that binds to platelets via GP Ib (its major receptor) and to subendothelium. Laboratory models show that platelets do not adhere in the absence of vWF. Prolonged bleeding time in patients with vWF deficiency also suggests a relation to platelet function. A second site on the vWF is now known to bind to GP IIb-IIIa.
   - **d. Other constituents**
     - **(1)** Various other factors (e.g., **fibronectin, thrombospondin**) also play a role in platelet adhesion, but the proteins do not correct the defect that results from diminished or absent vWF.
     - **(2) Calcium** also is necessary for adhesion, and in vitro models require the presence of **red blood cells**.

B. Aggregation. Platelet aggregation is induced by exposure to a variety of stimuli, such as ADP, thrombin, or epinephrine, and in vivo it appears to be stimulated by adhesion.

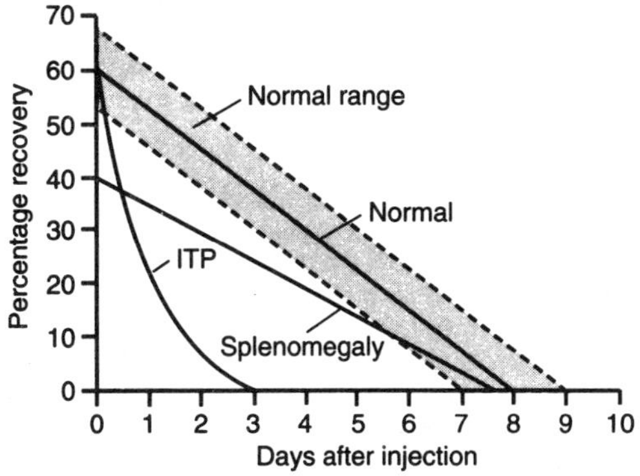

Figure 13-4. Platelet survival. Idealized chromium 51 (^{51}Cr)–labeled platelet survival curves are illustrated. The ordinate represents the percentage of injected radioactivity recovered upon sampling at the time intervals noted. The first sample is drawn shortly after the injection of radiolabeled platelets; the amount lost by the time of the first sample usually is attributable to the splenic pool. This effect is magnified in splenomegaly. *ITP* = idiopathic thrombocytopenic purpura.

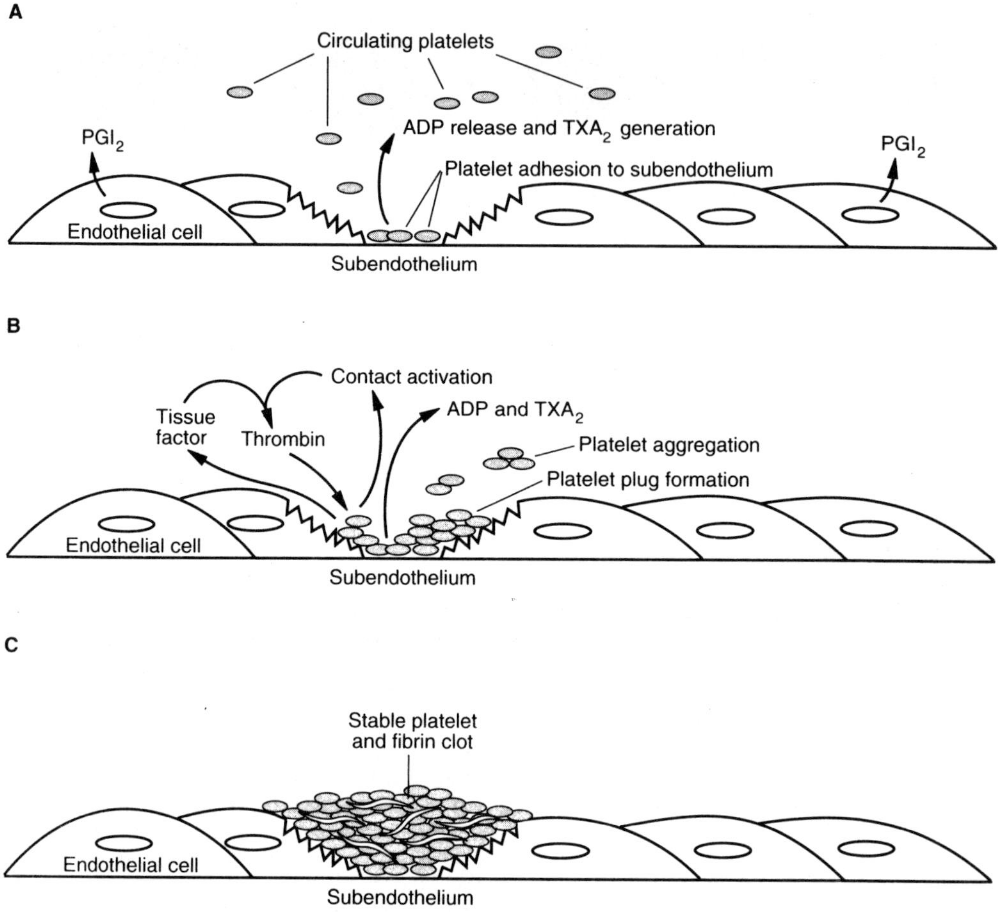

Figure 13-5. Sequence of events after disruption of the endothelium of a blood vessel. (*A*) Clot formation begins with the adhesion of platelets to the subendothelium. Surface properties of the intact endothelium plus the effect of prostacyclin (*PGI_2*) prevent platelets from adhering to the intact endothelium, but platelets adhere to the collagen in the subendothelium at the site of the disruption. This adhesion triggers platelet activation and aggregation, with subsequent release of adenosine diphosphate (*ADP*) and generation of thromboxane A_2 (*TXA_2*). (*B*) Generation of TXA_2 and further release of ADP both serve as stimuli for additional aggregation at the site of injury until the formation of a platelet plug that spans the disruption. The release of tissue factor and contact activation also initiates extrinsic and intrinsic coagulation, resulting in the formation of thrombin, another potent platelet agonist. (*C*) Fibrin strands generated as a result of the coagulation process become entwined in and stabilize the platelet plug.

1. **Aggregation in vitro**
   a. **Technique.** Platelet aggregation is evaluated in vitro by measuring the transmission of light through stirred platelet-rich plasma. The platelets are stimulated by the addition of an exogenous aggregating agent (e.g., ADP, thrombin). As the platelets change shape and aggregate, the continuous change in light transmission is recorded, resulting in an aggregation curve (Figure 13-6).
   b. **Major events of in vitro aggregation**
      (1) **Platelet morphologic change and fibrinogen binding.** Initial stimulation, triggered by the binding of an agonist to its platelet receptor, causes platelets to convert from disks to spiny spheres, decreasing light transmission through the mixture. Fibrinogen binding is necessary for aggregation to proceed. Binding of the agonist also activates assembly of the **GP IIb-IIIa complex,** which in turn forms the **fibrinogen receptor**.
      (2) **Primary aggregation** begins after the platelets change shape, as evidenced by increased light transmission through the platelet-rich medium (see Figure 13-6). If only a low dose of an agonist such as ADP is used or if the platelet cyclooxygenase pathway is blocked with aspirin, aggregation is limited and **reversible**.

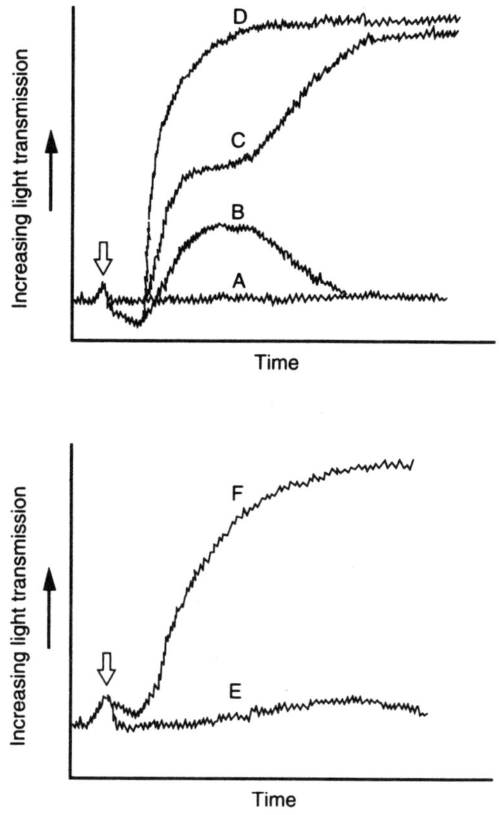

Figure 13-6. Platelet aggregation is determined by measuring the transmission of light through stirred, platelet-rich plasma to which agonist has been added (*open arrows*). As platelets aggregate over time, the medium in which they are suspended becomes clearer and light transmission increases. *A* = platelets that are unresponsive, such as control platelets (no agonist) or platelets from a thrombasthenic patient; *B* = first-wave, reversible aggregation, such as that induced by a low dose of adenosine diphosphate (ADP) or that which might be seen with higher doses of ADP if the platelets have been inhibited by aspirin; *C* = normal biphasic aggregation after stimulation with moderate doses of ADP; *D* = prompt, irreversible aggregation stimulated by high doses of ADP or other potent agonists, such as thrombin; *E* = platelets unresponsive to the addition of ristocetin, as seen in von Willebrand disease and Bernard-Soulier syndrome; *F* = control platelets with normal responsiveness to ristocetin.

(3) **Granule secretion.** After initial stimulation, platelets release the contents of their centralized granules through the open canalicular system. This secretory function of platelets requires energy from the metabolically active cellular stores of adenosine triphosphate (ATP).
   (a) **ADP** in the granules is released into the plasma, stimulating further aggregation.
   (b) **Fibrinogen, vWF,** and **other coagulation and adhesive proteins** also are released, providing a further stimulus for aggregation and adhesion and a link to the coagulation cascade.

(4) **Arachidonic acid metabolism** (Figure 13-7)
   (a) Platelet stimulation activates platelet **phospholipases,** causing the liberation of arachidonic acid from the platelet membrane.
   (b) Arachidonic acid is metabolized via the enzyme **cyclooxygenase** (present in the dense tubular system) to a variety of **prostaglandins** and **thromboxane A_2;** these metabolic products are released coincident with platelet secretion. Thromboxane A_2 is a potent stimulus for further platelet aggregation.
   (c) Aspirin and other nonsteroidal anti-inflammatory agents inhibit cyclooxygenase, causing a specific platelet function defect.

(5) **Secondary aggregation.** A second, more extensive, and **irreversible** wave of platelet aggregation follows arachidonic acid metabolism (see Figure 13-6). It is this second wave of aggregation that is inhibited when the action of cyclooxygenase is blocked by aspirin or other medications.

c. **Ristocetin aggregation.** A unique form of platelet aggregation is induced by the antibiotic ristocetin, which stimulates vWF to bind to platelets at the GP Ib receptor. Ristocetin aggregation can be used to test the interaction between GP Ib and vWF, since aggregation does not occur if either is missing or dysfunctional.

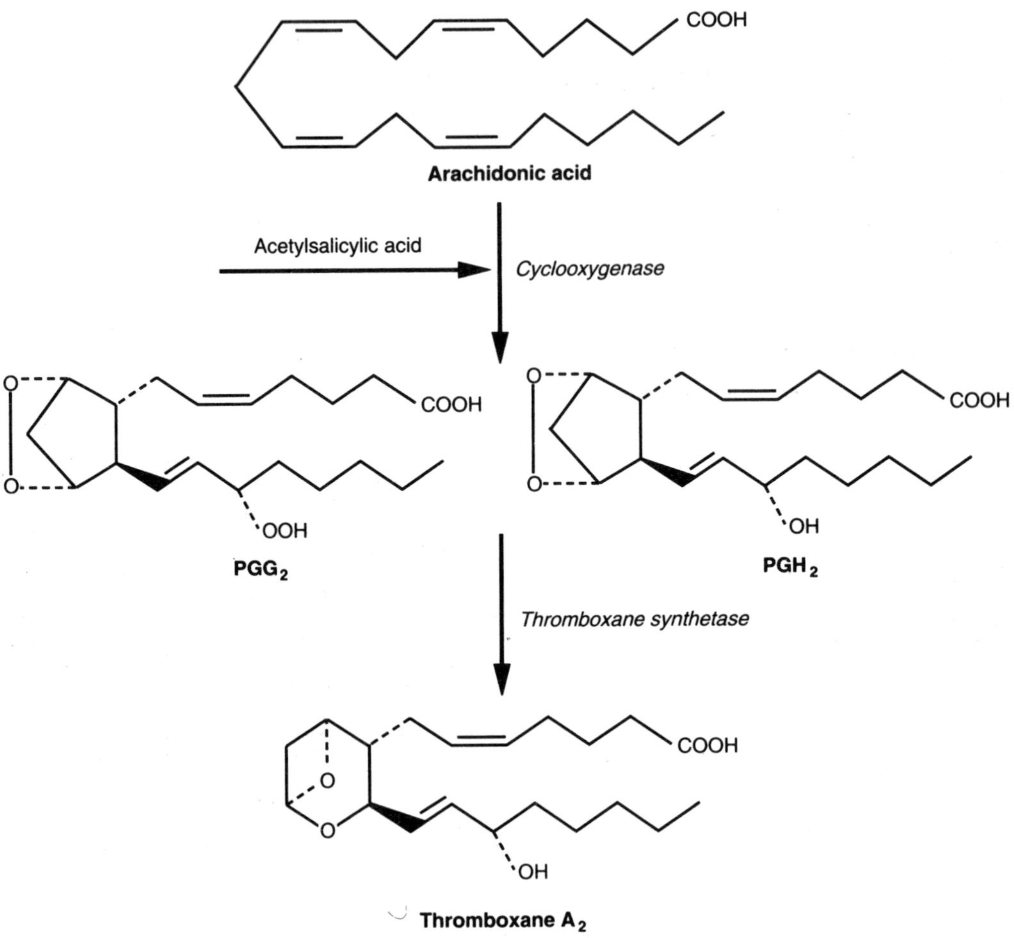

Figure 13-7. Platelet arachidonic acid metabolism. Arachidonic acid is converted to a variety of cyclic intermediates [prostaglandin G_2 (*PGG_2*), prostaglandin H_2 (*PGH_2*)] by the enzyme cyclooxygenase. Subsequently, these intermediates can be converted via thromboxane synthetase to thromboxane A_2, an important platelet intermediary in platelet function. Aspirin irreversibly inhibits cyclooxygenase, thus preventing the production of thromboxane A_2.

2. **Aggregation in vivo.** There is no direct way to study in vivo aggregation. The following sequence of events has been deduced from the in vitro model.
   a. **Platelet adhesion to the subendothelium** of the disrupted vessel is thought to be the stimulus for aggregation.
   b. **Fibrinogen binding** to the receptor on the platelet formed by the **GP IIb-IIIa complex** then stimulates platelet aggregation.
   c. **ADP is released and thromboxane A_2 is produced,** both of which enhance aggregation and provide positive feedback, until a platelet plug is formed and intrinsic coagulation is initiated.
   d. **Further stimulation** of aggregation is provided by **thrombin,** a potent platelet agonist that is produced through the coagulation system.
   e. The irreversible platelet aggregates formed by **secondary aggregation** ultimately become enmeshed in the network of the fibrin clot.

C. Platelet interaction with the coagulation system

1. **Coagulation factors.** It is likely that coagulation factors released during the secretory phase interact not only with platelets but also with the intrinsic coagulation system. Coagulation factors contained in the platelets include **fibrinogen, vWF, factor V, high-molecular-weight kininogen (HMWK),** and **factor XIII.**

2. **Coagulation cascade.** Platelets also participate in the coagulation cascade.
   a. Platelets provide a **negatively charged surface** that appears to facilitate the activation of factor XII by kallikrein and HMWK, the first step of the coagulation cascade.
   b. Platelets bind **factor Xa,** greatly increasing the rate of prothrombin activation by this factor. Substantial evidence suggests that the receptor for factor Xa on the platelet actually is factor Va.
   c. **vWF,** in addition to its role in platelet adhesion, has an important association with the coagulant portion of the **factor VIII complex** and stabilizes the coagulant activity of factor VIII.

D. **Tests of platelet function.** The **bleeding time** is used clinically as an overall measure of platelet function, since platelet plug formation is what stops the bleeding from an incision in a very small blood vessel.

1. This is a relatively crude test that must be scrupulously controlled for subtle variations in performance technique, and it has recently been criticized as insensitive.

2. Nonetheless, prolongation of the bleeding time in the patient with thrombocytopenia or platelet function abnormalities is well recognized, and many platelet function defects have been discovered because of the observation of a prolonged bleeding time.

IV. DISORDERS OF PLATELET NUMBER

A. **Thrombocytopenia.** A **decrease in the number of platelets** is the result of a disorder that either decreases the production or increases the destruction of platelets.

1. **Decreased production.** Findings of decreased or absent megakaryocytes in the bone marrow and a normal platelet survival suggest decreased platelet production. Unfortunately, quantitation of megakaryocytes by examination of the bone marrow smear is somewhat subjective, and it may not be possible to establish a definitive platelet survival for each patient. However, diagnosis usually can be made on clinical grounds.
   a. **Congenital disorders** that cause thrombocytopenia purely as a result of decreased production are extremely rare.
      (1) **Thrombocytopenia with absent radii (TAR)**
         (a) **Diagnosis.** Thrombocytopenia combined with the striking skeletal abnormality of absent radii usually is accompanied by decreased or absent megakaryocytes in the bone marrow. The etiology and mechanism are unknown.
         (b) **Therapy.** Serious bleeding may occur, and patients often require platelet transfusion. As with any lifelong disease, transfusion with platelets needs to be reserved for the treatment of serious bleeding episodes: Sensitization and refractoriness to platelet transfusion should be anticipated.
      (2) **Other congenital hematologic disorders. Fanconi's anemia** may manifest early in its course primarily as thrombocytopenia with decreased megakaryocytes. Other disorders, such as the **May-Hegglin anomaly,** may combine elements of decreased or ineffective thrombopoiesis with increased destruction.
   b. **Acquired disorders.** Many acquired disorders are associated with thrombocytopenia as the result of decreased production, but rarely is thrombocytopenia an isolated manifestation of the disorder. Platelet transfusion is frequently required in these patients.
      (1) **Aplasia.** Decreased production is the mechanism of thrombocytopenia in **aplastic anemias**. Rarely, thrombocytopenia may be an early manifestation of a more generalized hematologic disorder such as preleukemia or aplastic anemia. Therapy is supportive, and platelet transfusions may be necessary for bleeding episodes.
      (2) **Neoplasms.** Both primary hematologic malignancies and carcinomas that have metastasized to the bone marrow can be associated with thrombocytopenia of any severity. Often the other blood cell lines are affected as well, and the etiology is usually obvious.
         (a) **Pathophysiology.** Malignancy causes thrombocytopenia presumably by displacement. In the presence of widespread disease, this is a logical conclusion. However, in some instances marrow suppression may be mediated by more complex mechanisms such as fibrosis or other disturbances of marrow architecture or controls, resulting in unfavorable conditions for normal cell production.

(b) **Therapy** in this situation is directed at the underlying disease, and the prognosis varies accordingly. Support with prophylactic platelet transfusions is justified in patients in whom a response to chemotherapy can reasonably be anticipated (e.g., leukemics).

(3) **Deficiency states**

(a) **Megaloblastosis**

(i) Thrombocytopenia as part of the pancytopenia that can result from **vitamin B_{12} or folate deficiency** is unique, since the deficiency may actually be associated with an increased megakaryocyte mass. However, as with the other cell lines in this disorder, platelet maturation does not proceed normally, and decreased platelet production results from this ineffective thrombopoiesis.

(ii) Response to **replacement therapy** with the appropriate vitamin is usually prompt.

(b) **Iron deficiency.** Although most often accompanied by thrombocytosis, iron deficiency, paradoxically, only rarely causes thrombocytopenia. In such cases, megakaryocytes are found to be decreased. Platelet survival in animal models has been normal.

(4) **Toxins.** Thrombocytopenia can result from exposure to various substances; some of those most commonly seen are listed in Table 13-1.

(a) **Alcohol.** Thrombocytopenia is a common clinical problem in alcoholics.

(i) Alcohol can act as a direct marrow toxin and has been shown to depress the production of platelets. Alcohol appears to act through bone marrow suppression, and withdrawal of alcohol usually results in return of a normal platelet count within a few days.

(ii) More often, thrombocytopenia in an alcoholic patient is the result of multiple mechanisms. In addition to the toxic effect, **hypersplenism** may cause some peripheral destruction, and concomitant **deficiency states** may contribute as well.

(b) **Thiazide diuretics**

(i) Thrombocytopenia of varying degrees occurs in a small percentage of patients treated with these commonly used drugs. Studies of the mechanism of thrombocytopenia generally indicate that bone marrow suppression results from a direct toxic effect of the drug.

(ii) The onset of thrombocytopenia after institution of the drug usually is gradual, as is the recovery after drug withdrawal. As a consequence, evaluation of patients who have been receiving thiazides in addition to other drugs may be difficult. Although rechallenge with the drug has confirmed the relationship in some patients, this is obviously potentially risky.

(c) **Antineoplastic chemotherapeutic agents.** Almost all such agents have some suppressive effects on thrombopoiesis, especially those used specifically for their myelosuppressive effects, such as cytarabine (cytosine arabinoside). Recovery usually is prompt, depending on the pharmacokinetics of the specific agent, although long-term chronic marrow suppression can result from some agents, especially the nitrosoureas.

Table 13-1. Drugs That Commonly Cause Thrombocytopenia

Marrow-suppressing agents	Miscellaneous agents*
Chemotherapeutic agents	Quinidine
Doxorubicin	Quinine
Cytarabine (cytosine arabinoside)	Heparin
Cyclophosphamide	Aspirin
Nitrosoureas	Sulfonamides
Busulfan	Rifampin
Methotrexate	Aminosalicylic acid
Etoposide	Methyldopa
	Gold salts
Other marrow-suppressing agents	
Chloramphenicol	
Phenylbutazone	
Thiazide diuretics	
Alcohol	
Estrogens	

*These may induce thrombocytopenia by an immunologic mechanism.

(d) **Estrogens,** especially diethylstilbestrol, have been associated with thrombocytopenia. Although the mechanism is unknown, animal models have shown suppression of hematopoiesis, and bone marrow examination in patients has been consistent with decreased platelet production.

(5) **Radiotherapy.** The bone marrow is characteristically sensitive to the effects of ionizing radiation. Some myelosuppression, including megakaryocyte suppression, can be anticipated in patients undergoing radiotherapy. The degree of severity usually is proportional to the amount of active marrow exposed and, therefore, varies with the circumstances.

(6) **Other causes.** A variety of conditions and agents have been associated with decreased thrombopoiesis, although both suppressive and destructive mechanisms may be occurring in some cases. **Infections** (e.g., rubella, cytomegalovirus, other viral illnesses), **paroxysmal nocturnal hemoglobinuria,** and even **renal failure** have been reported to be associated with thrombocytopenia that at least in some cases may be the result of bone marrow suppression.

2. **Increased destruction.** Thrombocytopenia resulting from increased peripheral destruction of platelets is associated with increased numbers of megakaryocytes in the bone marrow. The platelet life span in these disorders is demonstrably short.

a. **Congenital disorders**

(1) **Neonatal alloimmune thrombocytopenia (NAIT; isoimmune neonatal purpura)**

(a) **Pathophysiology.** NAIT occurs when a woman whose platelets congenitally lack a specific platelet alloantigen (usually **PlA1**) becomes pregnant with a child whose platelets contain the antigen. In a small percentage of such pregnancies, the mother becomes sensitized to the antigen and produces antiplatelet antibodies that can cross the placenta, causing thrombocytopenia in the infant.

(b) **Diagnosis.** NAIT is suspected when a mother whose platelet count is normal gives birth to a thrombocytopenic infant. The diagnosis is confirmed when the mother's platelets are tested and found to lack a platelet alloantigen that is present in the infant and the father.

(c) **Therapy.** Because the antibodies that cause the neonatal thrombocytopenia are passively acquired, the disease is self-limited and improves as the maternal antibodies are gradually cleared from the infant's plasma. Treatment is necessary only when thrombocytopenia is severe or accompanied by clinically significant bleeding.

(i) The infant may need supportive transfusions of washed maternal platelets, which do not contain the alloantigen and, thus, are unaffected by the antibody.

(ii) Intravenous immunoglobulin (IVIG) has been used both for the treatment of infants and as prenatal prophylaxis, although the latter needs further study.

(2) **Structural disorders associated with increased platelet destruction** may affect not only platelet function but their life span as well.

(a) In **Bernard-Soulier syndrome** (see V A 1 a), the major defect is lack of a membrane glycoprotein, which results in an inability to bind vWF. Studies have shown that these platelets generally have a shortened survival.

(b) The same is true of the platelets of patients with **Wiscott-Aldrich syndrome** and some other, rarer platelet abnormalities. The result may be a thrombocytopenia of mixed etiology, with elements of both decreased production and increased destruction.

b. **Acquired disorders**

(1) **Idiopathic ("immune") thrombocytopenic purpura (ITP)** is the most common cause of isolated thrombocytopenia. It occurs in two forms: an acute, self-limited disease in children and a chronic form seen in adults, most commonly in women age 20–40.

(a) **Pathophysiology.** ITP is an autoimmune disorder in which thrombocytopenia results from the action of antiplatelet antibodies. Platelets coated with these antibodies have a shortened life span and are rapidly cleared from the circulation (see Figure 13-4). In severe cases, the antibody may also affect megakaryocytes, causing ineffective platelet production.

(b) **Clinical features.** The patient usually presents with petechiae, mucous membrane bleeding, or menorrhagia and is found to have isolated thrombocytopenia with no other hematologic abnormalities. Physical examination is entirely normal except for bruises or petechiae.

(c) **Diagnosis.** There is no single diagnostic test for ITP, and ultimately the diagnosis is made on clinical grounds.

(i) Bone marrow examination reveals normal or increased numbers of megakaryocytes. Other potential causes (e.g., drugs, concomitant immune disorders) must be excluded.

(ii) Demonstration of antiplatelet antibodies in the serum or, more significantly, on the platelet also is supportive.

(iii) Platelet survival studies can be confirmatory, especially when the platelet count is only moderately decreased and the adequacy of bone marrow megakaryocytes is difficult to judge. Unfortunately, this test is rarely available for clinical evaluations.

(d) **Therapy.** Acute ITP in children is almost invariably a self-limited disease that, in many cases, appears to be triggered by a preceding viral illness. In adults, however, treatment should be instituted in symptomatic or severely thrombocytopenic patients.

(i) Corticosteroids are the mainstay of therapy for ITP, and most patients respond to treatment. Unfortunately, thrombocytopenia usually recurs when therapy is discontinued.

(ii) Splenectomy is the definitive therapy, with permanent responses in more than 70% of patients.

(iii) Vincristine, danazol, or high doses of IVIG will often produce responses when the above therapies fail or when they are impractical or contraindicated.

(e) **ITP during pregnancy.** ITP is a disease often seen in young women, and consequently it is occasionally seen in pregnant women. Infants born to mothers with ITP often (but not invariably) are thrombocytopenic because the antiplatelet antibody can cross the placenta. This can also occur when the mother is in clinical remission after splenectomy but antiplatelet antibodies are still present.

(i) Treatment of the pregnant ITP patient is similar to treatment of the nonpregnant patient, except that splenectomy should be postponed if possible until after delivery.

(ii) Cesarean section may be a consideration, because delivery poses the threat of intracranial bleeding in the infant. Determination of the fetal platelet count may aid in making this therapeutic decision.

(iii) Thrombocytopenia in the infant is transient. Treatment may be required until antiplatelet antibodies are cleared. Steroids, platelet transfusions, and even exchange transfusion have been used for this purpose, depending on the urgency of the situation and the response of the infant.

(2) **ITP-like syndromes.** A variety of conditions are associated with immunologically mediated thrombocytopenia indistinguishable from ITP. A careful evaluation of patients with apparent ITP is critical so as not to overlook these associated conditions.

(a) **Human immunodeficiency virus (HIV) infection** frequently is associated with an ITP syndrome.

(i) **Incidence.** As many as 25% of acquired immune deficiency syndrome (AIDS) patients may develop ITP at some time in the course of their illness. Even patients with lymphadenopathy syndrome or otherwise asymptomatic HIV-positive patients may develop thrombocytopenia. Perhaps because of the permanent nature of HIV infection, the illness behaves like chronic ITP.

(ii) **Therapy** is similar to that for ITP. Splenectomy may be required, although the advantage of treatment with less immunosuppressant therapy (e.g., IVIG) must be considered.

(b) **Other viral infections.** Thrombocytopenia with shortened platelet survival has been reported with infectious mononucleosis, rubeola, mumps, and other viral illnesses.

(i) Antiplatelet antibodies may result from platelet-virus interactions; in some cases, the platelets may be "innocent bystanders" acted upon by the antiviral antibodies.

(ii) Thrombocytopenia of variable severity can result and, although usually self-limited, may persist for weeks or months.

(c) **Lymphoproliferative disorders.** ITP-like thrombocytopenia can be a systemic manifestation in a few patients with Hodgkin's disease, non-Hodgkin's lymphoma, or chronic lymphocytic leukemia (CLL).

(i) **Presentation.** Usually, the lymphoproliferative disorder is already diagnosed or obvious when thrombocytopenia occurs. Rarely, thrombocytopenia may be the presenting problem; thus, lymphoproliferative disorders must be considered in the evaluation of all patients with ITP.

(ii) **Therapy.** The thrombocytopenia usually responds to treatment of the underlying disease, but in severe cases treatment with appropriate doses of steroids may be required for support until the lymphoproliferative disorder is controlled.

(d) **Systemic lupus erythematosus (SLE)**

(i) **Presentation.** Immunologically mediated thrombocytopenia affects 15%–20% of patients with SLE. In a few patients, thrombocytopenia may be the first manifestation of SLE.

(ii) **Therapy** is similar to that for uncomplicated ITP; however, the role of splenectomy is controversial, with a low frequency of long-term response in some studies.

(3) **Thrombotic thrombocytopenic purpura (TTP)** presents as a complex of findings that includes consumptive thrombocytopenia, microangiopathic hemolytic anemia, fever, and neurologic and renal abnormalities. Although rare, TTP often has a dramatic presentation, and severe cases are associated with a high rate of mortality.

(a) **Pathophysiology** of TTP is complex and poorly understood. There may be precipitating factors (e.g., infection, drug exposure); approximately 10% of cases occur during pregnancy. Whether endothelial or platelet injury is the first event is unknown, but microvascular hyalin thrombi develop and apparently cause the resulting constellation of clinical findings.

(b) **Diagnosis** is made on clinical grounds, by demonstrating a destructive thrombocytopenic process in the presence of the other clinical features. Demonstration of hyaline thrombi on gingival biopsy may be useful in some cases.

(c) **Therapy** is controversial. Currently, the most useful modality is believed to be plasma infusions or plasma exchange transfusion. Corticosteroids, antiplatelet drugs, and, occasionally, splenectomy also are used.

(4) **Drug-induced thrombocytopenia.** A wide spectrum of drugs can cause thrombocytopenia; some of those most commonly reported are included in Table 13-1. Four of the most common agents whose mechanisms are better understood are as follows.

(a) **Quinidine-induced thrombocytopenia** has been extensively studied.

(i) **Pathophysiology.** Usually the onset is after 1 or more weeks of therapy. It is thought that quinidine induces antibody formation and then the drug–antibody complex attaches to the cell, which is subsequently cleared from the circulation—a so-called **innocent bystander** mechanism.

(ii) **Therapy.** The antibody is primarily directed at the drug, and there is little binding to the platelet in the drug's absence. Therefore, thrombocytopenia resolves quickly when the drug is discontinued, although antibody can be demonstrated in the patient's serum for several weeks thereafter.

(b) **Penicillin-induced thrombocytopenia** is much less common than thrombocytopenia due to quinine or quinidine. It is of interest, however, because penicillin binds to the cells, and it is this drug–cell complex that apparently induces the antibody, the penicillin acting as a true hapten. Again, thrombocytopenia resolves promptly with clearance of the drug.

(c) **Heparin-induced thrombocytopenia** has been reported in 2%–20% of patients treated with heparin; this probably is the most common drug-induced thrombocytopenia in hospitalized patients. Even small amounts of heparin used to flush venous access sites can result in thrombocytopenia. A few patients with heparin-induced thrombocytopenia also develop thromboembolic disease.

(i) **Pathophysiology.** The thrombocytopenia generally is believed to be immunologically mediated, with immune complexes binding to platelets, accelerating their degradation. It is also likely that antibodies in some way stimulate platelet aggregation, leading to both thromboembolism and platelet consumption. A second, nonimmunologic mechanism also appears to exist and to cause a mild, early-onset thrombocytopenia.

(ii) **Therapy** sometimes is difficult. Heparin must be discontinued, and patients may need alternative anticoagulation with warfarin preparations or, occasionally, with alternative forms of heparin or newer anticoagulants.

(d) **Gold-induced thrombocytopenia**

(i) **Pathophysiology.** The mechanism generally is believed to be immunologic, but evaluation of these patients is confounded by the autoimmune nature of the conditions for which the drug is administered (e.g., rheumatoid arthritis). Increased amounts of platelet-bound immunoglobulin have been found, but gold-dependent antiplatelet antibodies have not been clearly documented. Thrombocytopenia persists while gold is present, suggesting that it is either acting as a hapten or perhaps damaging the platelets directly.

(ii) **Clinical features.** Patients usually present with gradual onset of thrombocytopenia weeks to months after institution of gold therapy. Megakaryocytes are adequate or increased, and in some patients, platelet life span is shortened.

(iii) **Therapy** consists of discontinuation of the drug. Steroid administration and splenectomy also are effective and are necessary in some cases, further reinforcing the concept that this is an immunologically mediated disorder. Because gold salts remain in the body for long periods of time, chelation therapy sometimes is necessary to hasten the course of the illness.

(5) **Post-transfusion purpura**

(a) **Pathophysiology.** This rare condition occurs when a PlA1-negative individual (whose platelets congenitally lack the PlA1 antigen) is exposed to blood products from a PlA1-positive donor. PlA1 is present in 97% of the population. The mechanism is not entirely clear, since the anti-PlA1 antibodies that result from this exposure destroy the recipient's PlA1-negative platelets, but this may be the result of immune complexes binding to the recipient platelets. In most patients, a history compatible with previous sensitization can be documented.

(b) **Clinical features.** Thrombocytopenia occurs approximately 1 week after the transfusion. Although the course is self-limited, with recovery over 3–4 weeks, the thrombocytopenia often is severe and life-threatening bleeding may occur.

(c) **Therapy** with exchange transfusion or IVIG is, therefore, often necessary in the most severe cases.

(6) **Disseminated intravascular coagulation (DIC)** [see Ch 15 III A]. Thrombocytopenia may be the dominant feature in DIC. Therefore, DIC must be considered in the differential diagnosis of patients with apparently isolated consumptive thrombocytopenia.

B. Thrombocytosis. An **increased number of platelets** in the peripheral blood can be the result of primary bone marrow disorders or may accompany an apparently unrelated process such as iron deficiency.

1. Thrombocytosis resulting from myeloproliferation

a. Essential thrombocythemia (essential thrombocytosis)

(1) **Pathophysiology.** Essential thrombocythemia is caused by a clonal proliferation that involves all the myeloid cells, but for unknown reasons, it is manifested primarily as an increase in platelets. In addition to their increased number, the platelets produced by this clone may be functionally abnormal.

(2) **Clinical features.** Patients may be asymptomatic or may have symptoms related to microvascular occlusions, the most threatening of which may produce neurologic symptoms. Bruising and bleeding secondary to platelet dysfunction also are common, and the bleeding time may actually be prolonged.

(3) **Diagnosis.** Because essential thrombocythemia is strikingly similar to polycythemia vera, differentiating the two disorders may be difficult. Therefore, the Polycythemia Vera Study Group has defined diagnostic criteria (Table 13-2).

(4) **Therapy.** Once the diagnosis is confirmed, the goal of therapy is reduction of the platelet count to normal with myelosuppressive therapy, usually hydroxyurea.

b. Polycythemia vera (PV) [see Ch 3 III A]

(1) **Pathophysiology.** Like essential thrombocythemia, PV is caused by a clonal proliferation at the myeloid stem cell level, and patients may have a striking thrombocytosis in addition to the increased white cell counts and red cell mass. Platelet dysfunction may be present.

(2) **Diagnosis.** The criteria presented in Table 13-2 are essential for differentiating PV from essential thrombocythemia. Patients may have either thrombotic episodes or bleeding as a result of the thrombocytosis.

(3) **Therapy.** Reduction of the platelet count is important in patients with PV, and thrombocytosis may influence whether a patient can be managed with phlebotomy alone

Table 13-2. Polycythemia Vera Study Group Diagnostic Criteria for Essential Thrombocythemia*

Platelet count > 600,000/μl
Hemoglobin ≤ 13 g/dl or normal red cell mass
Stainable iron in bone marrow or failure of 1 month trial of iron therapy
No Philadelphia (Ph) chromosome
Collagen fibrosis of marrow: Absent, or Less than one-third of biopsy without both splenomegaly and leukoerythroblastic reaction
No known cause for reactive thrombocytosis

*All of these criteria must be met to make a diagnosis of essential thrombocythemia.

or whether hydroxyurea therapy will be necessary. Unfortunately, attempts to prevent thrombotic episodes with drugs that inhibit platelet function have been associated with significant increases in serious bleeding episodes.

c. **Other myeloproliferative disorders. Chronic myelogenous leukemia (CML), myelodysplasia,** and some **chromosome abnormalities** (e.g., 5q − syndrome) have been associated with thrombocytosis and must be considered in the evaluation of patients with increased platelet counts.

2. **Secondary thrombocytosis.** Increased platelet counts may occur in association with a variety of clinical conditions, but the pathophysiology is not understood. Except after splenectomy, the platelet count in these situations seldom exceeds 600,000 μl, and thrombotic events rarely occur.
   a. **Iron deficiency.** Although thrombocytopenia has been reported with iron deficiency, thrombocytosis is far more common. Platelet counts can occasionally exceed 1,000,000 μl. The mechanism is not understood, but treatment with iron results in a prompt decrease in the platelet count, often before the anemia responds.
   b. **Postsplenectomy.** The platelet count increases dramatically immediately after splenectomy, presumably due, in part, to removal of this site of platelet pooling and of senescent platelet clearing. The magnitude and duration of the thrombocytosis, however, suggest that additional mechanisms may be involved.
      (1) This is a self-limited phenomenon, and thrombocytosis gradually resolves within weeks to months with no associated thrombotic tendency.
      (2) One exception, however, is when the splenectomy is performed because of a hemolytic anemia that persists after splenectomy. In this setting, thrombocytosis usually persists and may be associated with thrombotic events.
   c. **Other disorders** such as **chronic inflammatory conditions, hemolytic anemias, malignancy,** and **hemorrhage** are also occasionally accompanied by thrombocytosis. The mechanism is not understood. Treatment is directed at the underlying condition.

V. DISORDERS OF PLATELET FUNCTION

A. **Congenital disorders** of platelet function are uncommon but must be considered in the evaluation of a patient with a prolonged bleeding time and a lifelong history of bruising or bleeding.

1. **Disorders of membrane receptors**
   a. **GP Ib deficiency (Bernard-Soulier syndrome)**
      (1) **Pathophysiology.** Bernard-Soulier syndrome is an autosomal recessive disorder in which platelets are deficient in GP Ib. The resultant inability to bind vWF causes defective platelet adhesion.
      (2) **Clinical features and diagnosis.** The severity of the bleeding is variable, but bleeding can be significant. Laboratory findings include a prolonged bleeding time, mild thrombocytopenia, and strikingly large platelets on the peripheral smear. Platelets from patients with this disorder do not aggregate when stimulated with ristocetin despite the presence of normal amounts of vWF.

(3) **Therapy.** Bleeding episodes can be treated with platelet transfusions, although this should be done very selectively because of the possible development of sensitization and refractoriness to platelets.

b. **GP IIb-IIIa deficiency (Glanzmann's thrombasthenia)**

(1) **Pathophysiology.** Glanzmann's thrombasthenia is an autosomal recessive disorder in which platelets are deficient in GP IIb-IIIa, the fibrinogen-binding site through which platelet aggregation is mediated.

(2) **Clinical features and diagnosis.** The severity of the bleeding varies, but significant bleeding can occur. The bleeding time is prolonged, and the diagnosis is made when platelet aggregation studies demonstrate an absence of any response to ADP, collagen, or epinephrine. Ristocetin-induced agglutination is normal.

(3) **Therapy.** Bleeding episodes may be controlled with platelet transfusions. Concerns regarding long-term sensitization are similar to those for patients with Bernard-Soulier syndrome.

2. **Disorders of platelet secretion** are characterized by mild bleeding and absence of the second wave of aggregation when ADP-induced aggregation is tested.

a. **Abnormalities of platelet granules (storage pool disease)**

(1) **Pathophysiology.** Storage pool disease actually refers to a group of disorders in which platelet storage granules are deficient. These disorders are rare but appear to be autosomally transmitted.

(a) **Dense granules.** In **δ storage pool disease,** there is a deficiency of dense granules and their contents (i.e., ADP, ATP, calcium, and serotonin). This deficiency is sometimes associated with other inherited disorders, such as albinism.

(b) **α Granules.** In α **storage pool disease ("gray platelet" syndrome),** the α granules and their contents are deficient. Platelets have a characteristic degranulated appearance.

(2) **Clinical features and diagnosis**

(a) Patients with either form of storage pool disease usually have a mild bleeding disorder and a prolonged bleeding time.

(b) The diagnosis can be suspected based on platelet aggregation studies, combined with the finding of reduced platelet ADP content (in the case of δ storage pool disease) or with reduced platelet factor 4 content and altered platelet morphology (in the case of α storage pool disease).

(3) **Therapy.** Some patients respond to treatment with the vasopressin analog desmopressin [1-desamino-8-D-arginine vasopressin (dDAVP)] for unknown reasons. Since the alternative therapy is platelet transfusions, it may be useful to determine if a patient will respond to dDAVP by measuring the bleeding time before and after a therapeutic trial.

b. **Abnormalities of the prostaglandin pathway** are rare. Deficiencies of cyclooxygenase and of thromboxane synthetase have been reported, as have disorders that result in abnormal arachidonic acid release and diminished platelet responsiveness to thromboxane.

c. **Other abnormalities** of platelet response to various stimuli (e.g., epinephrine, collagen) have been described, which may be the result of receptor defects.

3. **Abnormalities of platelet procoagulant activities** are extremely rare, but an abnormality of platelet factor Va has been described.

B. **Acquired disorders** of platelet function are common. They are more readily classified according to the underlying disease than by the nature of the functional defect, because multiple functional abnormalities may occur as the result of one underlying disease.

1. **Myeloproliferative disorders.** Platelet function abnormalities commonly occur in conjunction with **PV** and **essential thrombocythemia** and have been described in **CML and acute myelogenous leukemia (AML)** and in association with **myelodysplastic syndromes**.

a. **Pathophysiology.** Multiple defects have been described, including abnormalities in arachidonic acid release and metabolism, acquired storage pool deficiency, and abnormalities of membrane receptors.

b. **Clinical features and diagnosis.** Not all patients with myeloproliferative disorders have a demonstrable platelet function defect; some patients even have an increased tendency to thrombotic events. Nonetheless, significant bleeding attributable to platelet function disorders is not uncommon in these patients and may occur even in the face of significant thrombocytosis. Thus, the bleeding time and a high index of suspicion are useful as part of the baseline evaluation of such patients.

c. **Therapy** should be directed at the underlying disease, if possible. Cytoreduction in patients with thrombocytosis may improve the coagulation abnormalities.

2. **Functional defects with immunologic mechanisms**
   a. **ITP.** Some patients with ITP have a prolonged bleeding time disproportionate to the platelet count. This finding usually is presumed to be the result of platelet-bound immunoglobulin interfering with platelet membrane receptor function. In a few cases, antibody specificity for membrane receptors has been demonstrated.
   b. **Dysproteinemias.** Patients with **multiple myeloma** or **macroglobulinemia** may have a prolonged bleeding time, especially when the serum paraprotein level is high. As in ITP, the mechanism may be nonspecific coating of the platelets with the immunoglobulin (especially IgA and IgM), hyperviscosity, or, rarely, the myeloma protein may be specific for a particular platelet receptor.

3. **Functional defects associated with nonhematologic conditions**
   a. **Uremia**
      (1) **Pathophysiology.** Multiple platelet function defects have been reported to occur in uremia, including abnormalities of adhesion, aggregation, and secretion. The exact mechanism of these abnormalities is not known.
      (2) **Therapy.** Dialysis usually improves clinical bleeding and platelet function. Administration of dDAVP may shorten the bleeding time, but it should be used with caution, since there may be a relationship between dDAVP and thrombotic events in some patients.
   b. **Severe liver disease** is associated with multiple coagulation defects, most prominently decreased coagulation factor synthesis and thrombocytopenia, although some investigators have also reported platelet function abnormalities. The prolonged bleeding time in this situation reportedly responds to dDAVP, but the mechanism is unknown.
   c. **Cardiopulmonary bypass** is associated with severe platelet dysfunction that often requires platelet transfusion support.

4. **Drug-induced abnormalities.** The administration of drugs is by far the most common cause of platelet function abnormalities. The degree to which certain drugs contribute to bleeding is variable, but the drug history must always be evaluated in patients with acquired bleeding diatheses.
   a. **Drugs that affect the prostaglandin pathway**
      (1) **Aspirin** prolongs the bleeding time, although not necessarily outside the normal range.
         (a) Aspirin irreversibly acetylates cyclooxygenase (see Figure 13-7), rendering platelets unable to make new cyclooxygenase. Thus, aspirin's effect on platelets lasts for the life span of the cells. Platelet aggregation may be abnormal for as long as 1 week after aspirin ingestion, and the bleeding time may be prolonged for 3 or 4 days.
         (b) Aspirin is a very common and often overlooked medication and a frequent ingredient in over-the-counter medicines.
      (2) **Other nonsteroidal anti-inflammatory agents** (e.g., indomethacin, sulfinpyrazone, ibuprofen, phenylbutazone) reversibly inhibit cyclooxygenase. The resultant inhibition of platelet aggregation is transient, normalizing with clearance of the drug.
      (3) **Thromboxane receptor antagonists** are being studied for their possible use in prophylaxis for ischemic heart disease.
   b. **Phosphodiesterase inhibitors** (e.g., dipyridamole) inhibit the degradation of cyclic adenosine 3′,5′-monophosphate (cAMP). The significance of this effect on platelet function is currently controversial, but drugs of this class may also potentiate the platelet inhibitory effect of PGI_2 (see III A 1 a).
   c. **Antibiotics.** Many of the **penicillins** and some of the **cephalosporins** appear to inhibit platelet function. The mechanism is unknown but may be related to interference with normal platelet receptors. High doses of penicillins are associated with prolonged bleeding times but are seldom associated with bleeding events.
   d. **Other drugs.** A wide spectrum of drugs have been reported to interfere with platelet function. Therefore, it is imperative that the evaluation of a patient with an acquired platelet function defect include a review of concomitantly administered drugs. **Heparin, tricyclic antidepressants,** cardiovascular agents (e.g., **calcium channel blockers**), and even volume expanders (e.g., **dextran**) are some of the more commonly used agents associated with platelet function defects, but many others have been reported.

STUDY QUESTIONS

Directions: Each of the numbered items or incomplete statements in this section is followed by answers or by completions of the statement. Select the **one** lettered answer or completion that is **best** in each case.

1. A severe congenital deficiency of fibrinogen would be expected to have which of the following effects on platelets?

(A) Decreased response to aggregating agents
(B) Decreased adhesion
(C) Shortened survival
(D) Aspirin-like defect
(E) No effect

2. In addition to petechiae and bruises, a patient with ITP is most likely to present with which one of the following findings on physical examination?

(A) Splenomegaly
(B) Lymphadenopathy
(C) Hepatomegaly
(D) A normal physical examination
(E) Fever

3. A 55-year-old patient with polycythemia vera (PV) presents with a hemoglobin level of 16 g/dl, a hematocrit of 52%, a white cell count of 16,000/μl, and a platelet count of 1,500,000/μl. Except for itching after a hot shower, the patient is entirely asymptomatic. All of the following statements regarding this patient are correct EXCEPT

(A) this patient is at risk for hemorrhage
(B) this patient is at risk for thrombosis
(C) phlebotomy should adequately resolve the problem
(D) iron deficiency may be contributing to the thrombocytosis
(E) cytoreductive chemotherapy should decrease the patient's risk for thrombosis

4. A 70-year-old woman is hospitalized on the orthopedic service for elective total hip replacement. The procedure is accomplished without complication, and she is recovering in the hospital. After 1 week, her white cell count is 9000/μl, but her platelet count is 40,000/μl. The most likely cause of the thrombocytopenia is

(A) heparin-induced thrombocytopenia
(B) idiopathic thrombocytopenic purpura (ITP)
(C) bone marrow failure
(D) oxycodone administration
(E) an underlying myelodysplastic process

1-A
2-D
3-C
4-A

Directions: Each item below contains four suggested answers of which **one or more** is correct. Choose the answer

A if **1, 2, and 3** are correct
B if **1 and 3** are correct
C if **2 and 4** are correct
D if **4** is correct
E if **1, 2, 3, and 4** are correct

5. A patient with a normal platelet count is evaluated for a prolonged bleeding time. All tests of platelet aggregation are normal except for an absent ristocetin-induced aggregation. Possible causes of prolonged bleeding in this patient include

(1) ingestion of aspirin
(2) von Willebrand disease
(3) absent fibrinogen receptor
(4) absent GP Ib

6. A patient is evaluated for isolated, severe thrombocytopenia (platelet count = 10,000/μl). Tests that are likely to provide useful information about this patient include

(1) bone marrow examination
(2) bleeding time
(3) platelet survival
(4) platelet aggregation studies

7. A 43-year-old man is admitted to the hospital for control of newly diagnosed diabetes mellitus. He has a history of alcohol and intravenous drug abuse. His platelet count is 15,000/μl, and he reports occasional nosebleeds. Physical examination shows occasional bruises, petechiae only on the lower extremities, and marked splenomegaly. The only medications he is taking at this time are insulin and methadone. Possible causes of the thrombocytopenia include

(1) hypersplenism
(2) HIV infection
(3) alcohol-induced marrow suppression
(4) diabetes

8. A patient with multiple myeloma presents with gastrointestinal bleeding. Possible contributing factors include

(1) thrombocytopenia
(2) uremia
(3) hyperviscosity
(4) platelet function abnormalities

9. Idiopathic thrombocytopenic purpura (ITP) in a pregnant woman typically is associated with

(1) antiplatelet antibodies
(2) splenomegaly
(3) birth of a thrombocytopenic child
(4) a self-limited course

10. Aspirin's effect on platelets is

(1) secondary to aspirin's effect on cyclooxygenase
(2) proportional to the amount of aspirin taken
(3) irreversible
(4) clinically significant for 10 days

5-C 8-E
6-B 9-B
7-A 10-B

ANSWERS AND EXPLANATIONS

1. The answer is A *[III B 1 b (1)].*
Fibrinogen must bind to the platelet via its glycoprotein receptor in order for aggregation to occur. Without fibrinogen, even primary aggregation does not occur. Thus, fibrinogen deficiency is different from an aspirin-like defect, which inhibits only the second wave of aggregation. Fibrinogen is not a mediator of adhesion and does not affect platelet survival.

2. The answer is D *[IV A 2 b (1)].*
Idiopathic thrombocytopenic purpura (ITP) is notable for presenting as isolated thrombocytopenia, without other systemic manifestations (e.g., fever) and with a normal physical examination except for bruises or petechiae. A finding of splenomegaly should prompt investigation into the possibility of an underlying condition such as systemic lupus erythematosus (SLE). Hepatomegaly would suggest underlying liver disease, and lymphadenopathy would suggest an associated lymphoma.

3. The answer is C *[IV B 1 b, 2 a].*
Thrombocytosis that is the result of a myeloproliferative disorder [e.g., polycythemia vera (PV)] can be complicated by either bleeding or thrombotic events, and very occasionally by both. Most patients with PV become iron-deficient, which is a cause of secondary thrombocytosis. Normalization of the platelet count and control of the polycythemia both decrease the likelihood of bleeding. Phlebotomy would lower the hemoglobin level but not the platelet count.

4. The answer is A *[IV A 2 b (4) (c)].*
Virtually all patients undergoing elective hip replacement are now treated prophylactically with heparin, and heparin in all forms is a common cause of thrombocytopenia. It is probably safe to assume that this patient had a normal preoperative platelet count, as evidenced by the uneventful procedure; therefore, it is unlikely that she has an underlying disorder such as myelodysplasia or idiopathic thrombocytopenic purpura (ITP). Bone marrow failure could develop for a variety of reasons, but that would be most unusual given the normal white cell count. The patient may well have received oxycodone for pain, but this drug is not likely to cause thrombocytopenia.

5. The answer is C (2, 4) *[III B 1 c; V A 1 a (2)].*
Ristocetin-induced aggregation reflects the interaction of von Willebrand factor (vWF) with its receptor, glycoprotein Ib (GP Ib). An abnormality or deficiency of either vWF or GP Ib would result in abnormal platelet aggregation in response to ristocetin. Aspirin inhibits the cyclooxygenase pathway of arachidonic acid metabolism, leading to an absence of thromboxane. This deficiency manifests as decreased secondary aggregation, normally stimulated by platelet agonists such as adenosine diphosphate (ADP) and epinephrine; ristocetin-induced aggregation, however, is not affected. Similarly, fibrinogen receptor deficiency would manifest as a lack of platelet response to ADP, to collagen, and to epinephrine, but not to ristocetin.

6. The answer is B (1, 3) *[IV A 1, 2].*
In patients with severe thrombocytopenia, it is critical to examine the bone marrow in order to determine whether megakaryocytes are increased or decreased, since the implications for treatment are quite different. If megakaryocytes are increased, a destructive mechanism is the likely cause of platelet loss; if megakaryocytes are absent, decreased platelet production is the probable cause. The mechanism of thrombocytopenia can be further pinpointed by studying platelet survival, if the technique is available; it is usually reserved for unusual cases of equivocal bone marrow findings. Bleeding time is seldom helpful, since it would be expected to be long in a severely thrombocytopenic patient. Platelet aggregation studies cannot be performed in a severely thrombocytopenic patient.

7. The answer is A (1, 2, 3) *[II B 1 b; IV A 1 b (4) (a), 2 b (2) (a)].*
Splenomegaly can produce both altered distribution of platelets and some enhanced destruction. Alcohol is a known bone marrow suppressant. Human immunodeficiency virus (HIV) infection, for which this patient is at risk, is associated with a thrombocytopenia indistinguishable from idiopathic thrombocytopenic purpura (ITP). Diabetes is not associated with thrombocytopenia.

8. The answer is E (all) *[IV A 1 b (2); V B 2 b, 3 a].*
Many problems can result in bleeding in patients with multiple myeloma. The underlying bone marrow disease as well as the chemotherapy can result in thrombocytopenia, and when myeloma kidney disease

develops, uremia can cause platelet function abnormalities, including abnormalities of adhesion, aggregation, and secretion. Even without uremia, platelet function may be altered by nonspecific interaction with the myeloma protein. A very high monoclonal protein level can also result in hyperviscosity, which is associated with bleeding.

9. The answer is B (1, 3) *[IV A 2 b (1)].*
Platelet destruction in idiopathic thrombocytopenic purpura (ITP) is induced through the actions of antiplatelet antibodies, and it is these antibodies that can cross the placenta and cause thrombocytopenia in infants of mothers with ITP. Splenomegaly is usually seen only if there is an underlying condition associated with the ITP, such as systemic lupus erythematosus (SLE) or lymphoma. Childhood ITP usually is characterized by a self-limited course, but the disease in adults has a chronic, relapsing nature.

10. The answer is B (1, 3) *[II C 2 c; V B 4 a (1)].*
Aspirin irreversibly acetylates cyclooxygenase, the enzyme necessary for the production of thromboxane, which is important for platelet function. The platelet has no nucleus and is an end-stage cell without the ability to make new cyclooxygenase; thus, aspirin's effect on platelet cyclooxygenase lasts for the life of the cell. Platelets normally live for 7–9 days; however, they are produced at a rate needed to maintain a steady state. Therefore, by 3 or 4 days after a single dose of aspirin, about half of the body's circulating platelets have been produced in the absence of aspirin and, thus, are functionally normal. This level of normal platelets is sufficient to compensate clinically for platelets that are functionally abnormal. Platelets are so susceptible to inhibition by aspirin that a single 80-mg dose can block thromboxane production as completely as can a 650-mg dose.

14
Coagulation Physiology and Hemorrhagic Disorders

Patricia M. Catalano

I. COAGULATION PHYSIOLOGY

A. Overview. When a blood vessel wall is ruptured, platelets adhere to the exposed subendothelium and become activated, beginning the process of aggregation. The **platelet plug** thus formed provides a surface on which certain **coagulation factors** can become activated and initiate the **coagulation cascade**. This complex series of reactions ultimately results in the formation of a **fibrin clot** to seal the vessel until new cell growth can replace the damaged tissue.

B. Coagulation factors (Table 14-1)

1. **Biochemical nature.** Most coagulation factors are glycoproteins that normally exist in inactive, pre-enzymatic forms (**zymogens**). These must undergo activation to **serine proteases** in order to participate in coagulation. Several cofactors, calcium ion (Ca^{2+}), and phospholipids also contribute to coagulation.

2. **Nomenclature.** Coagulation factors are identified by Roman numeral (e.g., factor V, factor X); the addition of "a" (e.g., factor Xa) indicates that the zymogen has been activated. Coagulation factors were numbered in the order of their discovery; this does not always correspond to the order of their participation in the coagulation cascade.

3. **Sites of biosynthesis**
   a. **Hepatic synthesis.** The liver is the primary site of synthesis for the coagulation factors except for von Willebrand factor (vWF), which does not participate directly in the coagulation cascade. However, factor VIII, which is tightly bound to vWF, is synthesized in the liver, as demonstrated by the normalization of factor VIII levels in hemophiliacs who have undergone liver transplantation.
   b. **Extrahepatic synthesis**
      (1) Extrahepatic cell lines contribute to the production of some coagulation factors, such as **megakaryocytes** (synthesis of vWF, fibrinogen, factors V and XIII), **macrophages** (synthesis of factors V, VII, IX, and X), and **endothelial cells** (synthesis of vWF).
      (2) Except for vWF, which appears to have an entirely extrahepatic synthesis (see III B 1 b), the degree to which extrahepatic sites contribute to the plasma levels of coagulant proteins is unknown.

4. **Requirements for vitamin K.** The activities of prothrombin (factor II) and of factors VII, IX, and X require the binding of Ca^{2+} by the γ-carboxy residues in these factors. The γ-carboxylation of these glutamic acids is a post-translational event that depends on vitamin K (Figure 14-1). In the absence of vitamin K, these factors are formed, but they are inactive.

5. **Plasma half-life** of coagulation factors (see Table 14-1) must be known to calculate an effective replacement therapy and to understand the dynamics of anticoagulation.

C. Coagulation cascade (Figure 14-2)

1. **General considerations**
   a. **Overview.** The coagulation cascade is the serial activation of coagulant factor zymogens to their active enzymatic forms. Each enzyme catalyzes the conversion of the next zymogen in the series to its active enzymatic form and so on until thrombin converts fibrinogen to fibrin. Fibrin monomers rapidly polymerize to fibrin strands, and the resultant clot is further stabilized by the cross-linking action of factor XIII.

Table 14-1. Plasma Coagulation Factors

Factor	Alternative Name	Pathway	Half-life* (hours)
I	Fibrinogen	C	90–120
II†‡	Prothrombin	C	48–120
III	Tissue factor	I	Not available
V	Proaccelerin	C	12–24
VII†‡	Proconvertin	E	2–6
VIII	Antihemophilic factor	I	10–12
IX†‡	Christmas factor	I	18–30
X†‡	Stuart-Prower factor	I,E,C	24–60
XI†	Plasma thromboplastin antecedent	I	45–80
XII†	Hageman factor	I	40–70
XIII	Fibrin-stabilizing factor	I	72–200
High-molecular-weight kininogen	Fitzgerald factor	I	150
Prekallikrein†	Fletcher factor	I	48–52

C = common pathway; E = extrinsic pathway; I = intrinsic pathway.
*Ranges are approximate: estimates vary widely for some factors.
†Active form functions as serine protease.
‡Vitamin K–dependent.

b. Pathways. The coagulation cascade can be initiated and proceed along either the **extrinsic pathway** (system) or the **intrinsic pathway**. The two systems converge at the activation of factor X, and the final sequence of events—the **common pathway**—is the same for both systems. The extrinsic and intrinsic systems probably are interrelated in vivo, and at times, coagulation probably proceeds along both systems simultaneously.

(1) In the intrinsic pathway, factors XII, XI, IX, and VIII are sequentially activated when factors XII and XI and high-molecular-weight kininogen and prekallikrein contact an appropriate surface (the **contact phase**).

(a) A negatively charged surface (glass or kaolin) can initiate the contact phase in vitro.

(b) The in vivo initiator is not known but is presumed to be the platelet surface or exposed basement membrane.

(2) The extrinsic pathway is an additional clotting mechanism initiated by trauma to the tissues with release of tissue factor.

2. Factors in the intrinsic system

a. Factor XII (Hageman factor) undergoes initial activation by an unknown mechanism. However, factor XIIa can activate more XII and can activate prekallikrein to kallikrein; **kallikrein** greatly accelerates the activation of factor XII.

b. Prekallikrein and **factor XI** are complexed to **high-molecular-weight kininogen,** which binds to negatively charged surfaces, enhancing their availability to factor XIIa and accelerating the activation of factor XI.

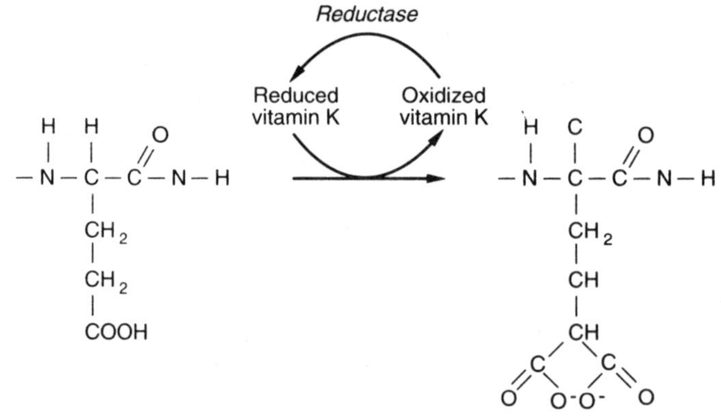

Glutamic acid **γ- Carboxyglutamic acid**

Figure 14-1. Vitamin K–dependent carboxylation of calcium ion (Ca^{2+})–binding coagulation factors. Carboxylation at the gamma (γ) position of glutamic acid requires the action of reduced vitamin K. Warfarin inhibits the reduction of oxidized vitamin K, resulting in a functional deficiency of the vitamin. As a result, factors II, VII, IX, and X are synthesized but are inactive because their glutamate residues cannot be γ-carboxylated and, hence, cannot bind Ca^{2+}.

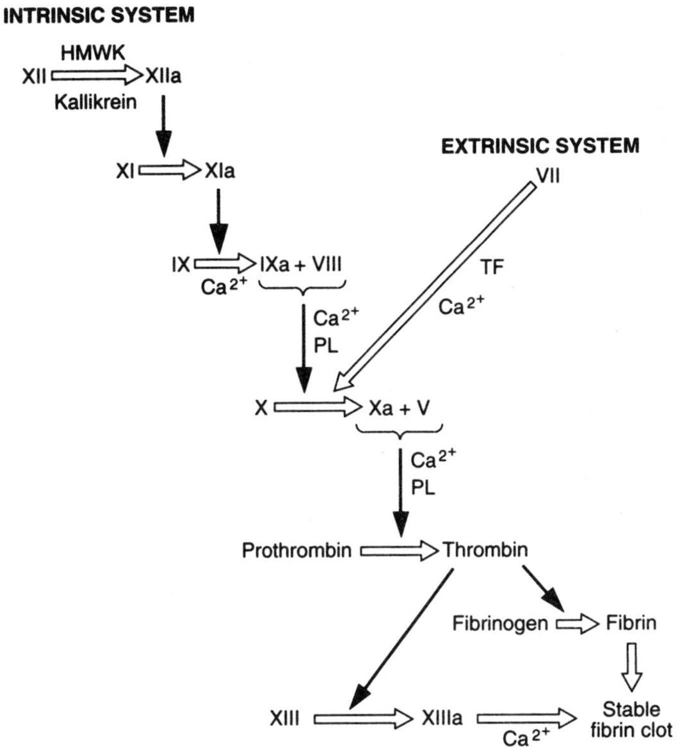

Figure 14-2. The coagulation cascade. Each coagulation factor, when activated, activates the next factor in the series. (Factors are numbered in order of their discovery, not in order of activation.) In the intrinsic system, factor XII is initially activated by an unknown mechanism and subsequently by kallikrein during the contact phase. Alternatively, factor VII and tissue factor can initiate the extrinsic system. Intrinsic and extrinsic pathways each end with activation of factor X, setting off a final, common pathway that ends with formation of the fibrin clot. *Open arrows* indicate conversion of a substrate or a reactant to a product. *HMWK* = high-molecular-weight kininogen; *TF* = tissue factor; *PL* = phospholipid.

c. **Factor IX** activation by factor XIa is greatly enhanced by the binding of factor IX to phospholipid and Ca^{2+}. Platelets provide a convenient phospholipid surface for this reaction.
d. **Factor VIII** is a cofactor that forms a catalytic complex with factor IXa bound (in the presence of Ca^{2+}) to phospholipid. This complex then activates **factor X**. Although factor VIII is not a serine protease, its activity is considerably enhanced when it is activated by thrombin or factor Xa. Factor VIII circulates bound to vWF, which stabilizes it.

3. **Factors in the extrinsic system**
   a. **Tissue factor** is a glycoprotein that is associated with many cellular membranes. It functions as a cofactor for factor VII, forming a catalytic complex with it in the presence of Ca^{2+}.
   b. **Factor VII,** unlike the other coagulation factors, has some inherent serine protease activity. Activation greatly enhances this activity and may be accomplished by factor IXa, factor Xa, or thrombin.
   c. Complexes of factor VII or VIIa with tissue factor in the presence of Ca^{2+} initiate coagulation by activating **factor X**. In addition, there is now some evidence that these complexes can also activate **factor IX**.

4. **Factors in the common pathway**
   a. **Factor X** can be activated either by the IXa–VIII–Ca^{2+} complex formed in the intrinsic pathway, or by VIIa enhanced by tissue factor and Ca^{2+} in the extrinsic pathway. In either case, factor X activation is marked by the release of a small portion of the X molecule called an **activation peptide**.
   b. **Factor V** acts as a cofactor to factor Xa. It also exists as a pro-cofactor that can be activated by thrombin and probably by platelet proteases. Factor V can be found in platelets, and factor Va appears to act as a receptor on the platelet for factor Xa.
   c. **Factor Xa** converts **prothrombin** to **thrombin** through two sequential proteolytic events.
      (1) A fragment referred to as **F1 + 2** is first released.
      (2) Next, the remaining portion of the molecule is cleaved into the two-chain, disulfide-linked thrombin molecule.
   d. **Thrombin** can further hydrolyze prothrombin and may also split F1 + 2 into fragments 1 and 2.

e. **Fibrin and fibrinogen** (Figure 14-3)

(1) **Structure. Fibrinogen** is composed of three pairs of polypeptide chains (Aα, Bβ, γ) covalently linked at their amino terminal portions, forming a central area called the **E domain**. The polypeptide chains form coils that extend out from both sides of this central domain, with the carboxy terminal portions of the Bβ and γ chains forming the terminal **D domain**.

(2) **Fibrin monomer formation.** Thrombin acts on fibrinogen by cleaving a small peptide from the Aα chain (**fibrinopeptide A**) and one from the Bβ chain (**fibrinopeptide B**), thus converting fibrinogen to fibrin monomer.

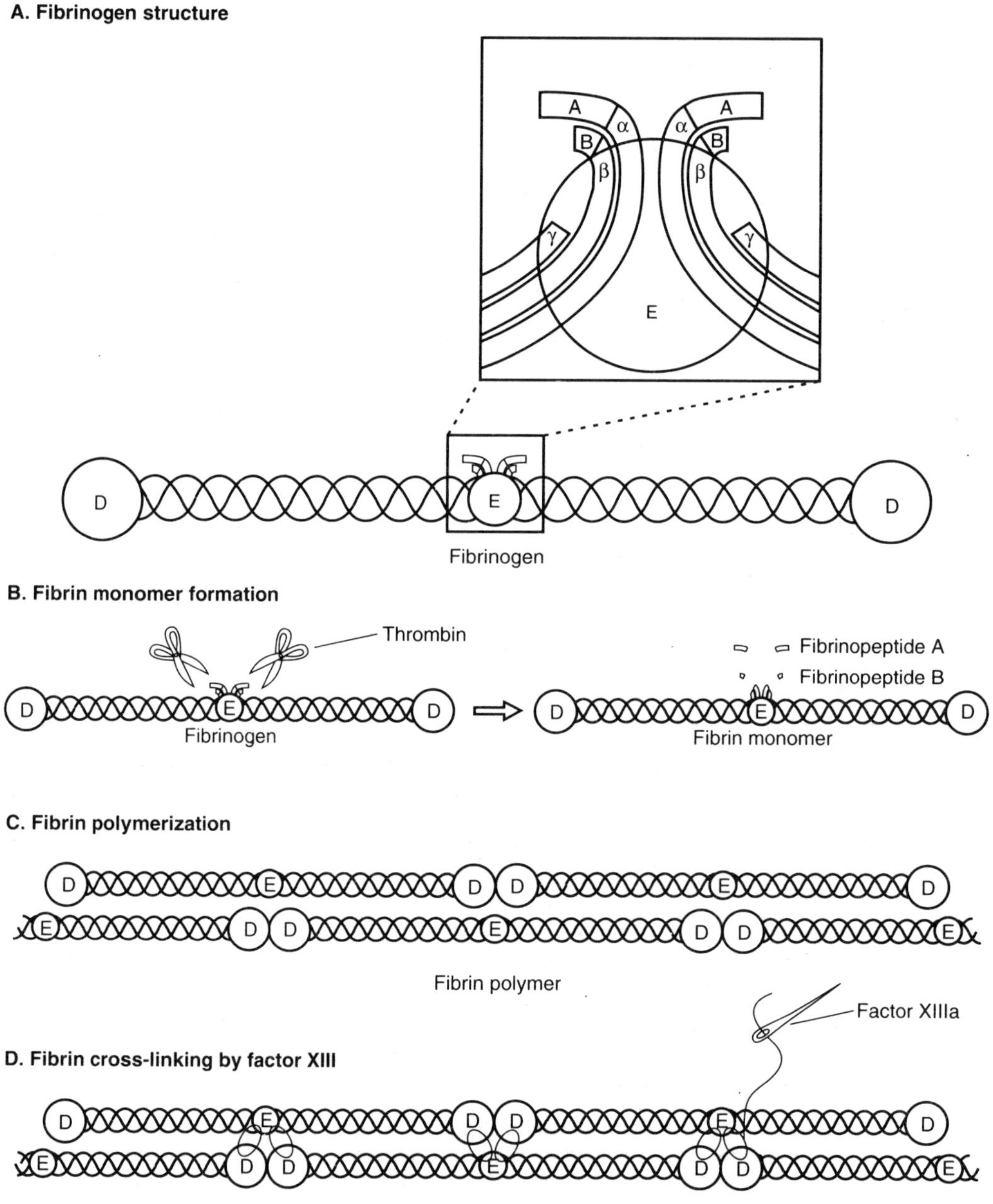

Figure 14-3. (*A*) Structure of fibrinogen. Six polypeptide chains, two each of the Aα, Bβ, and γ chains, are covalently linked to form a central E domain. The remainder of the chains coil outward to form the terminal D domain. (*B*) Thrombin cleavage releases fibrinopeptides A and B, thus transforming fibrinogen to fibrin monomer. (*C*) Fibrin monomers rapidly polymerize and form the fibrin gel. (*D*) Factor XIII acts to stabilize the fibrin by the formation of lysine–glutamine covalent bonds.

(3) **Fibrin polymerization.** Fibrin monomers rapidly polymerize, aligning both end-to-end (D–D) and side-to-side (D–E), forming an insoluble fibrin gel.

(4) **Stabilization by factor XIII.** Factor XIII, activated to XIIIa by thrombin, acts as a transaminase in the presence of Ca^{2+}, forming covalent bonds between lysine and glutamine residues on the fibrin polymers, thus stabilizing the fibrin clot.

II. TESTS OF THE COAGULATION SYSTEM

A. **Screening tests** are important for assessing the overall integrity of the coagulation system and for determining where in the cascade a defect may exist.

1. **Partial thromboplastin time (PTT)** and **activated partial thromboplastin time (APTT)** screen the intrinsic and common coagulation pathways.
   a. **Purpose.** The PTT and APTT are used to detect significant deficiencies of all the **intrinsic and common coagulation factors except XIII**. The PTT and APTT are commonly used to monitor heparin therapy.
   b. **PTT method.** Phospholipid is added to platelet-poor plasma taken from blood that is anticoagulated with citrate. Clotting is then initiated by the addition of Ca^{2+}. The time to formation of the first fibrin strands is the PTT.
   c. **APTT method.** The APTT is performed in the same manner as the PTT except for the addition of an activating agent such as kaolin or ellagic acid before recalcification.

2. **Prothrombin time (PT)**
   a. **Purpose.** The PT measures the function of the **extrinsic and common coagulation pathways**. It is commonly used to monitor oral anticoagulant therapy.
   b. **Method.** A source of phospholipid and tissue thromboplastin (rabbit or human brain extract) is added to platelet-poor plasma, and Ca^{2+} is added to initiate coagulation. The time to the appearance of fibrin strands (the PT) is measured and compared with that of a control.

3. **Quantitative fibrinogen**
   a. **Purpose.** It must be emphasized that fibrinogen quantitation measures **quantities of protein,** not function. Quantitative fibrinogen determination is useful in interpreting functional tests of fibrinogen. In addition, the fibrinogen level may be slightly low without detectable abnormalities of the PT or PTT.
   b. **Method.** Fibrinogen can be quantitated by a variety of techniques, including protein precipitation and immunologic methods.

4. **Thrombin time**
   a. **Purpose.** Thrombin time screens the **thrombin–fibrinogen reaction**.
      (1) Because thrombin acts on fibrinogen directly, the time it takes for a clot to form in plasma to which thrombin has been added is directly related to the amount of functional fibrinogen in the sample.
      (2) This test is affected not only by the amount of fibrinogen in the sample but also by inhibitors to fibrin formation (e.g., fibrin split products) or by the presence of functionally abnormal fibrinogen. In addition, the test is very sensitive to the antithrombin effect of heparin.
   b. **Method.** Thrombin is added to the patient's platelet-poor plasma, and the time to fibrin strand formation is measured. The normal range is influenced by the amount of thrombin added, and a **"dilute thrombin time"** is sometimes used for its added sensitivity.

5. **Screening test for factor XIII**
   a. **Purpose.** A **deficiency of factor XIII** cannot be detected by the above tests. A simple screening test for the presence of factor XIII is based on the fact that fibrin that has not been cross-linked will dissolve in urea, whereas fibrin that has been cross-linked by the action of factor XIII will not.
   b. **Method.** A small amount of plasma that has been clotted is placed in a solution of urea, and an identical clot is placed in saline as a control; both are incubated overnight and compared. Dissolution of the clot in the urea solution confirms factor XIII deficiency.

6. **Limitations of screening tests.** It is important to recognize that subtle factor deficiencies may not cause abnormalities in the screening tests. For example, the PTT may be normal if the factor VIII level is above 30%.

B. Specific factor assays. Once a defect has been localized to the extrinsic, intrinsic, or common pathway, specific assays can be performed for any of the coagulation factors. These assays may be based on the ability of the patient's plasma to correct clotting in a known factor-deficient plasma or on the ability of the patient's plasma to act on a synthetic substrate in a colorimetric assay.

III. CONGENITAL HEMORRHAGIC DISORDERS

A. Hemophilia A (factor VIII deficiency) and hemophilia B (factor IX deficiency). The clinical manifestations of hemophilias A and B are virtually indistinguishable. However, it is critical to differentiate between them for treatment purposes.

1. Pathophysiology

a. The genes for factor VIII and for factor IX both reside on the X chromosome. As a result, hemophilia only occurs in males who have inherited the abnormal gene, whereas females who inherit the gene are carriers (Figure 14-4). Although a family history of hemophilia can be documented for most patients, the frequency of de novo mutations has been estimated to be as high as 30%.

b. It is now known that the genetic defects that result in hemophilia are actually quite heterogeneous, as deletions, insertions, and point mutations have all been described but the resultant clinical manifestations of these defects are similar.

2. Clinical features. The severity of the clinical manifestations is directly related to the degree of factor deficiency.

a. Mild disease. Patients with mild disease (factor levels > 0.05 U/ml) usually are asymptomatic except when stressed by trauma or surgery. Serious bleeding after a relatively minor surgical procedure (e.g., a dental extraction) may be the first clue to the diagnosis.

b. Moderate disease. Patients with moderate disease (factor levels between 0.02 and 0.05 U/ml) often are asymptomatic, but occasional bleeding can occur without a defined trauma. Most commonly, bleeding is associated with minor trauma. Some patients experience spontaneous episodes of soft tissue bleeding and even hemarthrosis. Rarely, neurologic events, such as intracranial bleeds, can occur spontaneously.

c. Severe disease

(1) Patients with severe disease (factor levels < 0.01 U/ml) experience frequent spontaneous bleeding, most commonly hemarthrosis in large joints (see III A 5 a).

(2) Soft tissue bleeding can result in nerve compression syndromes, and central nervous system (CNS) bleeding has been estimated to occur in as many as 1% of hemophiliacs each year.

(3) Bleeding associated with trauma or surgery is life-threatening unless properly treated.

3. Diagnosis

a. Screening tests of the intrinsic system, namely the PTT or APTT, are abnormal in patients with hemophilia, although the prolongation of these tests may be minimal in patients with very mild disease. The bleeding time and PT are unaffected.

b. Specific factor assay provides a definitive diagnosis. Factor levels range from less than 0.01 U/ml (< 1% of normal) in patients with severe disease to as high as 0.40 U/ml (40%

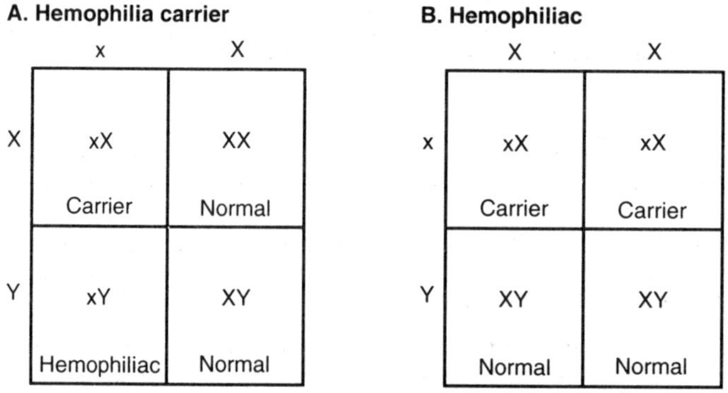

Figure 14-4. Mode of inheritance of hemophilia. (*A*) Hemophilia results when a woman who carries the abnormality on one X chromosome (represented by *x*) transmits that chromosome to a son. If she transmits it to a daughter, that daughter will be a carrier. (*B*) A hemophiliac transmits the abnormal gene to all of his daughters, who are, therefore, carriers. His sons receive only the normal Y chromosome from him and are, therefore, unaffected.

of normal) in those with very mild disease. Unless an inhibitor develops, the factor level for an individual patient remains essentially constant throughout the course of the disease.

4. Therapy. The goal of therapy is to raise the deficient factor to a level that will control bleeding. The method used depends on many variables.

a. Pharmacologic therapy

(1) Hemophilia A. The vasopressin analog **desmopressin** (1-desamino-8-D-arginine vasopressin; **dDAVP**) stimulates the release of body stores of factor VIII, effectively increasing the factor VIII level by three to four times the baseline level.

(a) In patients with very low baseline levels (< 0.05 U/ml), this may not be enough to control bleeding.

(b) However, in patients with higher baseline levels, this increase usually is enough to prevent bleeding related to many surgical procedures or minor trauma.

(2) Hemophilia B has no effective pharmacologic therapy.

b. Replacement therapy

(1) General principles

(a) All blood products used for replacement therapy have potentially adverse effects ranging from allergic reactions to the transmission of viral diseases. The technology of blood product preparation has changed dramatically in response to the acquired immune deficiency syndrome (AIDS) epidemic and continues to evolve.

(b) The choice of blood product for replacement therapy is a critical one and must be made by a physician who has experience and expertise in issues related to the currently available preparations.

(2) Dosage calculation

(a) The increase in factor level that can be achieved by a given dose of the factor depends on the **plasma volume** in which the factor is distributed. Normal factor levels are, by definition, 1 U/ml (100%), and the normal plasma volume can be estimated to be 40 ml/kg.

(i) Therefore, a patient who receives 20 U/kg of factor should have an increase in factor level of approximately 0.5 U/ml, or 50%.

(ii) The increase may be somewhat less for factor IX, which is a smaller molecule than factor VIII, and has some extravascular distribution.

(b) The **duration** of the increased factor level depends on the half-life of the factor being replaced.

(3) Treatment options (see Ch 17 I B 6, 7, 11, 12)

(a) Fresh frozen plasma (FFP) contains all the clotting factors and can be used for the treatment of mild hemophilia B.

(i) Advantages. Each unit of FFP comes from a single donor; thus, FFP is statistically less likely to contain undetected viral contaminants.

(ii) Disadvantages. The major limitations in its usefulness are the relatively large volume of plasma that needs to be given to raise the factor level significantly and the possibility of viral contamination.

(b) Cryoprecipitate is prepared by thawing FFP at 4° C, which results in the precipitation of a large percentage of factor VIII, vWF, and fibrinogen from the plasma. Cryoprecipitation does not concentrate factor IX and, thus, is not used for the treatment of hemophilia B.

(i) Advantages include its small volume and the fact that it is prepared from a relatively small number of donors.

(ii) Disadvantages include the risk of viral infection inherent in any fresh blood product, and the possibility of hyperfibrinogenemia in patients requiring repeated administration over long periods.

(c) Factor concentrates. Lyophilized, highly purified concentrates of **factor VIII** and **factor IX** are made commercially from plasma pooled from thousands of donors.

(i) Advantages. These preparations are ideal for home therapy and for chronic treatment when high doses are necessary for extended periods of time.

(ii) Disadvantages. In the past, transmission of hepatitis and human immunodeficiency virus (HIV) through these products was almost inevitable, but advances in product preparation (e.g., pasteurization, monoclonal purification) have now greatly decreased these risks. In addition, recombinant products are currently under development that should eliminate the problem of viral contamination.

5. **Complications of hemophilia and its treatment**
   a. **Arthropathy**
      (1) **Repeated bleeding into the joints (hemarthrosis)** results in an inflammatory reaction and eventual destruction of cartilage, narrowing of the joint space, and bony spur formation. The resultant arthropathy is characterized by chronic painful enlargement and limitation of motion of the affected joints.
      (2) Fortunately, the advent of products such as factor concentrates that facilitate the early treatment of hemarthrosis has helped to decrease the extent of the arthropathy that most patients now develop.
   b. **Inhibitors**
      (1) From 10% to 15% of patients with severe hemophilia A and approximately 5% of those with severe hemophilia B develop **antibodies** that act as inhibitors of the missing factor, thus greatly complicating the treatment of these patients.
      (2) Various treatments are used, such as the administration of **overwhelming doses of factor** in patients with low titers of inhibitors or the administration of products that bypass the missing factor (e.g., **activated prothrombin complex concentrate**) if the antibody titer is too high to be overwhelmed.
   c. **Liver disease** is among the most frequent causes of death in patients with hemophilia.
      (1) Essentially all multitransfused hemophilia patients have been exposed to hepatitis at some time, and many have chronic persistent or chronic active hepatitis.
      (2) Liver transplantation has been performed in hemophilia patients with hepatic failure and, when successful, is accompanied by normalization of the factor VIII level.
   d. **HIV infection.** HIV transmission from pooled blood products has resulted in the seroconversion of as many as 90% of patients with severe hemophilia A. As a result, many of the medical problems in patients with hemophilia are now a result of this devastating complication of blood product therapy, and AIDS is now the leading cause of death in patients with severe hemophilia.

6. **Interdisciplinary care.** Comprehensive care of patients with hemophilia requires expertise from many medical disciplines. The development of **hemophilia centers** has made such a comprehensive approach possible.
   a. **Medical care.** Patients with hemophilia need access not only to physicians with experience in replacement therapy (including home care) but also to specialists in orthopedics, physical medicine, and dentistry who are experienced in treating patients with bleeding disorders. Increasingly, these physicians must also have experience in the treatment of HIV-related illnesses.
   b. **Psychosocial care.** In addition to issues related to any chronic, painful, disabling disease, the treatment of hemophilia is very expensive, and most patients will at some time need support or guidance related to one or more of these problems. AIDS-related psychosocial issues must also be addressed.
   c. **Genetic counseling.** With the increasing availability of gene probe analyses, carrier testing and prenatal diagnosis have become an integral part of the care of the hemophiliac and his family.

B. **von Willebrand's disease,** the most common inherited bleeding disorder, should be considered in the diagnosis of patients with a lifelong history of bruising or excessive bleeding. von Willebrand's disease is now recognized to be a heterogeneous disorder, with variability in the severity of the bleeding manifestations among the different subtypes as well as in the same patient over time.

1. **Physiology of vWF**
   a. **Structure**
      (1) vWF is a high-molecular-weight glycoprotein composed of multimers of a basic subunit (see III B 3 d) with a molecular weight of approximately 250 kilodaltons. The subunit is coded for on chromosome 12.
      (2) vWF is present both in plasma and in platelets. A distribution of multimers of varying size can be visualized by specialized electrophoretic techniques (Figure 14-5).
   b. **Synthesis.** Both endothelial cells and megakaryocytes synthesize vWF by the multistep processing of a precursor molecule. Endothelial cells produce plasma vWF, whereas megakaryocytes appear to be the source of platelet vWF.
   c. **Function.** vWF serves as a carrier protein for coagulation factor VIII. It is also important for

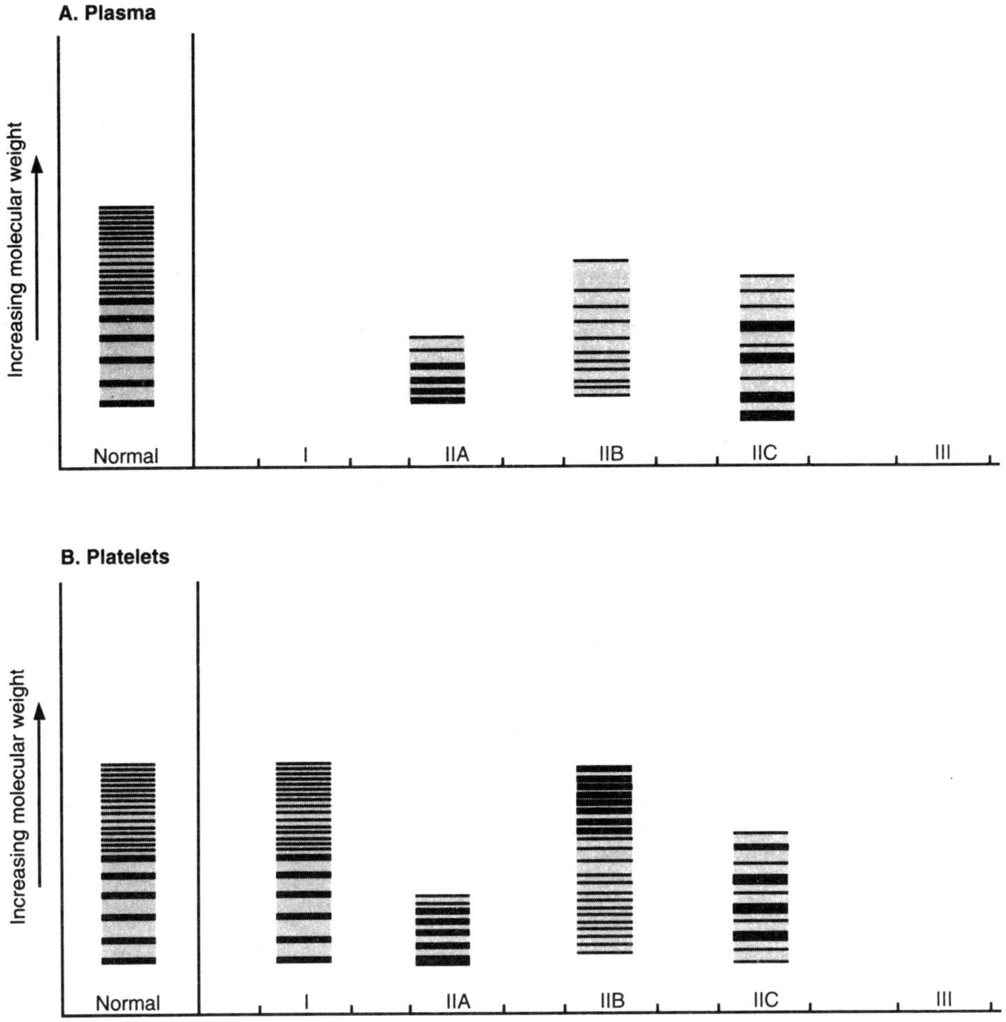

Figure 14-5. Multimeric structure of von Willebrand factor (vWF) in four different variants of von Willebrand's disease, as visualized by electrophoretic techniques. Shown are schematic representations of the multimer distributions (*A*) in plasma and (*B*) in platelets.

primary hemostasis. vWF mediates adhesion of platelets to the subendothelium. This function depends on the binding of vWF to glycoprotein Ib (GP Ib) on the platelet. In addition, some binding to GP IIb-IIIa (the fibrinogen binding site) may also occur (see Ch 13 I A).

d. The vWF–factor VIII complex has until recently been referred to collectively as **"factor VIII,"** and the terminology for various laboratory parameters of this complex can be confusing. The most commonly used terms are defined below.

(1) Factor VIII:C (factor VIII:coagulant) is the plasma factor that is greatly reduced in patients with hemophilia A.

(2) Factor VIII:Ag (factor VIII:antigen; also called **vWF** and **factor VIII:vWF**) is the large, multimeric glycoprotein needed for the adhesion of platelets to the subendothelium. It is the major antigenic determinant of the vWF–factor VIII complex and can be detected by a variety of immunologic assays using heterologous antibodies.

(3) Factor VIII:Cag is the antigenic activity attributable to the VIII:C portion of the vWF–factor VIII complex.

(4) **Factor VIII:RCof** (factor VIII:ristocetin cofactor activity; also called **vWF activity**) is a measure of the ability of vWF in plasma to support ristocetin-induced platelet aggregation.

2. **Clinical features.** Mucous membrane bleeding predominates; epistaxis and menorrhagia are common problems. Except in severe disease, bruising and bleeding are usually mild unless induced by trauma. Because spontaneous bleeding is rare in patients with mild disease, these patients often come to diagnosis only after excessive bleeding has occurred during surgery.

3. **Diagnosis**

a. Classically, the combination of a **prolonged bleeding time and a decreased VIII:C level** is considered the hallmark of von Willebrand's disease. Bleeding time is not a test of vWF alone: It also depends on normal platelet numbers and function. Nonetheless, it is an important screening test of the ability of the patient's vWF to support the platelet-subendothelium interaction at the time of vessel disruption.

b. It is now recognized that any **combination of abnormalities of the functional measures of the vWF–factor VIII complex** may be seen in the many variants of von Willebrand's disease. A common combination of findings is a prolonged bleeding time and a decreased ristocetin cofactor activity (VIII:RCof); but for diagnostic purposes, bleeding time, VIII:C, VIII:Ag, and VIII:RCof tests should all be performed. Rarely is the VIII:C sufficiently low to prolong the PTT, so a **normal coagulation screening profile** does not exclude the diagnosis. The different findings that would be anticipated in von Willebrand's disease and in hemophilia A are summarized in Table 14-2.

c. **Ristocetin aggregation,** the aggregation of platelets by the addition of ristocetin to platelet-rich plasma, requires the presence of adequate amounts of functional vWF in the plasma (see Ch 13 III B 1 c).

(1) In **classic von Willebrand's disease,** ristocetin aggregation is absent or markedly reduced. However, in the **IIB subtype** [see III B 3 d (3) (b)], ristocetin aggregation occurs even at ristocetin doses lower than those inducing aggregation in normal platelet-rich plasma.

(2) This is not a very sensitive test for von Willebrand's disease but can be a useful tool for investigating the possibility of type IIB disease.

d. **Differentiation of subtypes.** Although not widely available, **factor VIII multimer analysis** has proved extremely useful in defining subtypes of von Willebrand's disease (Table 14-3). Ideally, patients with von Willebrand's disease should be typed because of the therapeutic implications of this classification.

(1) **Type I.** The plasma is severely depleted of all multimers, but the platelets from these patients contain all the normal multimers.

(2) **Type IIA.** Both plasma and platelets have decreased amounts of high- and intermediate-molecular-weight multimers.

(3) **Type IIB**

(a) High-molecular-weight multimers are decreased in plasma, but not in platelets, from these patients.

Table 14-2. Laboratory Findings in Hemophilia A and Severe von Willebrand's Disease

	Finding	
Laboratory Test	**Hemophilia A**	**von Willebrand's disease***
Bleeding time	Normal	Prolonged
VIII:C	Decreased	Decreased
VIII:Ag	Normal	Decreased
VIII:RCof	Normal	Decreased

VIII:C = factor VIII:coagulant; VIII:Ag = factor VIII:antigen; VIII:RCof = factor VIII: ristocetin cofactor activity.

*These findings are typical in classic, severe von Willebrand's disease; they could vary in milder disease (see III B 3 d).

Table 14-3. von Willebrand's Disease Classification

	von Willebrand Factor	
Type	**In Plasma**	**In Platelets**
I	↓ All multimers	Normal multimers
IIA	↓ Large and intermediate multimers	↓ Large and intermediate multimers
IIB	↓ Large multimers	Normal multimers
IIC	Abnormal multimers	Abnormal multimers
III	↓ All multimers	↓ All multimers

(b) Platelet-rich plasma is very sensitive to ristocetin; aggregation is induced at ristocetin concentrations lower than the lowest dose that induces normal platelet-rich plasma to aggregate because the abnormal multimers have a higher than normal affinity for platelets. It is this avidity for platelets that results in depletion of the plasma high-molecular-weight multimers.

(4) **Type IIC.** The multimers are evenly distributed but are of an abnormal pattern in both platelets and plasma.

(5) **Type III** (sometimes referred to as **type I severe**). Both plasma and platelets are severely deficient in all the vWF multimers.

4. **Therapy**

a. **dDAVP.** Patients with mild von Willebrand's disease will respond to dDAVP with a several-fold increase in vWF–factor VIII–related activities. This increase represents a relief of stores of the multimers normally made by the patient.

(1) Consequently, patients with **type I** disease respond best, whereas patients with **type III** disease cannot be treated with dDAVP.

(2) Patients with **type II** disease will respond by producing their abnormal multimers. This could be dangerous in the case of **type IIB** disease, since the increased amounts of abnormal multimers would be likely to cause in vivo platelet aggregation.

(3) Ideally, patients with mild disease (except those with type IIB) should be tested for their responsiveness to dDAVP. In those who respond, the increase usually is sufficient to treat bleeding episodes or for expectant treatment before surgery.

b. **Cryoprecipitate.** Because it contains large amounts of vWF, cryoprecipitate has traditionally been the treatment of choice for the patient with severe disease or with type IIB disease. The risks are those outlined in III A 4 b (3) (b).

c. **Factor VIII concentrates.** Some of the newer lyophilized factor VIII concentrates contain some vWF. These are now used in some circumstances because they have undergone extensive purification and viral inactivation and may, therefore, be safer than a fresh product such as cryoprecipitate.

C. Other inherited factor deficiencies

1. **Factor XII, prekallikrein, and high-molecular-weight kininogen.** Deficiencies of these factors result in prolongation of the PTT, but they are not associated with clinical bleeding disorders and are of unknown clinical consequence.

2. **Factors I, II, V, VII, X, XI, and XIII.** Inherited deficiencies of each of these factors have been reported; of these, **factor XI deficiency** is the most common. All are autosomally transmitted and result in bleeding disorders of various severity. Factor XIII deficiency can be particularly subtle as it does not prolong the PT or the PTT screening test but can cause a disorder in which the onset of bleeding is often delayed. Afibrinogenemia or dysfibrinogenemia (factor I abnormalities) can be treated with cryoprecipitate; all the other deficiencies can be treated with FFP.

IV. ACQUIRED HEMORRHAGIC DISORDERS

A. **Vitamin K deficiency.** Vitamin K is a fat-soluble vitamin that is necessary for the functional integrity of factors II (prothrombin), VII, IX, and X (see I B 4). The major source of vitamin K is dietary, especially leafy green vegetables, but some intestinal bacteria also produce a form of vitamin K.

1. **Etiology**
   a. **Dietary deficiency.** Vitamin K reserves can be depleted over a period of several weeks. Such dietary deficiency is not uncommon in chronically ill, severely malnourished patients.
   b. **Malabsorption.** Because vitamin K is fat-soluble, its absorption depends on biliary and pancreatic secretions. Cholestasis, therapy with bile acid–binding resins, or any fat-losing enteropathy can result in malabsorption of vitamin K.
   c. **Antibiotic therapy.** Although the amount of vitamin K that intestinal bacteria normally contribute is unknown, alteration of this flora with broad-spectrum antibiotics appears to enhance the likelihood of development of vitamin K deficiency.
   d. **Vitamin K antagonists.** Oral anticoagulants (e.g., warfarin) act by interfering with the reduction of vitamin K, thus depleting the active form of the vitamin.
   e. **Hemorrhagic disease of the newborn.** Neonates who have not yet been colonized with normal intestinal flora can develop a severe hemorrhagic disorder if their dietary intake of vitamin K is inadequate. This condition is now generally prevented with prophylactic administration of vitamin K.

2. **Clinical features.** Patients may present with severe bruising or excessive bleeding following a surgical procedure, or they may be asymptomatic. Vitamin K deficiency is frequently found as a result of routine screening of coagulation parameters in chronically ill, hospitalized patients.

3. **Diagnosis.** Severe vitamin K deficiency prolongs both the PT and PTT. The PT alone may be prolonged in early or milder deficiencies, such as that induced by administration of therapeutic doses of warfarin.

4. **Therapy**
   a. Parenteral vitamin K therapy should result in normalization of the PT within 12–24 hours, and such a response confirms the etiology of the abnormality.
   b. FFP can be used for immediate replacement of vitamin K–dependent factors, but this is only justified when severe deficiency is accompanied by life-threatening bleeding.

B. **Liver disease.** The coagulopathy associated with liver disease is complex and multifactorial. In addition to the factors discussed below, bleeding may result from or be complicated by thrombocytopenia (see Ch 13 V B 3 b).

1. **Etiology**
   a. **Decreased synthesis of coagulation factors** is the primary cause of coagulation abnormalities in severe liver disease, since all the coagulation factors except vWF are made by hepatocytes.
   b. Cholestatic liver disease can cause **vitamin K deficiency** that may only be distinguished from decreased synthesis of coagulation factors after a successful trial of vitamin K replacement.
   c. **Functionally abnormal fibrinogens** have been described in patients with severe liver disease.
   d. Clearance of activated coagulation factors from the blood by the liver also is impaired in severe liver disease, and the result may be **disseminated intravascular coagulation (DIC)** and consequent **consumption of coagulation factors** (see Ch 15 III A 1).

2. **Clinical features** vary with the course of the patient's liver disease, but, in general, evidence for decreased synthesis of coagulation factors is an ominous prognostic sign. Gastrointestinal bleeding is common in patients with liver disease and often originates from complicating coincident lesions (e.g., esophageal varices). A coexisting coagulopathy of liver disease may make this bleeding extremely difficult to control.

3. **Diagnosis.** Laboratory findings also are variable.
   a. Early in the course of liver disease, the PT is most commonly prolonged, but abnormalities of all the coagulation screening tests can be anticipated in patients with severe disease because the liver synthesizes all coagulation factors except vWF.
   b. These findings may be accompanied by other abnormalities of coagulation such as thrombocytopenia or evidence of fibrinolysis.

4. **Therapy**
   a. Because vitamin K deficiency in liver disease can be hard to distinguish from decreased

synthesis of coagulation factors, an initial **trial of parenteral vitamin K therapy** is appropriate, not only for diagnostic assessment but also for its potential therapeutic benefit if an element of vitamin K deficiency exists.

b. Replacement therapy with FFP can be used in patients who are unresponsive to vitamin K when life-threatening bleeding occurs. Prothrombin complex concentrates, however, should not be used, since they contain activated coagulation factors that cannot be cleared by a seriously diseased liver and, as a result, can initiate DIC.

C. Clotting factor inhibitors are **autoantibodies** (usually IgG) that inactivate coagulation factors and, therefore, act as **anticoagulants**.

1. Inhibitors in hemophilia (see III A 5 b)

2. Inhibitors in patients without preexisting bleeding disorders. Rarely, previously normal individuals develop circulating inhibitors to specific coagulation factors.

a. Etiology. Such inhibitors may be associated with a variety of **drugs,** especially penicillin, sulfonamides, and isoniazid (isonicotinylhydrazine; INH). Anticoagulant antibodies also are seen occasionally in patients with **autoimmune or lymphoproliferative disorders**. **Spontaneous anticoagulants** have also been seen during pregnancy and in previously healthy elderly patients without apparent associated drugs or conditions.

b. Diagnosis. A circulating anticoagulant is confirmed when addition of an equal volume of normal plasma to a patient's plasma (**mixing study**) fails to correct the abnormal coagulation test (PT or PTT). Factor assays can also be performed to determine the specific factor at which the antibody is directed.

c. Therapy is supportive. Any suspect drugs should be discontinued. The usefulness of blood products in the treatment of bleeding episodes depends on the titer and kinetics of the specific antibody; as in hemophilia, blood products that bypass the affected factor may be necessary for bleeding episodes. Treatment with immunosuppressive drugs is of variable success.

3. Lupus anticoagulant. The so-called lupus anticoagulant is an antibody directed against phospholipid, often **cardiolipin** (the antigen used in serologic tests for syphilis), but without factor specificity. Lupus anticoagulant often is seen in patients with autoimmune disease, and its presence may be the only finding suggestive of such a disorder.

a. Laboratory findings include a prolonged PTT and, often, a false–positive serologic test for syphilis.

b. Lupus anticoagulant is associated with recurrent spontaneous abortions, an increased incidence of thrombotic events, but not usually with a bleeding diathesis. It is important to distinguish this inhibitor from one with clotting factor specificity, because a specific clotting factor inhibitor usually results in a serious bleeding diathesis.

STUDY QUESTIONS

Directions: Each of the numbered items or incomplete statements in this section is followed by answers or by completions of the statement. Select the **one** lettered answer or completion that is **best** in each case.

1. When activated, each of the following coagulation factors acts as a serine protease EXCEPT factor

(A) II
(B) VII
(C) VIII
(D) IX
(E) XI

2. Vitamin K is required for synthesis of each of the following coagulation factors EXCEPT factor

(A) II
(B) V
(C) VII
(D) IX
(E) X

3. The likelihood that a son of a patient with severe hemophilia A will have hemophilia is

(A) 0%
(B) 25%
(C) 50%
(D) 75%
(E) 100%

4. Which of the following signs or symptoms would be expected in a patient with a factor VII level of 0.15 U/ml (15%)?

(A) Severe bleeding
(B) Joint deformities
(C) Prolonged PTT
(D) Prolonged PT
(E) Prolonged thrombin time

5. A deficiency of which of the following factors will prolong the PTT and result in a bleeding disorder?

(A) High-molecular-weight kininogen
(B) Prekallikrein
(C) Factor VII
(D) Factor XI
(E) Factor XII

6. Twenty-four hours after a 10-mg dose of warfarin, a patient has a PT of 1.25 times the control. A decrease in the function of which of the following factors is most likely to produce this finding?

(A) II
(B) VII
(C) IX
(D) X

7. A 17-year-old patient with well-documented hemophilia A has a factor VIII level of 15% of normal. The patient was diagnosed because of a positive family history but has never required treatment. He is scheduled to have a wisdom tooth extracted. The treatment of choice is

(A) fresh frozen plasma (FFP)
(B) cryoprecipitate
(C) factor VIII concentrate
(D) desmopressin (dDAVP)
(E) no treatment

8. A woman with a prolonged bleeding time and a factor VIII:C level of 0.35 U/ml (35%) is scheduled for breast biopsy and possible mastectomy. Multimer analysis of factor VIII is not done by the hospital laboratory, and results from a referral laboratory could take several months. Which of the following tests would be most useful in helping to make a recommendation for the treatment of excessive bleeding?

(A) VIII:RCof
(B) Ristocetin aggregation (low and high titer)
(C) VIII:Ag
(D) PTT
(E) Platelet aggregation with adenosine diphosphate (ADP)

1-C	4-D	7-D
2-B	5-D	8-B
3-A	6-B	

Questions 9–10

A hematologist is asked to see a 52-year-old man who has been hospitalized for 6 weeks because of various complications beginning with a bowel obstruction. The patient has had several operative procedures, one of which required transfusion of 3 units of packed red cells. He has been unable to eat and has been receiving broad-spectrum antibiotics almost continuously. Recently performed tests show a prolonged PT and PTT, which were corrected when the patient's plasma was mixed with an equal volume of normal plasma. Quantitative fibrinogen, thrombin time, and platelet count all are normal.

9. The most likely cause of the coagulation abnormality is

(A) an acquired inhibitor
(B) dilution of coagulation factors secondary to transfusions
(C) vitamin K deficiency
(D) folate deficiency
(E) von Willebrand's disease

10. If the patient is not actually bleeding, which of the following therapeutic measures would be best?

(A) Watch and wait
(B) Give fresh frozen plasma (FFP)
(C) Give parenteral vitamin K
(D) Give cryoprecipitate
(E) Discontinue the antibiotics

Directions: The group of items in this section consists of lettered options followed by a set of numbered items. For each item, select the **one** lettered option that is most closely associated with it. Each lettered option may be selected once, more than once, or not at all.

Questions 11–12

For each set of laboratory findings listed below, select the disorder that is most likely to be associated with them.

(A) von Willebrand's disease
(B) Severe liver disease
(C) Factor VIII deficiency
(D) Factor IX deficiency

11. Normal PT, normal PTT, prolonged bleeding time

12. Prolonged PT, prolonged PTT, normal bleeding time

9-C
10-C
11-A
12-B

ANSWERS AND EXPLANATIONS

1. The answer is C *[I C 2 d; Table 14-1].*
Activated factor VIII does not act as a serine protease. It is a cofactor that forms a catalytic complex with factor IXa to activate factor X. Factors II (prothrombin), VII, IX, and XI are glycoproteins that exist in inactive, pre-enzymatic forms (zymogens) and must undergo catalytic activation to serine proteases in order to participate in coagulation.

2. The answer is B *[I B 4, C 4 b; Table 14-1].*
Vitamin K is not required for synthesis of factor V, a cofactor to factor Xa in the common pathway of the coagulation cascade. Factors II, VII, IX, and X all must bind calcium ion (Ca^{2+}) via γ-carboxyglutamic acid residues in order to function. It is the γ-carboxylation of glutamic acid that is dependent on vitamin K. In the absence of vitamin K, these factors are formed but are inactive because their glutamic acid residues have not undergone this γ-carboxylation.

3. The answer is A *[III A 1; Figure 14-4].*
The son of a hemophilia patient cannot be a hemophiliac. Hemophilia A results from a deficiency of factor VIII, which is coded for on the X chromosome. Since a male offspring would have received only the Y chromosome from his father, the genetic defect would not be transmitted.

4. The answer is D *[I C 3 b; II A 2; IV A].*
Decreased levels of factor VII seldom result in symptomatic bleeding but will, at the level described (0.15 U/ml), prolong the prothrombin time (PT). This apparent lack of anticoagulation in the face of decreased factor VII is an important observation that should be kept in mind when evaluating the anticoagulant effect of warfarin-type vitamin K antagonists.

5. The answer is D *[II A 1; III A, C 1, 2; IV A].*
The partial thromboplastin time (PTT) can be prolonged by a deficiency of factor XII, factor XI, high-molecular-weight kininogen, or prekallikrein, but of these, only factor XI deficiency is associated with a bleeding disorder. Factor VII deficiency does not prolong the PTT, which measures only factors of the intrinsic and common pathways.

6. The answer is B *[II A 2; IV A 1 d; Table 14-1].*
Warfarin inhibits the vitamin K–dependent γ-carboxylation that is necessary for the functional activity of factors II, VII, IX, and X. However, these factors have very different half-lives. Factor VII has by far the shortest half-life, only about 6 hours. As a result, by 24 hours (5 or 6 half-lives after the action of vitamin K has been inhibited), factor VII will be functionally inactive. The other factors will not be significantly decreased, because they have longer life spans: not much more than one of their half-lives will have expired in the 24 hours since the administration of warfarin.

7. The answer is D *[III A 4 a (1)].*
This patient is an ideal candidate for pharmacologic treatment of his hemophilia: His factor VIII level is relatively high, and the increase that would be anticipated with desmopressin (1-desamino-8-D-arginine vasopressin; dDAVP) should be adequate for his scheduled procedure. A dental extraction without treatment in this patient would inevitably be followed by bleeding that would require treatment. Transfusion with blood products should be avoided whenever possible because of the risks of hepatitis and human immunodeficiency virus (HIV) transmission as well as such lesser risks as allergic reactions.

8. The answer is B *[III B 3 c].*
This patient might be a candidate for treatment with desmopressin (dDAVP), but before it is tried, the possibility of type IIB von Willebrand's disease should be excluded. Platelets in the plasma from patients with this variant will aggregate at lower than normal concentrations of ristocetin. If the patient does have the type IIB variant, dDAVP should not be used because it might stimulate in vivo aggregation. This very specific functional abnormality is not reflected in the other measures of von Willebrand factor (vWF), such as ristocetin cofactor activity (VIII:RCof) or antigenic level (VIII:Ag), or by its ability to stabilize factor VIII [indirectly measured by the partial thromboplastin time (PTT)]. Platelet aggregation with adenosine diphosphate (ADP) would not be affected by von Willebrand's disease.

9–10. The answers are: 9-C *[IV A 1 a, c, 3],* **10-C** *[IV A 4].*
This patient's coagulation abnormality most likely is the result of vitamin K deficiency. A prolonged pe-

riod of malnutrition with administration of broad-spectrum antibiotics is a common combination that frequently results in vitamin K deficiency. Correction of the prothrombin time (PT) and partial thromboplastin time (PTT) in the mixing test excludes the possibility of an acquired inhibitor. Coagulation factors would not have been diluted by the transfusion of 3 units of packed red cells; only massive transfusions might cause this effect. Folate deficiency is not associated with abnormalities of the coagulation cascade, and von Willebrand's disease does not affect the PT.

Replenishment of vitamin K is simple and without significant adverse effects, and it usually normalizes the PT within 12–24 hours. Although the patient is not bleeding, he is at increased risk for bleeding, and so treatment is justified. Fresh frozen plasma (FFP) and cryoprecipitate carry significant risks, and cryoprecipitation does not concentrate the necessary factors. A decision to discontinue the antibiotics must be based on the patient's infection; discontinuation would do little acutely to alter the established deficiency.

11–12. The answers are: 11-A *[III B 3 b]*, **12-B** *[IV B 3]*.

Factor VII deficiency is most likely to be associated with prolonged prothrombin time (PT), normal partial thromboplastin time (PTT), and normal bleeding time. The PT measures the extrinsic coagulation system, whereas the PTT measures the intrinsic coagulation system. Factor VII participates in the extrinsic system but not in the intrinsic system. Therefore, a deficiency of factor VII would be expected to cause a prolongation of the PT but not the PTT. The bleeding time is a measure of platelet function and is unaffected by an isolated deficiency of factor VII.

von Willebrand's disease results from an abnormality of von Willebrand factor (vWF), which is necessary to support platelet adhesion. The bleeding time is an in vivo measure of the ability of platelets to adhere to and form a platelet plug at the site of interrupted blood vessels, and bleeding time is frequently prolonged in von Willebrand's disease. vWF is also necessary for the stabilization of factor VIII, and factor VIII coagulant activity, therefore, may be low enough to prolong the PTT in some patients with von Willebrand's disease; however, more frequently the PTT is normal. Because vWF does not participate in the extrinsic system, the PT is normal in patients with von Willebrand's disease.

Most of the coagulation factors are manufactured in the liver; consequently, severe liver disease can result in abnormalities of both the intrinsic system (measured by the PTT) and the extrinsic system (measured by the PT). These abnormalities do not, however, necessarily affect platelet function, which is measured by the bleeding time. Unless the patient is also thrombocytopenic, the bleeding time would be expected to be normal.

15
Coagulation Regulation and Hypercoagulable States

Patricia M. Catalano

I. CONTROL MECHANISMS IN COAGULATION. Soon after coagulation is initiated, several regulatory mechanisms are activated, which ultimately inhibit coagulation. If left unchecked, the autoamplification mechanisms of coagulation would result in generalized thrombosis.

A. Naturally occurring anticoagulants

1. **Antithrombin III (AT III)** currently is regarded as the most important physiologic inhibitor of coagulation. AT III is a plasma protein that acts as a serine protease inhibitor.
   a. **Activation.** Although AT III inherently can inhibit the enzymatic activity of serine protease coagulation factors, the presence of **heparin** increases this ability as much as 1000-fold. (This is the predominant mechanism by which heparin acts as an anticoagulant.)
      (1) Rather than true activation, heparin's effect on AT III is more accurately regarded as **enhancement of preexisting activity**. Binding of heparin to AT III induces a conformational change that renders the serine protease inactivating site on AT III more accessible to its substrates, thus accelerating the rate of inactivation.
      (2) This effect can be seen in vitro and when heparin is administered therapeutically. In vivo, however, heparin does not naturally exist in plasma, which suggests that a heparin-like substance is responsible for enhancing the anticoagulant activity of AT III. This substance has been identified on the surface of endothelial cells and is called **heparan sulfate** (Figure 15-1).
   b. **Sites of action.** AT III can inhibit many serine protease enzymes (e.g., thrombin and factors Xa, IXa, and XIa) by forming one-to-one inactive complexes with them (see Figure 15-1); however, thrombin's central role in coagulation makes this the most critical site of inactivation.

2. **Protein C** is the inactive precursor form of the anticoagulant, **protein Ca,** which is a serine protease that acts on specific clotting factors in the presence of the cofactor **protein S**. Both protein C and protein S are vitamin K–dependent. About 40% of circulating protein S is free to act as a cofactor for protein C; the remaining 60% circulates in an inactive complex with complement component C4b.
   a. **Activation** of protein C requires **thrombin** and **thrombomodulin,** a protein receptor found on the surface of endothelial cells, and occurs by cleavage of a small activation peptide from the heavy chain of protein C. Interaction of thrombin and thrombomodulin causes a conformational change that greatly enhances thrombin's effect on protein C and inhibits its effects on fibrinogen and platelets (Figure 15-2).
   b. **Sites of action**
      (1) **Coagulation.** In the presence of phospholipid and with protein S as cofactor, protein Ca cleaves and inactivates factors Va and VIIIa, effectively disrupting the coagulation pathways.
      (2) **Fibrinolysis.** With protein S as cofactor, protein Ca enhances fibrinolysis by preventing the degradation of plasminogen activator by its inhibitors.
   c. **Inactivation.** Protein Ca activity is limited by another protein, **protein C inhibitor**.

3. **Other plasma protease inhibitors** exist, but their relative importance is unknown. These include:
   a. **Heparin cofactor II,** a heparin-activated protease inhibitor that acts on thrombin but not on factor Xa
   b. **α_2-Macroglobulin,** which inhibits thrombin and various other proteases

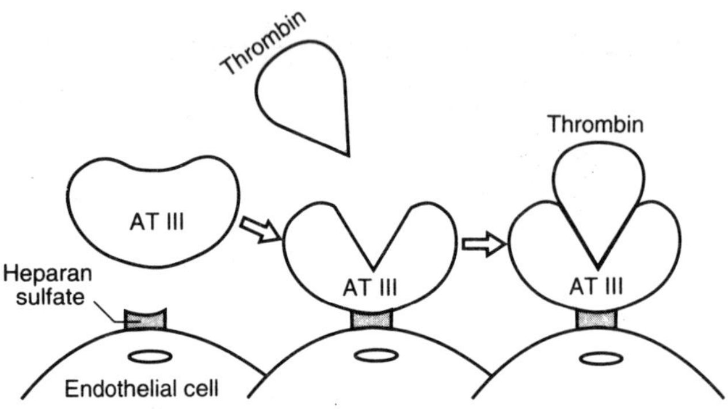

Figure 15-1. Antithrombin III (*AT III*) circulates in a form that is capable of inactivating serine proteases (e.g., thrombin, factor Xa). Binding of heparin or heparin-like substances (e.g., heparan sulfate) to AT III causes a conformational change in AT III, which greatly enhances its ability to bind to and inactivate serine proteases. Once these inactive complexes are formed, the affinity of the heparin or heparin-like substance for AT III decreases, making dissociation possible.

B. Fibrinolytic system. The body's system for dissolution of clots has similarities to the coagulation mechanism. In this system, the inactive precursor **plasminogen** is converted to **plasmin,** a serine protease with specific fibrinolytic activity. Unique structural features of plasminogen are shown in Figure 15-3A.

1. **Activation.** Inactive plasminogen is converted to plasmin when a plasminogen activator cleaves an arginine–valine bond between the heavy and light chains of the molecule, leaving the chains linked by a single disulfide bond (see Figure 15-3B). There are three mechanisms of activation and several plasminogen activators.
   a. **Intrinsic activation.** A poorly understood mechanism of activation appears to be related to the intrinsic system of coagulation. Specifically, plasmin appears to be generated as the result of contact activation, but it is not known which factor (or factors) is responsible.
   b. **Extrinsic activation**
      (1) **Tissue plasminogen activator (t-PA)** is a serine protease that is synthesized in endothelial cells and released in response to a variety of stimuli. t-PA has a high-affinity fibrin-binding site, and its activation of plasminogen is significantly enhanced by the presence of fibrin.
      (2) **Urokinase** is another serine protease that converts plasminogen to plasmin. It is normally found in urine, where it is believed to be important for thrombolysis in the collecting systems. Unlike t-PA, urokinase does not bind to fibrin, and fibrin does not enhance its activity.
   c. **Exogenous (therapeutic) activation**
      (1) **Streptokinase** does not by itself activate plasminogen, but it forms a one-to-one complex with plasminogen, which then activates other plasminogen molecules. As with urokinase, this process is not enhanced by the presence of fibrin.
      (2) **Urokinase and t-PA** may be administered therapeutically and, in this setting, are regarded as exogenous activators.

2. **Sites of action.** Although capable of degrading a variety of proteins, under physiologic conditions plasmin acts primarily on fibrin. In conditions of enhanced plasmin activity, fibrinogen also is degraded. Plasmin's effect on fibrinogen will be considered first.
   a. **Fibrinogen** degradation by plasmin (Figure 15-4) proceeds as follows.
      (1) First, plasmin removes a segment of the carboxy terminal ends of the Aα chain.
      (2) Next, a fragment from the amino terminal portion of the Bβ chain, the **Bβ 1–42 fragment,** is released. The remaining portion of the fibrinogen molecule is called **fragment X**.
      (3) Next, all three chains on one side of the molecule are split, resulting in **fragment Y** and **fragment D**.
      (4) Finally, fragment Y is lysed to form another fragment D plus **fragment E,** which is formed from the remains of the disulfide-linked core of the fibrinogen molecule.
   b. **Fibrin** degradation by plasmin (Figure 15-5) is essentially identical to that described for fibrinogen, with the following exceptions.
      (1) The rate of degradation is slower due to the resistance conferred by fibrin's extensive cross-link bonds.
      (2) The fragment cleaved from the amino terminal portion of the Bβ chain is the **Bβ 15–42 fragment**.
      (3) The end products are dimers or trimers of the fragments that result from fibrinogenolysis, because, although lysis occurs at the same points, the covalent and noncovalent

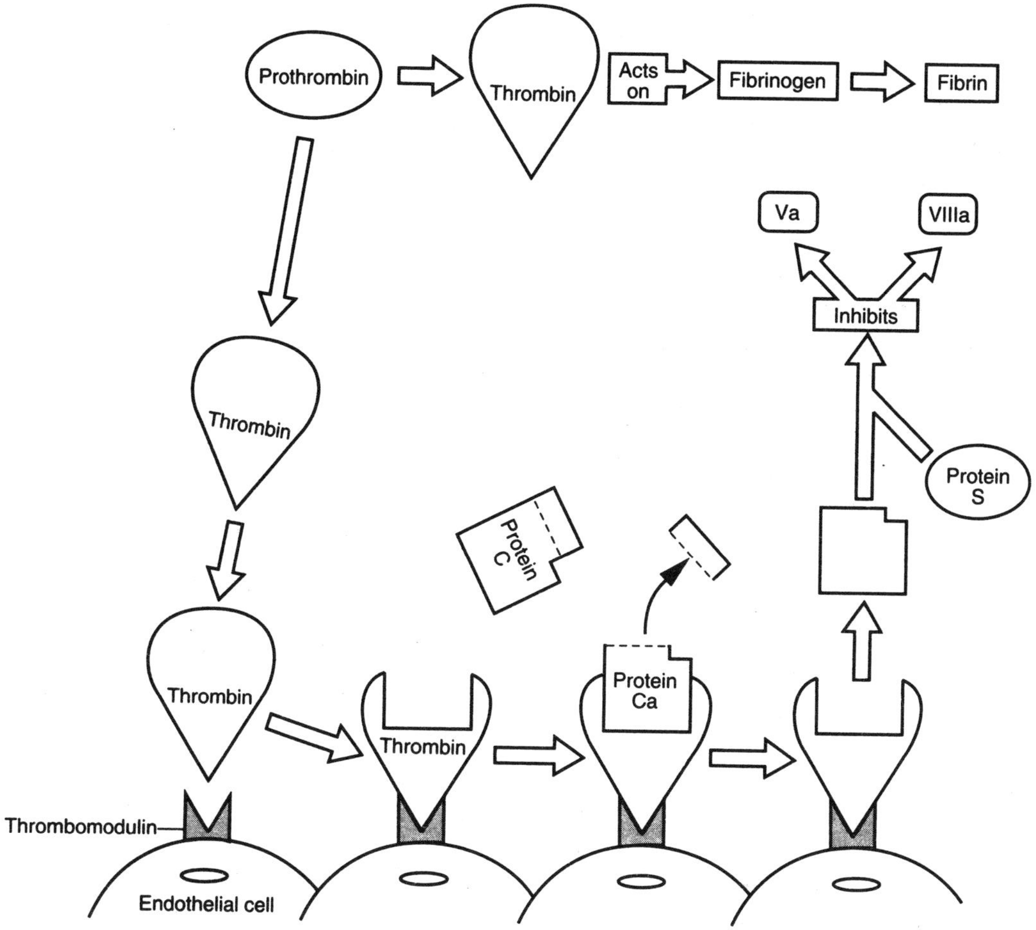

Figure 15-2. Thrombin has multiple effects on coagulation. When complexed with thrombomodulin, thrombin undergoes a conformational change that enhances its ability to activate protein C. In the presence of free protein S, activated protein C (*protein Ca*) inhibits coagulation by acting on factors Va and VIIIa. Without the conformational change, thrombin is able to act on fibrinogen to cause formation of a fibrin clot.

bonds that result from polymerization and the cross-linking action of factor XIII are maintained. Fibrin split products (FSPs) generated include **DD dimers** as well as **DD/E, YD/DY, and other fragments**.

c. **Inactivation.** Plasmin is inactivated when the protein, **α_2-antiplasmin,** binds to the active site of the light chain of plasmin, forming a one-to-one complex. The efficiency of this system is believed to be enhanced by α_2-antiplasmin's ability to cross-link with fibrin through the action of factor XIII.

II. THROMBOTIC DISORDERS

A. **Congenital thrombotic disorders.** Inherited abnormalities that predispose to thrombosis must be considered in patients who experience thromboembolic disease, especially if they are young, do not have other predisposing risk factors, or suffer from recurrent thrombosis.

1. **AT III deficiency** is an autosomal dominant disorder with an estimated prevalence of 1 in 2000 individuals.

   a. **Clinical features**

      (1) **Thrombosis.** Studies suggest that more than 50% of patients identified as AT III deficient experience at least one thromboembolic event.

         (a) Symptoms usually appear in the second or third decade, with venous thrombosis of the lower extremities the most common manifestation. Mesenteric thrombosis and upper extremity events may also occur.

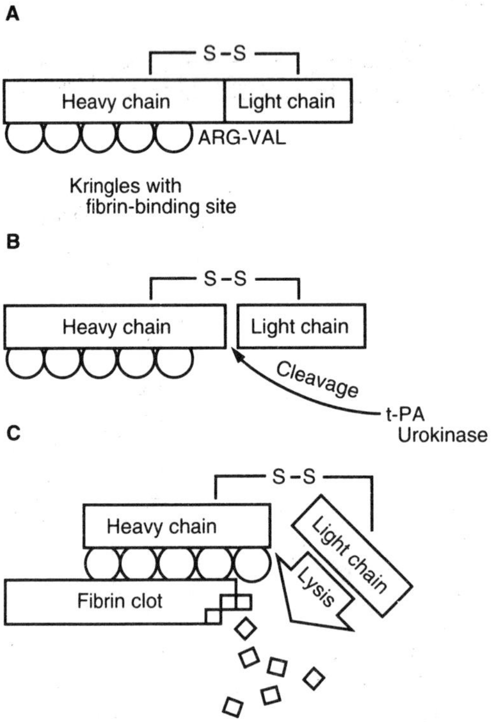

Figure 15-3. (*A*) Plasminogen is a single-chain glycoprotein composed of a heavy and a light chain. The heavy chain portion contains five kringle structures with lysin-binding sites that enable the molecule to bind fibrin. (*B*) Inactive plasminogen is converted to plasmin by cleavage of an arginine–valine (*ARG–VAL*) bond between the heavy and light chains. (*C*) Binding to fibrin occurs on the heavy chain, and fibrinolytic activity is localized on the light chain. *t-PA* = tissue plasminogen activator.

(b) Many patients have no obvious precipitating cause for thrombosis, but the first event sometimes is seen during pregnancy or after surgery.

(2) Heparin resistance. Because heparin's anticoagulant effect depends on AT III, heparin resistance may occur in patients with severe AT III deficiency.

b. Diagnosis

(1) The functional level of AT III should be measured, as a decrease is pathognomonic. In some individuals, quantitative levels of AT III are normal while functional levels are low; thus, measurement of functional levels is imperative.

(2) Measurement of AT III levels during a thrombotic event can be misleading; AT III levels may be decreased during the event and may also drop with heparin therapy. Warfarin therapy is associated with increases in AT III levels. Thus, patients in whom AT III deficiency is suspected should ideally be studied when they are well and not receiving treatment.

c. Therapy for acute events is the same as for any thromboembolic event (i.e., acute treatment with heparin followed by long-term warfarin therapy). Severely deficient patients may be resistant to heparin and, so, may benefit from fresh frozen plasma (FFP), which is a source of AT III. AT III concentrates also are available now and are potentially most useful for support in situations when anticoagulation would not be appropriate (e.g., surgery).

2. Protein C deficiency. This autosomal dominant disorder may be the most common of the inherited thrombotic abnormalities. An estimated 1 in 300 individuals are heterozygous for protein C deficiency.

a. Clinical features. Protein C deficiency is associated with three distinct clinical syndromes.

(1) Thromboembolic disease. As in AT III deficiency, thromboembolic events without obvious risk factors begin in early adulthood. Although there is no heparin resistance, administration of warfarin alone might initially worsen the disorder because protein C is vitamin K–dependent and has a relatively short half-life.

(2) Warfarin-induced necrosis is a syndrome characterized by extensive necrosis of the skin, especially over fatty areas (e.g., breasts, abdomen), 3–8 days after initiation of warfarin treatment. It is the result of extensive thrombosis of the veins and capillary blood supply to the skin, presumably due to further decreases in protein C in response to the warfarin. It is not known why the skin is the target for this syndrome.

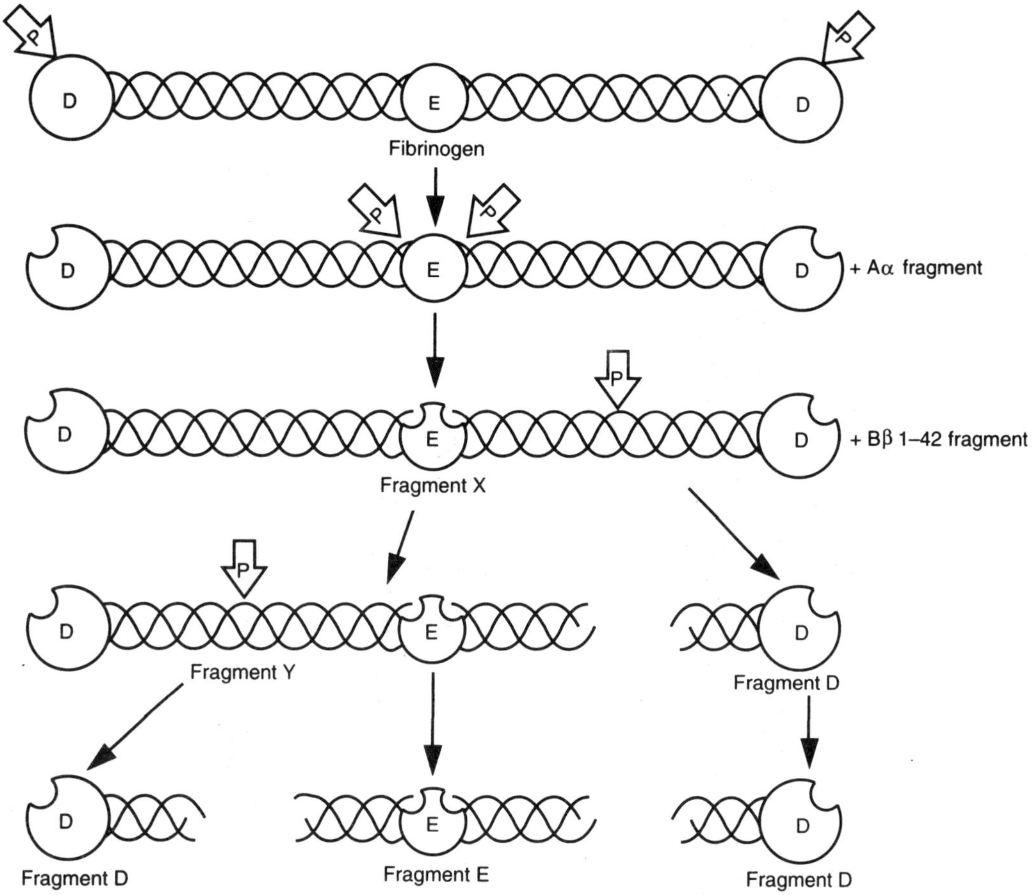

Figure 15-4. Fibrinogenolysis begins with plasmin-mediated degradation of a segment of the carboxy terminal ends of the Aα chain and release of the Bβ 1–42 fragment of the amino terminal end of the Bβ chain, which forms fragment X. Next, the coils between the E and D domains are cleaved; fragments Y and D are formed first, and then fragment Y is cleaved to form another fragment D and fragment E. *P* = plasmin; *E* = E domain; *D* = D domain.

(3) **Purpura fulminans neonatalis** is a potentially fatal condition characterized by the development of skin necrosis and systemic thrombosis in newborns homozygous for protein C deficiency. Not all homozygous individuals develop the syndrome; however, additional factors predisposing to its development are unknown.

b. **Diagnosis.** A decreased functional level of protein C is diagnostic. Vitamin K antagonists decrease the protein C level, so the measurement must be obtained when a patient is not receiving such treatment.

c. **Therapy.** Acute events are readily managed with heparin. Long-term warfarin therapy appears to be effective but must be begun while the patient is receiving heparin and must be closely monitored. Treatment of purpura fulminans neonatalis with a purified protein C concentrate has also been reported recently.

3. **Protein S deficiency**

a. **Clinical features** are similar to those of protein C deficiency and AT III deficiency. Affected individuals are predisposed to recurrent thromboembolic disease that begins relatively early in life.

b. **Diagnosis**

(1) Measurement of **free protein S activity** probably is the most clinically relevant test but may not be readily available.

(2) The more usual test measures **total protein S antigen**. When interpreting results of this test, it is important to keep in mind that normally 60% of circulating protein S is bound to C4b and, thus, is inactive; conditions that increase C4b may further decrease the

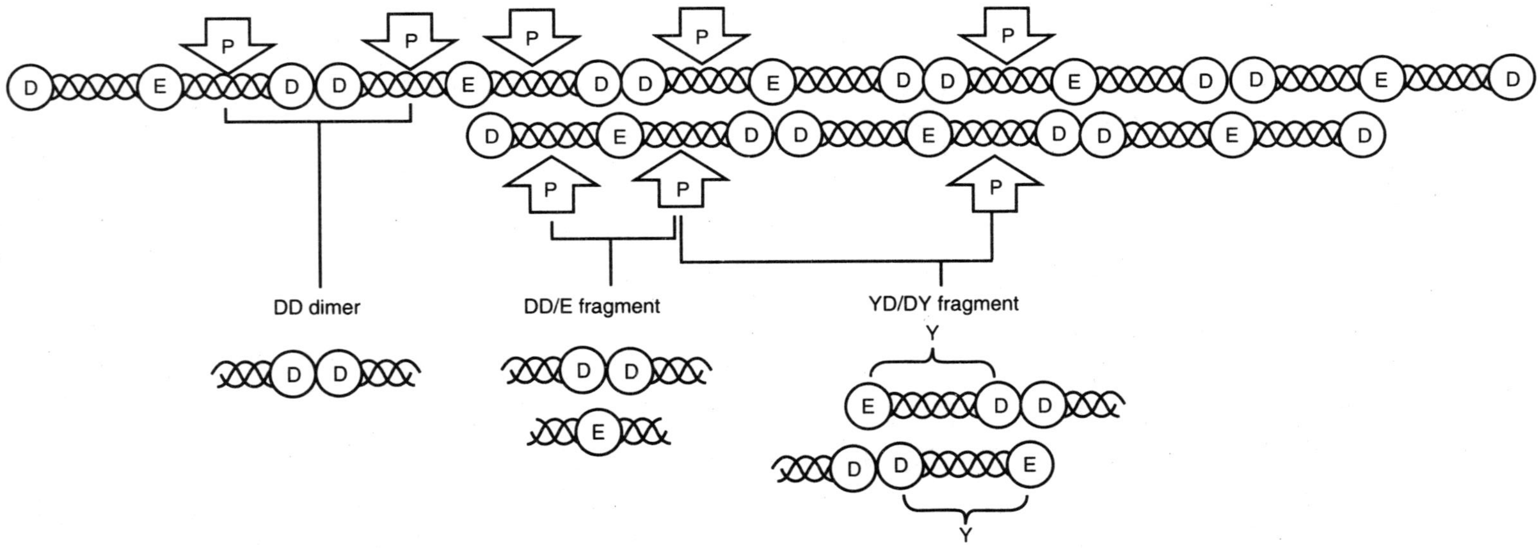

Figure 15-5. Fibrinolysis is similar to fibrinogenolysis, except that the covalent and noncovalent bonds resulting from fibrin polymerization and stabilization persist in fibrinolysis. As a consequence, the fragments formed in fibrinolysis are dimers and trimers of those formed in fibrinogenolysis. *P* = plasmin; *E* = E domain; *D* = D domain.

amount of functionally available protein C and, thus, may predispose to an acute thrombotic event. Unfortunately, functional assays of protein S activity are not commercially available.

c. **Therapy** is the same as for protein S deficiency. As with protein C, protein S is vitamin K–dependent, and vitamin K antagonists given alone may initially worsen the condition.

4. **Other.** Inherited abnormalities of plasminogen, fibrinogen, and other plasma proteins have also been reported to be associated with thrombotic disorders, but they appear to be much less frequent than the disorders discussed above.

B. **Acquired thrombotic disorders. Thromboembolic disease** is common even in patients without congenital deficiencies that predispose to these clinical problems.

1. **Risk factors** for the development of pathologic thrombosis can be grouped into abnormalities of blood flow, of the vasculature, or of coagulation. Important examples of clinical risk factors for thrombosis are noted here and in Table 15-1.
   a. **Abnormalities of blood flow.** A common predisposing factor is **stasis,** which can be localized or generalized. Generalized stasis can result from **prolonged bed rest;** localized stasis can result when blood flow from the extremities is compromised by pressure from an **intra-abdominal mass**. Intracardiac thrombi can result from a variety of conditions that alter flow (e.g., atrial fibrillation, aneurysms).
   b. **Abnormalities of the vasculature.** An important predisposing factor for arterial thrombosis is **atherosclerosis**.
   c. **Abnormalities of the coagulation system.** Factors that limit coagulation may be decreased in various conditions, and these deficiencies are believed to predispose to thrombosis. For example, **liver disease** is associated with decreased synthesis of the natural anticoagulants, and protein S may be depleted in the **nephrotic syndrome**.

2. **Pathophysiology** of thrombosis encompasses all of the elements of the coagulation system, regardless of the precipitating cause (Figure 15-6).
   a. The process begins at the endothelial cell and the subendothelium, where platelets adhere and undergo aggregation and release, and the coagulation cascade is initiated.
   b. A fibrin clot is formed, and the mechanisms that normally limit thrombosis are activated, as is the fibrinolytic pathway.
   c. A pathologic thrombus forms as a result of imbalances among coagulant, anticoagulant, and fibrinolytic processes. Once formed, all or part of the thrombus can embolize.

3. **Clinical manifestations.** Thrombosis can occur in any vessel, and the manifestations vary with location. Some of the most common clinical conditions resulting from pathologic thrombosis are the following.
   a. **Venous thrombosis** can be superficial or deep and most commonly affects the lower extremities.
      (1) **Superficial thrombosis** usually is accompanied by obvious signs of inflammation.

Table 15-1. Risk Factors for Thrombosis

Abnormal blood flow	**Abnormal coagulation**
Congenital risk factors	Congenital risk factors
Sickle cell disease	Antithrombin III (AT III) deficiency
Acquired risk factors	Protein C deficiency
Congestive heart failure	Protein S deficiency
Obesity	Acquired risk factors
Hyperviscosity	Malignancy
Abnormal vasculature	Nephrotic syndrome
Congenital risk factors	Lupus anticoagulants
Hyperlipidemia	Trauma
Acquired risk factors	
Atherosclerosis	
Hyperlipidemia	
Diabetes mellitus	
Estrogen therapy	
Prosthetic valves or vasculature	

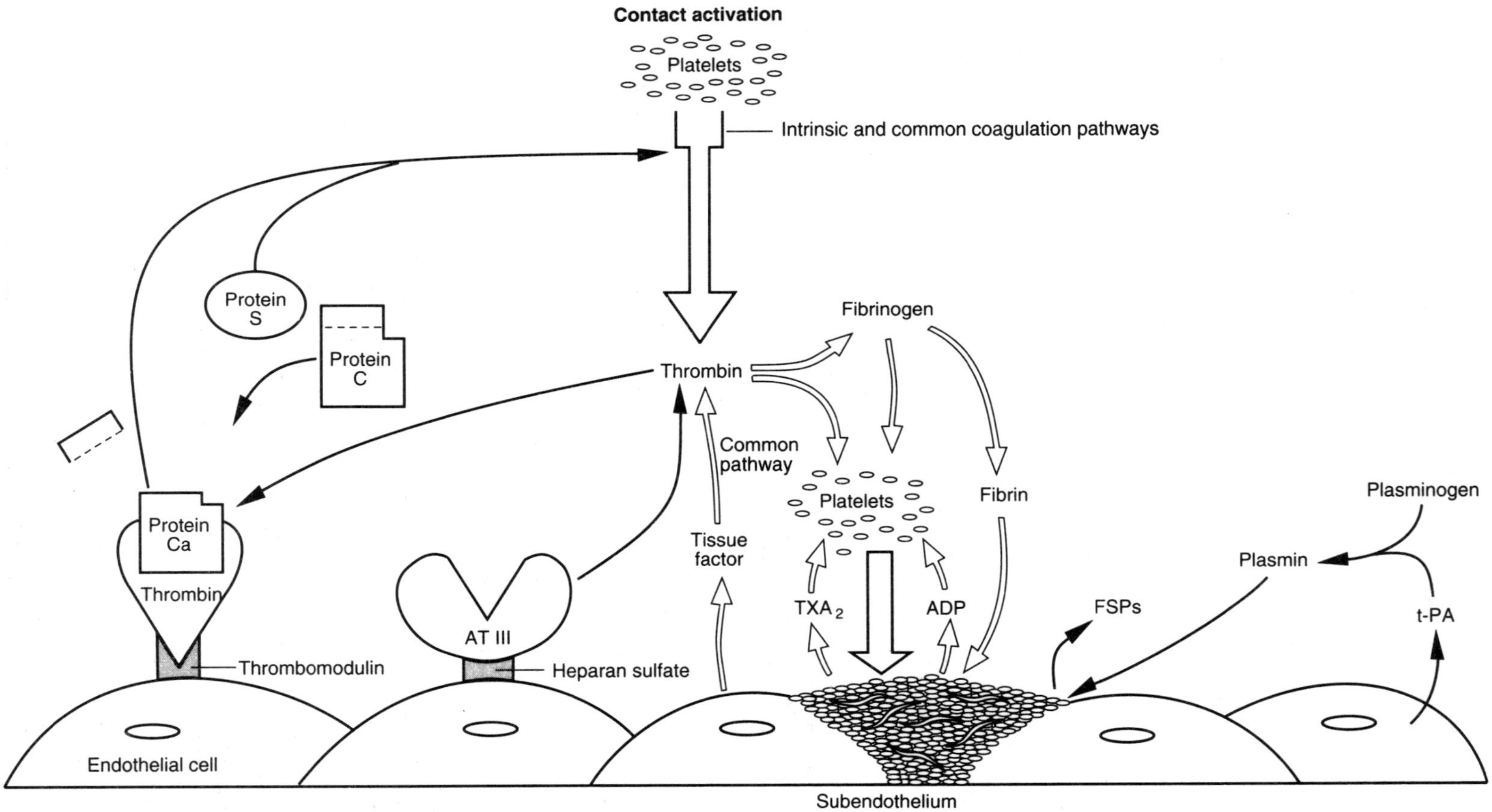

Figure 15-6. **The extent of thrombosis is determined** by the balance **among coagulant, anticoagulant, and fibrinolytic mechanisms.** The process begins with platelet adherence and aggregation **at the subendothelium. Platelet-produced adenosine diphosphate** (*ADP*) **and thromboxane** A_2 (*TXA_2*) stimulate further aggregation, and the coagulation system is activated, **resulting in fibrin deposition. The multiple positive feedback mechanisms, often mediated by thrombin,** would result in massive thrombosis in the absence of antithrombin III (*AT III*) **and the protein C–protein S** system, which **effectively inhibit coagulation at steps in the common pathway** (whether initiated through the intrinsic or extrinsic pathway). **Plasmin-mediated fibrinolysis acts** to dissolve **the thrombus once fibrin has been deposited.** *FSPs* = fibrin split products; *t-PA* = tissue plasminogen activator; *open arrows* = pathways that lead to clot formation; *closed arrows* = pathways that diminish clot formation.

(2) **Deep venous thrombosis,** or thrombosis of large vessels (e.g., femoral or iliac veins), can be more subtle but actually is more dangerous; it is from these large thrombi that life-threatening emboli arise.

b. Pulmonary embolism is the most threatening complication of venous thrombosis. It results when a fragment of thrombus breaks loose, travels up the inferior vena cava into the heart, and ultimately lodges in the lungs. Small emboli can be asymptomatic, and large ones can be fatal.

c. Arterial thrombosis. Thrombosis can occur in coronary, peripheral, cerebral, and mesenteric arteries, most often in the setting of atherosclerotic vascular lesions.

d. Other. Clinically important thrombi also occur in association with cardiac valve abnormalities, rhythm disturbances, vascular prostheses, and a variety of other conditions.

4. Therapy

a. Agents used in treatment and prevention of thrombotic disorders include anticoagulants (heparin, warfarin) as well as thrombolytic agents (streptokinase, urokinase, t-PA). As in congenital thrombotic disorders, heparin is the mainstay of treatment for acute thrombotic events, and warfarin is used for long-term therapy. In low doses, heparin provides prophylaxis when prolonged stasis is anticipated.

(1) Anticoagulants

(a) Heparin is a large polysaccharide molecule derived from bovine lung or porcine intestine. It is the mainstay of treatment for acute thrombotic events.

(i) Mechanism of action. Heparin binds to AT III, markedly enhancing its ability to inactivate serine proteases, especially thrombin. The immediate anticoagulation that results limits further clot formation.

(ii) Monitoring. Therapy is monitored using the partial thromboplastin time (PTT).

(iii) Adverse effects. Bleeding and **heparin-induced thrombocytopenia** are the major adverse effects of heparin treatment.

(b) Warfarin is used for long-term therapy, since it can be given orally and stable anticoagulant effects can be maintained for long periods of time.

(i) Mechanism of action. Warfarin inhibits the reduction of oxidized vitamin K, causing relative vitamin K deficiency; thus, its anticoagulant effect depends on depletion of functionally normal vitamin K–dependent factors (i.e., II, VII, IX, and X).

(ii) Administration and monitoring. Warfarin usually is begun while a patient is receiving heparin, with about a 3-day overlap of therapies. The dose of warfarin is adjusted by monitoring the prothrombin time (PT). Many drugs interfere with warfarin, either increasing or decreasing its effects; therefore, patients must be monitored closely when new drugs are added.

(iii) Adverse effects. Bleeding is the most common complication. **Fetal anomalies** also have been described; thus, warfarin therapy should be avoided in pregnancy. **Warfarin-induced necrosis** is a rare complication of therapy in patients with protein C deficiency [see II A 2 a (2)].

(2) Thrombolytic agents are the treatment of choice in many clinical situations, owing to the recent development of recombinant t-PA and to increasing experience with the use of streptokinase and urokinase.

(a) Commonly used agents. A variety of thrombolytic agents are available or under development. The most frequently used include the following.

(i) Streptokinase is a bacterial protein derived from group C β-hemolytic streptococci, which acts indirectly on plasminogen. Streptokinase and plasminogen form a one-to-one complex, which then converts other plasminogen to plasmin. Because it is highly antigenic, streptokinase has limited usefulness in some patients.

(ii) Urokinase is produced from human renal cell cultures and is rarely antigenic. It acts directly on plasminogen, converting it to plasmin. A new, single-chain urokinase preparation appears to have greater activity toward fibrin-bound plasminogen than toward free plasminogen.

(iii) t-PA is a recombinant product that has the theoretical advantage of enhanced activity toward fibrin-bound plasminogen.

(b) Administration and monitoring

(i) Thrombolytic agents are given intravenously. Heparin therapy usually is begun immediately after thrombolytic therapy is discontinued.

(ii) No laboratory tests are useful for predicting the risk of bleeding. A documented decrease in fibrinogen is adequate confirmation that a lytic state has been induced.

(c) Contraindications

(i) **Conditions that predispose to bleeding** are the major contraindications to thrombolytic therapy. The most important of these is evidence of a recent cerebrovascular accident.

(ii) **Other significant contraindications** include recent surgery, trauma, gastrointestinal bleeding, coagulopathies, and neoplasms.

(d) Complications. The most important complication of thrombolytic therapy is **bleeding**. Severe bleeding may require cessation of therapy and support with cryoprecipitate to replace fibrinogen and factor VIII. Rare cases may require ϵ-aminocaproic acid, which specifically inhibits the lysine binding site of plasmin.

b. Treatment approaches

(1) **Deep venous thrombosis.** Heparin remains the mainstay of treatment, but thrombolytic agents provide rapid symptomatic relief and cause early clot lysis—effects seen in few patients treated with heparin alone. Thrombolytic agents are most effective in recently developed lesions and appear to decrease the incidence of postphlebitic syndrome.

(2) **Pulmonary embolus.** Either heparin or thrombolytic therapy can be used. However, rapid improvement in pulmonary perfusion occurs with thrombolytic therapy. In patients who are treated for 7 days or more, however, heparin therapy may be equivalent to thrombolysis. Thrombolytic therapy is most useful in fresh and in massive emboli, where it may be life-saving.

(3) **Myocardial infarction.** Early administration of thrombolytic therapy appears to limit infarct size and may significantly improve mortality rates.

(4) **Peripheral artery and catheter thrombosis.** Local infusion of thrombolytic agents is used for peripheral vascular lesions, especially small distal emboli not amenable to surgery. Local infusions also are used to reestablish patency of thrombosed central venous catheters.

III. THROMBOHEMORRHAGIC DISORDERS.

Although bleeding usually is the most obvious clinical manifestation of these disorders, the initiating pathophysiologic events are thrombotic in nature.

A. Disseminated intravascular coagulation (DIC) probably is the most common thrombohemorrhagic disorder. DIC should be viewed as a secondary phenomenon; thus, the underlying and precipitating condition should be sought.

1. Pathophysiology. Various underlying conditions can precipitate DIC (Table 15-2). Once initiated, the balance among coagulant, anticoagulant, and fibrinolytic processes determines the clinical features of DIC in a given patient (Figure 15-7).

a. Initiation. DIC is initiated by pathologic activation of the coagulation cascade, which can occur by a variety of mechanisms at different points in the cascade. For example, endotoxin produced during septicemia can activate factor XII directly. It also can damage endothelial cells, causing the release of tissue factor and the destruction of thrombomodulin.

b. Thrombosis. If the stimulus persists, normal control mechanisms are overwhelmed and there is diffuse microthrombus formation.

c. Consumption. Continuation of the process leads to depletion of all elements of the coagulation system and development of hemorrhagic characteristics. AT III also seems to decrease, which may further enhance the thrombotic component of the disorder.

d. Fibrinolysis occurs soon after initiation of fibrin deposition. FSPs begin to be detectable and may be present in high titers. These products further aggravate the hemorrhagic component of the disorder by inhibiting platelet function and by interfering with normal fibrin polymerization.

e. Hemolysis. Trauma to red cells that are forced through vessels partially occluded by microvascular thrombi causes a microangiopathic hemolytic process.

2. Clinical features. The clinical picture of DIC varies widely over time and in different situations. The disorder may be so subtle that abnormal laboratory findings are the only signs. Conversely, life-threatening bleeding may occur. The balance among pathophysiologic processes and the resulting tempo of consumption determine the severity of manifestations.

Table 15-2. Conditions that Commonly Precipitate Disseminated Intravascular Coagulation (DIC)

Infectious conditions
Gram-negative septicemia
Other endotoxin-related conditions (e.g., toxic shock syndrome)
Obstetric conditions
Abruptio placentae
Amniotic fluid embolism
Retained dead fetus
Vascular conditions
Aneurysm
Giant cavernous hemangioma
Hematologic conditions
Massive hemolysis
Promyelocytic leukemia
Snake venom
Trauma

a. The presence of DIC often is heralded by the appearance of **diffuse bleeding from multiple sites.**
b. Careful evaluation usually reveals **thrombotic lesions** as well (e.g., skin infarctions, gastrointestinal ulcerations, abnormal renal function, pulmonary and CNS infarctions). The thrombotic nature of these lesions initially may not be apparent, as bleeding may supervene at these compromised sites.

3. **Diagnosis.** Laboratory findings vary with time and circumstances. In severe DIC, all of the following are present.
   a. **Thrombocytopenia.** The platelet count almost invariably is less than 100,000/μl, and, in severe DIC, commonly is less than 50,000/μl.
   b. **Prolonged PT** often is the result of factor VII depletion and consumption of factors in the common pathway. Prolongation may be severe, and vitamin K deficiency should be excluded, especially in patients in whom both DIC and vitamin K deficiency are likely.
   c. **Prolonged PTT.** PTT may be markedly prolonged, especially when most factors have been consumed by massive DIC. Prolonged PTT in combination with the other findings and with appropriate clinical features strongly suggests DIC.
   d. **Prolonged thrombin time** is a highly suggestive finding, which may be the result of decreased fibrinogen. However, thrombin time may be disproportionately long due to the anticoagulant effects of FSPs or to the inadvertent use of small amounts of heparin (e.g., to flush intravenous catheters).
   e. **Decreased fibrinogen.** Fibrinogen may be severely depressed but can also be normal or only mildly depressed because of a high fibrinogen level that may have existed prior to the onset of consumption (e.g., in an infected or ill patient).
   f. **FSPs.** The presence of FSPs strongly suggests DIC in the absence of other explanations (e.g., recent surgery). The absence of FSPs makes the diagnosis of DIC highly unlikely.
   g. **Microangiopathic hemolytic anemia.** Review of the peripheral smear is extremely important to confirm the suspected traumatic effect of small vessel thrombi on red cells. Findings such as schistocytes or helmet cells are supportive evidence.

4. **Therapy.** Foremost in treatment is elimination of the precipitating cause of DIC. This usually means treatment of sepsis or, in obstetric patients, emptying the uterus. Unfortunately, some situations are not immediately reversible. The need for additional treatment in these cases is determined by the tempo and clinical consequences of the coagulopathy.
   a. In **low-grade DIC without clinical evidence of bleeding or clinically significant thrombosis,** treatment may not be necessary, especially if the underlying cause is reversible.
   b. For **clinically significant bleeding,** replacement of depleted coagulation factors and cells with appropriate blood products (FFP, cryoprecipitate, platelets, red cells) is useful until treatment of the underlying process is successful.
   c. When **thrombosis** is a major manifestation, heparin therapy may be required. Rarely,

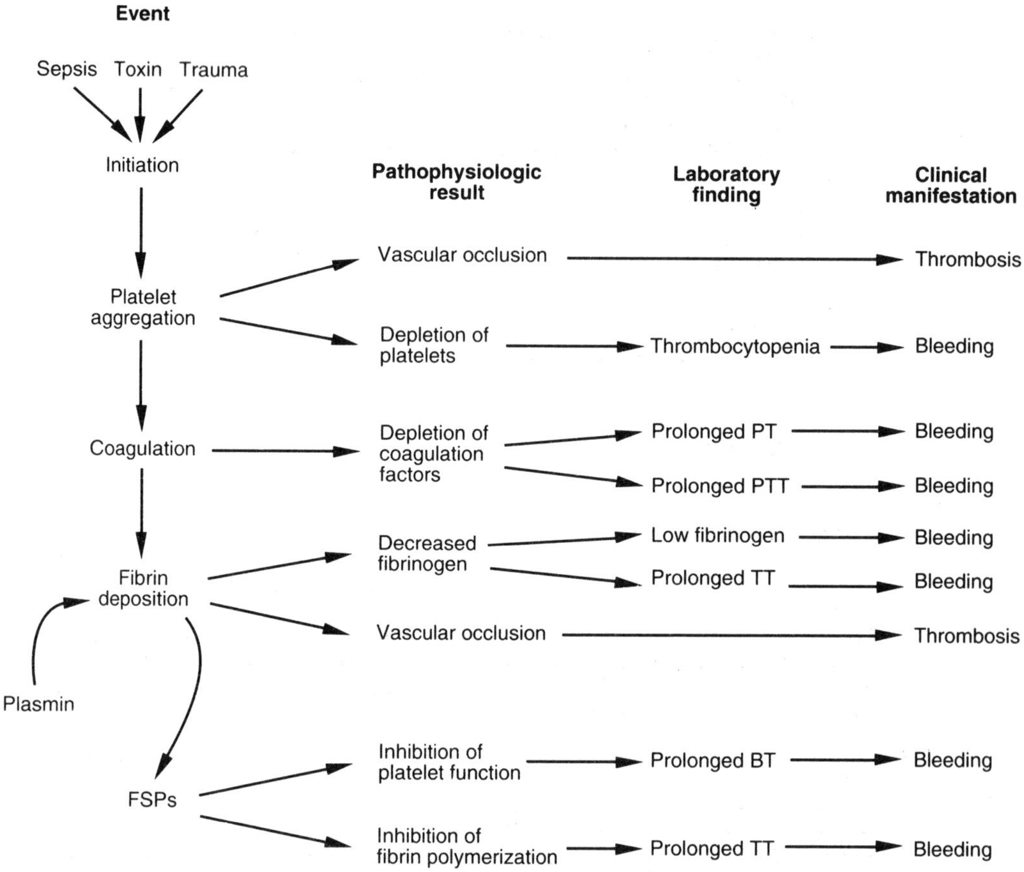

Figure 15-7. Disseminated intravascular coagulation (DIC) can be precipitated by a variety of conditions, not all of which necessarily act initially by stimulating platelets. However, the sequence of events that follows and the pathophysiologic, laboratory, and clinical consequences are the same regardless of the initial stimulus. For example, conditions that initiate coagulation by activating a coagulation factor at some point later in the coagulation cascade will trigger feedback mechanisms (e.g., thrombin production), causing platelet aggregation and producing the sequence of events and consequences summarized here. *BT* = bleeding time; PT = prothrombin time; *PTT* = partial thromboplastin time; *TT* = thrombin time; and FSPs = fibrin split products.

heparin may be used to interrupt the cycle of consumption when the precipitating cause cannot be readily treated. The added risk of bleeding, however, demands careful risk–benefit assessment before such a decision to give heparin is made.

B. Thrombotic thrombocytopenic purpura (TTP) and hemolytic-uremic syndrome (HUS)

1. **Definition.** TTP and HUS are such closely related syndromes that most hematologists consider them aspects of the clinical spectrum of a single disease.
   a. **TTP** is a rare clinical syndrome characterized by thrombocytopenia, microangiopathic hemolytic anemia, and fluctuating neurologic abnormalities. Fever and renal dysfunction also are common. Although it can occur at any age, TTP occurs most frequently in young and middle-aged adults.
   b. **HUS** is very similar to TTP but occurs most frequently in children. The predominant features are hemolysis, renal failure, and thrombocytopenia; neurologic manifestations are rare.

2. **Pathophysiology.** The characteristic lesion is occlusion of capillaries and small arterioles by platelet thrombi.
   a. The pathophysiologic mechanism appears to involve endothelial cell damage, which may

be immunologically mediated. This endothelial damage is associated with decreased prostacyclin production, t-PA deficiency, and release of high molecular weight von Willebrand factor (vWF) multimers (which has been demonstrated in this disorder), all of which contribute to the formation of platelet thrombi.

b. Passage of red cells through small vessels partially occluded by platelet thrombi results in the characteristic microangiopathic hemolytic anemia.

3. **Clinical features** are determined by the location of the microthrombi. It is unknown why neurologic problems are more common in adults with TTP and why renal failure is more common in children with HUS.

a. TTP is seen most frequently in young women and occasionally appears to be precipitated by pregnancy, infection, or chemotherapy. TTP usually has an acute onset and can progress to a rapidly fatal outcome as a result of hemorrhagic or neurologic events.

b. HUS occurs primarily in children and also can have a devastating course. Spontaneous remission is rare, and aggressive treatment is indicated. Relapses are seen occasionally in patients who do achieve remission.

4. **Diagnosis**

a. Severe thrombocytopenia and evidence of hemolytic anemia are the major laboratory findings. The peripheral blood smear reveals numerous schistocytes and helmet cells.

b. Evidence of renal dysfunction is variable and may include an abnormal urinalysis and elevation of blood urea nitrogen (BUN) and creatinine.

c. The PT and PTT usually are normal, which differentiates TTP and HUS from DIC.

5. **Therapy.** Because of differences in therapy, it is important to differentiate TTP from idiopathic thrombocytopenic purpura (ITP) with anemia of blood loss or with Coombs' positive hemolysis (Evan's syndrome).

a. Infusions of FFP have been found empirically to induce remissions. Plasmapheresis with aggressive plasma replacement is now the usual method of treatment. Steroids, inhibitors of platelet function, and splenectomy have been used in the past but with less consistent results.

b. Dialysis support often is necessary in HUS.

C. Heparin thrombocytopenia is a common clinical problem that must be considered in the context of thrombohemorrhagic disorders. In some cases, platelet thrombi contribute to the development of thrombocytopenia and to the clinical manifestations, with significant thromboembolic events in some patients. Heparin thrombocytopenia is discussed in more detail in Chapter 13 IV A 2 b (4) (c).

STUDY QUESTIONS

Directions: Each item below contains four suggested answers of which **one or more** is correct. Choose the answer

- **A** if **1, 2, and 3** are correct
- **B** if **1 and 3** are correct
- **C** if **2 and 4** are correct
- **D** if **4** is correct
- **E** if **1, 2, 3, and 4** are correct

1. The endothelial cell contributes to the control of coagulation by

(1) participating in the activation of protein C
(2) releasing t-PA
(3) producing prostacyclin
(4) enhancing AT III activity

2. Disseminated intravascular coagulation (DIC) is suspected in a patient with urosepsis. Helpful diagnostic studies would include

(1) prothrombin time (PT)
(2) platelet aggregation studies
(3) platelet count
(4) protein C level

Directions: The group of items in this section consists of lettered options followed by a set of numbered items. For each item, select the **one** lettered option that is most closely associated with it. Each lettered option may be selected once, more than once, or not at all.

Questions 3–8

For each functional characteristic described below, select the plasma protein or anticoagulant drug with which it is associated.

(A) AT III
(B) Heparin
(C) Protein C
(D) Warfarin
(E) Plasminogen

3. Forms one-to-one inactive complexes with thrombin

4. Inhibits factors Va and VIIIa

5. Is activated via thrombomodulin

6. Is indirectly activated by streptokinase

7. Enhances inactivation of thrombin and factor Xa

8. Interferes with vitamin K metabolism

1-E	4-C	7-B
2-B	5-C	8-D
3-A	6-E	

ANSWERS AND EXPLANATIONS

1. The answer is E (all) *[I A 1 a (2), 2 a, B 1 b (1); III B 2 a].*
The endothelial cell contributes in several ways to the control of coagulation. The endothelial cell surface receptor, thrombomodulin, is required for activation of protein C, a serine protease that acts on specific clotting factors in the presence of a cofactor. Endothelial cells also contain tissue plasminogen activator (t-PA), which is an important plasminogen activator, and heparan sulfate, which is a substance that greatly enhances the anticoagulant activity of antithrombin III (AT III). Prostacyclin produced by the arachidonic acid pathway in the endothelial cells is a potent inhibitor of platelet aggregation.

2. The answer is B (1, 3) *[III A 3].*
The consumption of platelets and coagulation factors in disseminated intravascular coagulation (DIC) could result in a prolonged prothrombin time (PT) and decreased platelet count. Although platelet aggregation studies might be abnormal, the platelet count might be too low for an accurate reading, and this expensive bit of information would not contribute to diagnosis or treatment of DIC. Similarly, levels of the naturally occurring anticoagulants (e.g., protein C) might vary in the course of DIC, but this information is not reliable for a diagnosis.

3–8. The answers are: 3-A *[I A 1 b],* **4-C** *[I A 2 b (1)],* **5-C** *[I A 2 a],* **6-E** *[I B 1 c (1)],* **7-B** *[I A 1],* **8-D** *[II B 4 a (1) (b)].*
Antithrombin III (AT III) is a naturally occurring anticoagulant that exists in plasma. AT III inhibits the activity of several serine proteases (e.g., thrombin, factor Xa) by binding them in one-to-one complexes. The presence of heparin or heparin-like substances (e.g., heparan sulfate) causes a conformational change in AT III, which enhances its inhibitory effect as much as 1000 times. This effect is the primary mechanism by which heparin acts as an anticoagulant drug.

Protein C is another naturally occurring anticoagulant, which must be activated before it can inhibit specific clotting factors (i.e., Va and VIIIa); it has no effect on the other coagulation proteins. Activation of protein C requires the interaction of thrombin and thrombomodulin. Once activated, protein C requires the presence of its cofactor, protein S, to inhibit factors Va and VIIIa.

Plasminogen is a single-chain glycoprotein that is the inactive precursor to plasmin, a serine protease with fibrinolytic activity. Streptokinase activates plasminogen indirectly; it forms a complex with plasminogen, which can then activate other plasminogen molecules. Urokinase directly cleaves the heavy and light chains of plasminogen, converting it to plasmin.

Warfarin is an anticoagulant drug that blocks the reduction of vitamin K, thus rendering a patient functionally deficient in vitamin K despite an adequate supply. Vitamin K is necessary for the post-translational addition of γ-carboxyglutamic acid residues to the vitamin K–dependent coagulation factors (i.e., II, VII, IX, and X). In the absence of vitamin K, the proteins are still made but, without these residues, are functionally inactive. Warfarin also decreases the levels of functional protein C and protein S, both of which are vitamin K–dependent.

Heparin enhances the natural ability of AT III to inhibit the activities of thrombin and factor Xa.

16
Approach to Patients with Coagulation Disorders

Patricia M. Catalano

I. BLEEDING DISORDERS are among the most common problems in hematology. A bleeding disorder may be obvious or so subtle that it is overlooked. Occasionally, the problem is identified by routine screening tests. The evaluation of a patient with a bleeding disorder should be performed in a logical sequence, as expediently as possible. A careful, detailed history is critical and may uncover clues to the nature of the disorder, thus facilitating the choice of laboratory studies.

A. History

1. **Bleeding history.** It is very useful to know if the bleeding disorder has been lifelong, although this may be difficult to ascertain.
   a. **Clues to a congenital bleeding disorder**
      (1) Specific questioning may uncover a history of excessive bleeding initiated by common childhood traumas or after dental extractions, which suggests that the disorder is lifelong.
      (2) A history of bleeding disorders in family members is extremely useful and, when the mode of inheritance can be determined, may even suggest a specific diagnosis.
         (a) Hemophilia (A or B) is suggested when the inheritance is X-linked.
         (b) von Willebrand's disease is suggested in a patient with a low level of factor VIII:C and a family history consistent with an autosomal inheritance.
   b. **Clues to an acquired bleeding disorder**
      (1) A patient who presents with a bleeding disorder and who gives a history of tolerating stress to the coagulation system (e.g., excessive bleeding after extraction of a permanent tooth) usually can be assumed to have an acquired disorder.
      (2) The time between exposure to potentially causative factors and the onset of the bleeding disorder may provide clues to the etiology and, particularly in medication-related disorders, the treatment of the bleeding problem.
   c. **Nature of bleeding**
      (1) **Sites** of bleeding may suggest where in the coagulation process the defect may be.
         (a) Mucous membrane bleeding and petechiae are often seen in platelet-related disorders.
         (b) Hemarthroses are common in hemophilia.
         (c) Soft tissue hematomas without petechiae or mucous membrane bleeding suggest a defect in the coagulation cascade.
      (2) **Severity** of the bleeding disorder influences therapeutic decisions and may be deduced from the degree of trauma necessary to induce excessive bleeding.
         (a) Spontaneous bleeding usually occurs only in the most severe disorders.
         (b) A history of bleeding only after major trauma or surgery suggests a mild bleeding disorder. In this case, factor levels should be evaluated even if screening test results are normal, because very mild decreases in factor levels may not prolong the prothrombin time (PT) or partial thromboplastin time (PTT).
      (3) **Timing of episodes.** Bleeding that is uncontrolled from the onset suggests a defect in primary hemostasis, whereas a history of bleeding after initial apparent hemostasis is more consistent with a factor deficiency. A marked delay in bleeding after the initiating event is sometimes seen in factor XIII deficiency.

2. **Medical history.** A review of all medical conditions, and their treatment, can provide insight into the possible nature of the bleeding disorder.

a. Malnourished, hospitalized patients who have been treated with multiple antibiotics are highly prone to vitamin K deficiency.
b. Systemic lupus erythematosus (SLE) and human immunodeficiency virus (HIV) infection are associated with syndromes of immune-mediated (idiopathic) thrombocytopenic purpura (ITP).
c. Septicemia is the most common underlying cause of disseminated intravascular coagulation (DIC).

3. **Medications.** Careful review of all medications is critical in evaluating a patient with a coagulation abnormality.
a. Aspirin is a common cause of altered platelet function.
b. Incidental heparin, which often is used for flushing intravenous access lines, can cause thrombocytopenia and inadvertent anticoagulation.
c. An extensive number of drugs are known to induce thrombocytopenia.
d. Acquired factor inhibitors have been associated with medications (e.g., penicillin).

B. **Physical examination** may provide valuable clues as to where in the coagulation system the abnormality is likely to be found.

1. **Petechiae** usually indicate bleeding at the level of the microvasculature and are associated with abnormalities of platelet number and function.

2. **Mucous membrane bleeding** can result from any defect in coagulation, but when mucous membranes are the only bleeding sites, thrombocytopenia, platelet function disorders, or von Willebrand's disease is likely.

3. **Hemarthrosis** or evidence of recurrent joint bleeding is almost always associated with a severe form of hemophilia, although this type of bleeding can occur in severe acquired factor deficiencies as well.

4. **Diffuse bleeding from multiple sites,** both mucous membrane and sites of trauma such as venipuncture sites, is often seen with severe combined coagulation defects, such as DIC, or severe liver disease.

5. **Other physical findings** may suggest underlying medical conditions that could predispose to the bleeding disorder, such as splenomegaly in a patient with SLE and thrombocytopenia or fever and evidence of sepsis in a patient with DIC.

C. **Laboratory studies** (Table 16-1). Ideally, the choice of laboratory studies is guided by the history and physical examination of the patient. However, for general screening purposes or when the history and examination provide no clues, a battery of appropriate tests often is the most expedient approach.

1. **Platelet tests**
a. **Platelet count** determination is the first step in evaluating disorders of primary hemostasis. Abnormal platelet counts must be confirmed by peripheral blood smear.
b. **Platelet function**
(1) **Bleeding time.** The **template bleeding time** is a crude test of the time it takes for a standardized incision to stop bleeding. When the test is done properly, this time should be dependent only on the presence of adequate numbers of normally functioning platelets. However, the test is extremely susceptible to variability introduced by the person performing the test and, therefore, must be interpreted with caution.
(2) **Platelet aggregation** studies require experience both to perform and to interpret.

Table 16-1. Screening Tests of Coagulation

Test	Interpretation
Platelet count	Platelet number
Peripheral blood smear	Cellular morphology and number
Bleeding time (BT)	Platelet function
Prothrombin time (PT)	Extrinsic pathway
Partial thromboplastin time (PTT)	Intrinsic pathway
Thrombin time (TT)	Fibrinogen conversion to fibrin

(a) **Aggregation with adenosine diphosphate (ADP), epinephrine, or collagen** will uncover abnormalities of fibrinogen binding (thrombasthenia) or of arachidonic acid metabolism (i.e., cyclooxygenase inhibition secondary to aspirin) or secretion (storage pool disease).

(b) **Aggregation with ristocetin** is abnormal in von Willebrand's disease and in Bernard-Soulier syndrome.

2. **Tests of coagulation**
   a. **Screening tests of coagulation** must always be interpreted in light of the clinical situation. In general, however, screening provides invaluable information.
      (1) **PTT** reflects the function of the intrinsic pathway from the contact phase through the common pathway.
      (2) **PT** reflects the function of the extrinsic pathway including the common pathway.
      (3) **Thrombin time (TT)** measures the ability of thrombin to convert fibrinogen to fibrin. It is abnormal in the setting of hypofibrinogenemia and dysfibrinogenemia and is markedly sensitive to the anti-thrombin effect caused by heparin.
      (4) **Urea clot lysis test** measures fibrin stabilization. Although factor XIII deficiency is rare, it should be considered in a patient with an appropriate history and normal results on the other screening tests; PT, PTT, and TT do not evaluate factor XIII activity.
   b. **Mixing test** is critical once a prolonged screening test is identified. The test is performed by mixing equal amounts of the patient's plasma and a known normal plasma and determining if the normal plasma corrects the defect. A 50% level of any plasma factor is usually associated with normal results on screening tests; therefore, correction implies a factor deficiency. However, failure of the admixed normal plasma to correct the clotting defect indicates that there is an antibody to a coagulation factor present, which inhibits that factor in both the normal and the patient's plasma. This factor inhibitor will need to be identified by further, specific tests.
   c. **Specific factor assays** can further define abnormalities of the coagulation cascade once they have been localized by means of screening tests. The choice of which factors to assay should be guided by such factors as family history and statistical likelihood. Factor assays may also be useful in patients with normal screening tests but compelling family or clinical evidence suggesting a mild factor deficiency.

3. **Peripheral blood smear.** In addition to tests of platelets and coagulation, the peripheral smear must be examined. Findings such as red cell fragmentation (suggesting a concomitant microangiopathic process), unusual platelet morphology, or other hematopoietic abnormalities would also influence the evaluation.

4. **Bone marrow evaluation** is used primarily to assess platelet production. If megakaryocytes are plentiful in the bone marrow of a patient with severe thrombocytopenia, peripheral destruction must be involved. If megakaryocytes are decreased, failure of production is the cause.

D. Approach to the patient with a bleeding disorder

1. **Patients with an isolated platelet abnormality**
   a. **Thrombocytopenia.** The evaluation of a patient in whom the only abnormality is isolated thrombocytopenia is summarized in Figure 16-1. An understanding of the role of the following tests is fundamental to this evaluation.
      (1) **Peripheral smear.** Because platelet counts almost universally are done by automated counter, it is important to examine the blood smear to confirm the presence of thrombocytopenia. Occasionally, platelets clump in the automated counter, causing an inappropriately low platelet count (pseudothrombocytopenia); but adequate numbers of platelets can be clearly discerned on the smear. Also, evaluation of other blood cell morphology may suggest an underlying disorder [e.g., fragmented red cells in thrombotic thrombocytopenic purpura (TTP)].
      (2) **Bone marrow examination** for the presence of megakaryocytes may be critical for determining the mechanism of the thrombocytopenia. An increased number of megakaryocytes suggests that thrombocytopenia is the result of a destructive mechanism and not decreased production.
      (3) **Antiplatelet antibodies.** Although the presence of antiplatelet antibodies supports a diagnosis of ITP or an ITP-like syndrome, this study usually is not necessary in straightforward cases. However, detection of antibodies to specific platelet antigens may be necessary to confirm certain diagnoses, such as post-transfusion purpura or neonatal alloimmune thrombocytopenia.

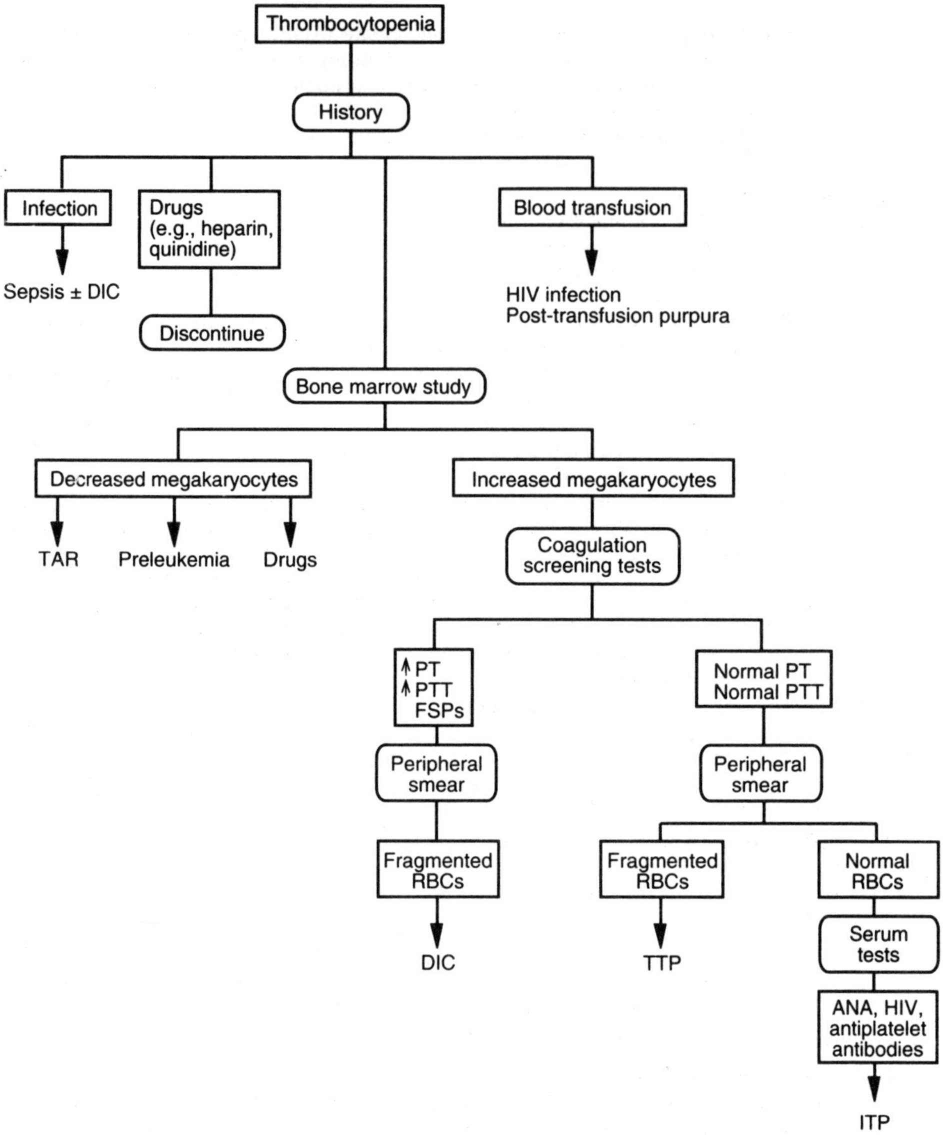

Figure 16-1. Algorithm for evaluation of a patient with isolated thrombocytopenia. *ANA* = antinuclear antibodies; *DIC* = disseminated intravascular coagulation; *FSPs* = fibrin split products; *HIV* = human immunodeficiency virus; *ITP* = idiopathic thrombocytopenic purpura; PT = prothrombin time; PTT = partial thromboplastin time; *RBCs* = red blood cells; *TAR* = thrombocytopenia with absent radii; TT = thrombin time; *TTP* = thrombotic thrombocytopenic purpura; ↑ = increased; ↓ = decreased.

b. Thrombocytosis. Much of the evaluation of a patient with isolated thrombocytosis is based on clinical findings and is aimed at excluding a cause for secondary thrombocytosis.

(1) Clinical features

(a) Thrombocytosis that results from a **myeloproliferative disorder** [e.g., essential thrombocythemia, polycythemia vera (PV)] may be associated with bleeding due to functional abnormalities of the platelets produced by the abnormal clone. However, it also can predispose to thrombosis. The presence of **splenomegaly** strongly suggests the presence of a myeloproliferative disorder.

(b) Thrombocytosis that is part of a **reactive process** does not predispose to bleeding, nor is it generally associated with thrombosis. Patients who have just undergone splenectomy or who have certain underlying disorders (e.g., iron deficiency) are likely to have reactive (secondary) thrombocytosis.

(2) **Laboratory findings**

(a) Support for the diagnosis of a myeloproliferative disorder can be obtained by testing the leukocyte alkaline phosphatase (LAP) activity and the vitamin B_{12} level. The bone marrow also should be evaluated for chromosome abnormalities, cellularity, and evidence of fibrosis.

(b) Platelet function tests often are abnormal when the thrombocytosis is the result of a myeloproliferative disorder and should be normal in secondary thrombocytosis.

c. **Prolonged bleeding time**

(1) Bleeding time should not be measured in the absence of a platelet count, as it generally is prolonged in the setting of thrombocytopenia. Ideally, the relationship between platelet count and the degree to which bleeding time is prolonged should be defined in the laboratory where bleeding time is measured, so the results can be interpreted in mildly thrombocytopenic patients. In general, platelet count and bleeding time are inversely related when the platelet count is 20,000–100,000/μl.

(2) When bleeding time is prolonged and platelet count is normal (Figure 16-2), additional studies may be indicated to define the nature of the disorder.

2. **Patients with a single abnormal screening test**

a. **Prolonged PTT** (Figure 16-3). An isolated abnormality of the PTT suggests an abnormality in the intrinsic coagulation pathway. The patient history and the context in which the patient presents may give clues as to the most likely etiology.

(1) **Inherited abnormalities** may be associated with a strong family history. If a sex-linked pattern is apparent, specific assays for factors VIII and IX can be chosen; if there is an autosomal pattern, an assay for factor XI can be used.

(2) **Acquired abnormalities** with bleeding manifestations or asymptomatic and previously unsuspected abnormalities may be the result of acquired inhibitors or contact factor abnormalities. A mixing test to screen for the presence of an inhibitor will guide the next steps of the evaluation. Correction of the PTT by admixed normal plasma would suggest a factor deficiency such as factor XII or prekallikrein deficiency, while lack of correction suggests an inhibitor, which would then need specific characterization.

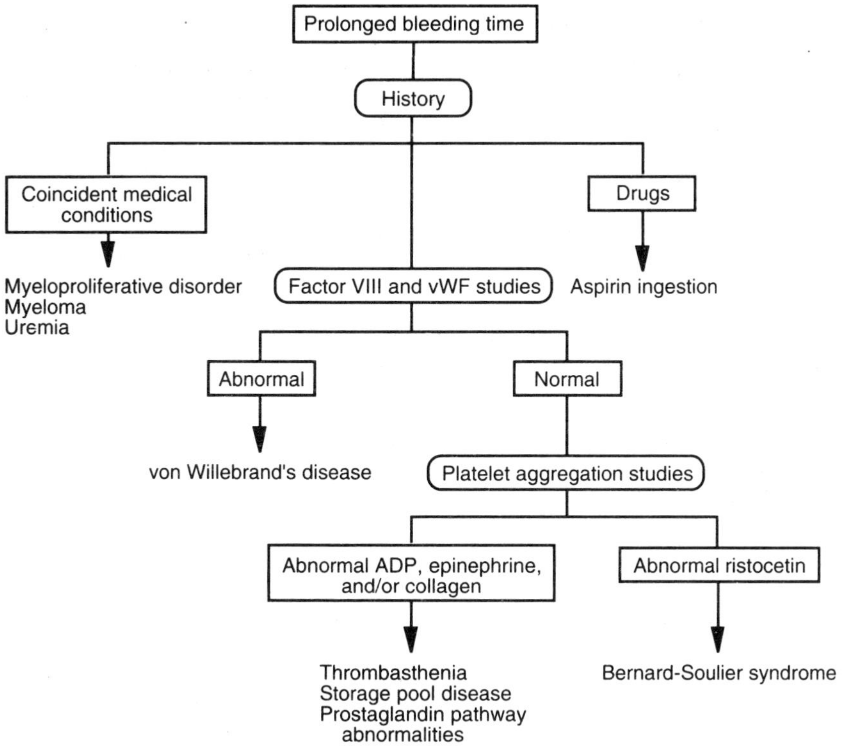

Figure 16-2. Algorithm for evaluation of a patient with a prolonged bleeding time and a normal platelet count. *ADP* = adenosine diphosphate; *vWF* = von Willebrand factor.

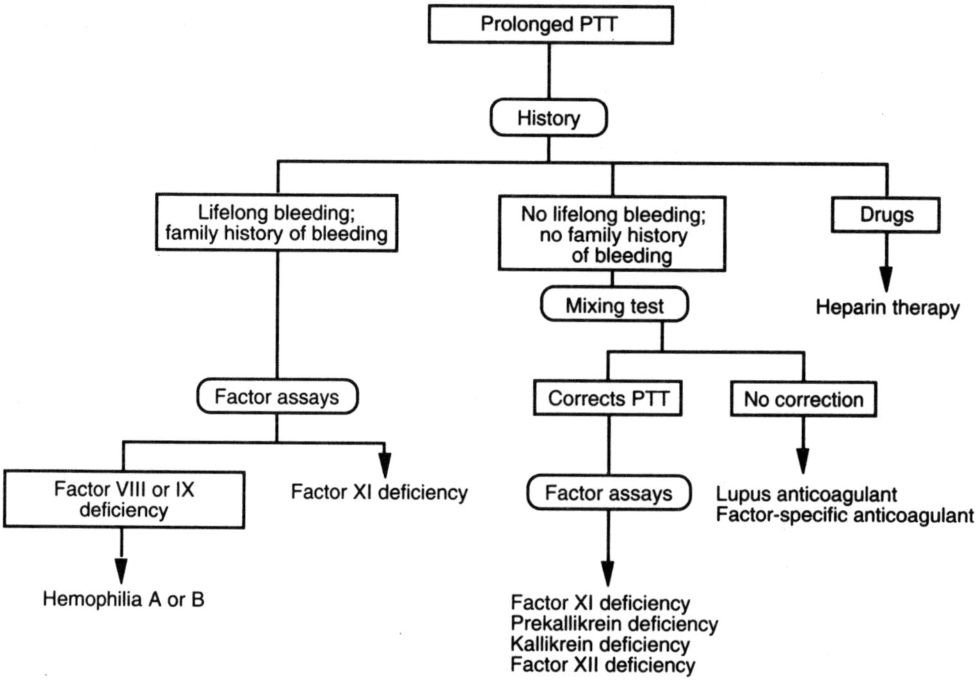

Figure 16-3. Algorithm for evaluation of a patient with isolated prolonged partial thromboplastin time (PTT).

(3) **Drugs,** especially **heparin,** may be the cause detected on a careful history or review of records.

b. **Prolonged PT** (Figure 16-4). An isolated prolonged PT suggests an abnormality of factor VII. This is seldom the result of a congenital deficiency but is often associated with liver disease, vitamin K deficiency, or therapy with vitamin K antagonists. Rarely, coagulation factor inhibitors occur that can cause this abnormality; these can be detected by a mixing test.

c. **Prolonged TT** should be evaluated along with the fibrinogen level, as prolongation occurs with hypofibrinogenemia. More commonly, however, the antithrombin action of small amounts of heparin prolongs the TT. Other conditions that can interfere with fibrin polymerization must also be considered, such as inherited dysfibrinogenemias, the presence of fibrin split products (FSPs), or even the presence of myeloma proteins.

3. **Patients with multiple coagulation defects.** When multiple defects of the coagulation system are found, a unifying diagnosis is likely (Table 16-2).

a. **Vitamin K deficiency** most commonly presents as an isolated prolongation of the PT, but PTT also may be prolonged. Coincident thrombocytopenia does not occur. The diagnosis usually is suggested by the clinical presentation and is easily tested by an empiric trial of vitamin K.

b. **DIC.** The combination of thrombocytopenia, prolonged PT, and prolonged PTT suggests consumption of coagulation factors and platelets, especially in the setting of a precipitating cause for DIC. Additional tests to support the diagnosis include fibrinogen levels, tests for FSPs, and examination of the peripheral smear for the presence of fragmented red blood cells.

c. **Liver disease** results in decreased production of most coagulation factors.

(1) The early stages of liver disease may be associated with only prolonged PT, and the possibility of vitamin K deficiency must be considered. With more severe liver disease, both PT and PTT are prolonged, but, again, vitamin K deficiency must be excluded. In either case, a therapeutic trial of vitamin K may be diagnostically useful.

(2) Prolonged TT usually results when fibrinogen production also is diminished, a finding not consistent with vitamin K deficiency.

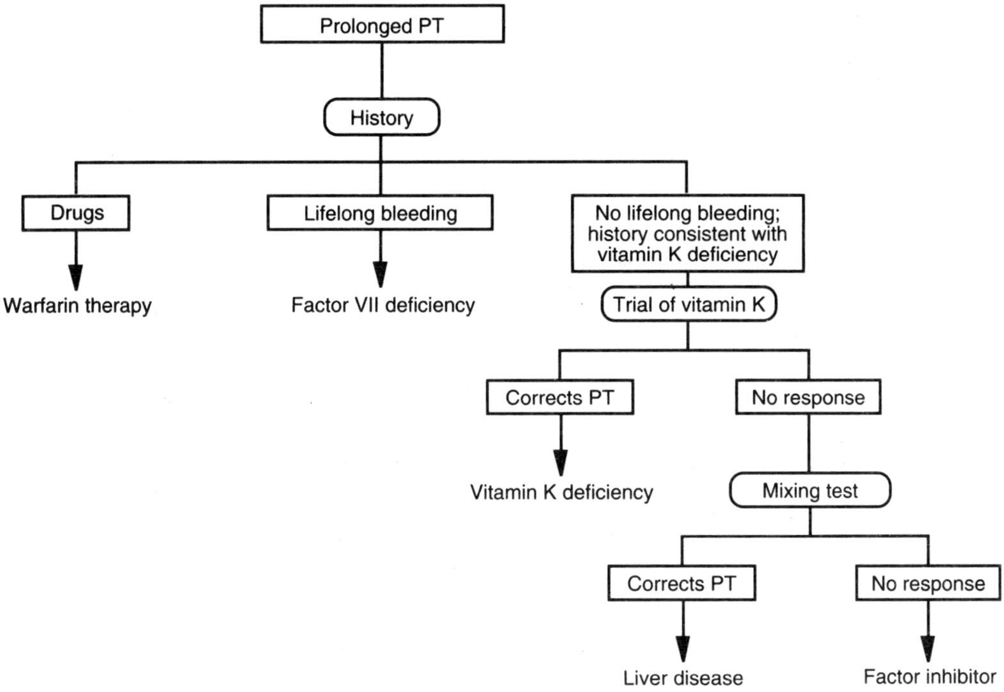

Figure 16-4. Algorithm for evaluation of a patient with isolated prolonged prothrombin time (PT).

(3) Thrombocytopenia in patients with liver disease can result from hypersplenism and sequestration of platelets. Thrombocytopenia in such a patient combined with prolonged PT, PTT, and TT may be difficult to differentiate from DIC. This may be compounded by finding elevated FSPs, since the diseased liver has a decreased ability to clear FSPs. Most often, the distinction can be made on clinical grounds.

4. Acquired clotting factor inhibitors may be suspected in a patient with recent marked prolongation of one or more screening tests. This suspicion should be confirmed by a **mixing test,** in which the prolonged screening test is not corrected when performed on a 1:1 mixture of the patient's plasma with normal plasma. Tests for the lupus anticoagulant (usually in patients without clinical bleeding) or, if this is negative, for specific factors will localize the action of the inhibitor.

II. THROMBOTIC DISORDERS.

Venous thrombosis is a common clinical problem. Usually the patient has characteristic risk factors for thrombosis, and no further evaluation is necessary. However, suspicious elements of the history or physical examination should be evaluated to identify a possible underlying hypercoagulable state.

Table 16-2. Common Conditions with Multiple Coagulation Defects

	Test Result			
Disorder	**Platelet Count**	**PT**	**PTT**	**TT**
Vitamin K deficiency	N	↑	N/↑	N
Liver disease	N/↓	↑	↑	↑
DIC	↓	↑	↑	↑

DIC = disseminated intravascular coagulation; N = normal; PT = prothrombin time; PTT = partial thromboplastin time; TT = thrombin time; ↑ = increased; ↓ = decreased.

A. History

1. **Recurrent thrombotic disorders.** Recurrence of a thrombotic event at the site of a previous thrombosis is not uncommon. However, when a young patient (age < 35 years) develops more than one thrombotic event, particularly at varied sites and without obvious risk factors, the likelihood of a hypercoagulable state must be considered.
   a. **Family history.** A history of thrombotic events at an early age in other family members strongly suggests an inherited abnormality [e.g., antithrombin III (AT III), protein C, or protein S deficiency]. Patients should be questioned specifically about a family history of the following events:
      (1) **Recurrent or unusual thromboses.** Multiple thrombotic events at an early age in family members suggest a familial hypercoagulable state.
      (2) **Anticoagulant intolerance.** In rare cases, questioning regarding anticoagulation of family members may uncover a history of warfarin-induced necrosis or refractoriness to heparin, both of which strongly suggest a familial anticoagulant deficiency.
      (3) **Thrombotic events during pregnancy.** Although there are mechanical and hormonal risk factors for thrombotic events during pregnancy, a strong family history of such events may suggest an inherited abnormality.
      (4) **Purpura fulminans neonatalis.** A documented history of this rare but dramatic condition in a family member is strong evidence for protein C deficiency in the family.
   b. **Past medical history.** Recurrent thromboses may simply be the result of **persistent risk factors** rather than a hematologic abnormality. Factors that may predispose to thrombosis include stasis, hyperlipidemia, pregnancy, smoking, and underlying diseases (e.g., malignancy).
   c. **Medications.** Patients with recurrent thromboembolic disease usually have a history of **prior anticoagulation**. Several aspects of this treatment may provide clues regarding the nature of the abnormality.
      (1) **Intolerance.** Patients with protein C deficiency may have a history suggestive of warfarin-induced necrosis, but a history of uneventful warfarin therapy does not exclude the diagnosis.
      (2) **Ineffectiveness.** Difficulty in obtaining therapeutic anticoagulation with heparin suggests the possibility of severe AT III deficiency.

2. **Isolated thrombotic events.** Whether or not an isolated thrombotic event should be evaluated for an underlying coagulation abnormality is debated. Factors that may be helpful in making this decision include the following.
   a. **Family history.** Similar events or recurrent events in other family members strongly suggest an inherited disorder.
   b. **History of onset.** A sudden thrombotic event in an otherwise healthy young person who is without risk factors for thrombosis is suspicious and should stimulate a careful search for more subtle risk factors in the patient's history. Unusual sites (axillary or mesenteric veins) are also suspicious.
   c. **Past medical history.** Medical conditions that predispose to thrombosis should be sought in patients with thrombotic events. Often these conditions are obvious, as in the immobilized, postoperative patient or the patient with a malignancy.
   d. **Medications and other risk factors.** Exogenous estrogens and some chemotherapeutic agents may predispose to thrombosis, as does cigarette smoking.

B. Physical examination

1. **Underlying disorder.** Physical examination seldom reveals specific findings in most hypercoagulable states; however, there may be findings of an underlying disorder. For example, splenomegaly in a patient with thrombocytosis may suggest an underlying myeloproliferative disorder.

2. **Differentiation of arterial from venous events.** Physical examination may help differentiate arterial from venous events. Arterial thrombi or emboli usually result in cold, pulseless extremities, while venous obstruction often results in swelling of the affected limb.

C. Laboratory studies are important to the evaluation of thrombotic disorders. However, laboratory results must be interpreted carefully, since variations in the naturally occurring anticoagulants may occur in relationship to acute events and their treatment.

1. **Platelet count**
   a. Persistent thrombocytosis in patients with myeloproliferative disorders can predispose to thrombosis. Evaluation of such patients is aimed at confirming the presence of a myeloproliferative disorder (see I D 1 b).
   b. Secondary thrombocytosis usually is transient and, in general, does not predispose to thrombosis.

2. **Tests of naturally occurring anticoagulants**
   a. **Functional AT III levels** should be measured in any patient with a history suggestive of a hypercoagulable state.
   b. **Functional protein C levels** also should be measured. It is important to emphasize that because protein C is vitamin K–dependent levels will be affected by warfarin.
   c. **Protein S levels.** This protein also is vitamin K–dependent, so measurements should be done at a time when the patient is not receiving warfarin.

3. **Lupus anticoagulants.** A prolonged PTT in a patient with a thrombotic event may suggest the presence of a lupus anticoagulant, and appropriate studies should be performed to document the nature of this "anticoagulant."

4. **Other tests.** Specific evaluation of the plasminogen system and other more subtle and rare abnormalities may be justified in some cases, but these studies seldom are performed routinely.

D. **Approach to the patient with a thrombotic disorder.** Unlike a bleeding disorder, a thrombotic disorder is almost never suspected based on laboratory screening tests but rather because the patient has endured a clinical thrombotic event. Thrombocytosis is the one exception.

1. **Thrombocytosis** (see I D 1 b) can be associated with thrombotic as well as hemorrhagic events.
   a. Thrombocytosis that is part of an underlying myeloproliferative process is often associated with thrombotic events. Therefore, a patient must be evaluated for conditions such as essential thrombocythemia and PV. Once such a diagnosis is established, treatment to lower the platelet count and, thus, limit the likelihood of thromboses can be instituted.
   b. Reactive thrombocytosis (e.g., secondary to removal of the spleen or associated with other medical conditions such as iron deficiency) is not associated with thrombotic events and is transient. It should just be watched. The goal of evaluating such a patient is, therefore, to exclude an underlying myeloproliferative process.

2. **Deficiencies of natural anticoagulants** are usually discovered because of the onset of thrombotic events in a patient at an early age. Rarely, warfarin necrosis suggests protein C or protein S deficiency, or a history of heparin resistance suggests AT III deficiency. More commonly, tests for all of these natural anticoagulants need to be conducted to exclude a deficiency.

3. **Abnormalities of the fibrinolytic system** are not as common as deficiencies of the natural anticoagulants. However, a patient with a strongly suggestive history and normal protein C, protein S, and AT III levels should undergo an euglobulin clot lysis test, which may suggest an abnormality of fibrinolysis, and plasminogen and plasminogen activators can be measured.

4. **Thrombohemorrhagic disorders,** such as DIC and TTP, are usually suspected because the hemorrhagic component of the disorder is often the most dramatic element. This is not the case in rare instances, and, therefore, coagulation tests in patients with unexplained thrombotic events must always be considered. Thrombocytopenia, for example, should not be overlooked as a clue to heparin thrombocytopenia or DIC.

5. **Other risk factors** for a thrombotic disorder should always be sought, as abnormalities of the vasculature or of blood flow are by far the most common cause of thrombosis. Multiple factors such as smoking, birth control pills, and obesity may explain the possibility of thrombosis in a young person, who might otherwise be suspected of having a primary hematologic abnormality. An underlying malignancy is another consideration in patients with hypercoagulable states that are otherwise unexplained.

STUDY QUESTIONS

Directions: Each of the numbered items or incomplete statements in this section is followed by answers or by completions of the statement. Select the **one** lettered answer or completion that is **best** in each case.

1. Which of the following conditions is NOT associated with a prolonged bleeding time?

(A) Uremia
(B) Thrombocytopenia
(C) Multiple myeloma
(D) Hemophilia
(E) von Willebrand's disease

2. A 54-year-old, previously well man is seen after preoperative blood screening reveals a platelet count of 70,000/μl. The man, who is to undergo elective angioplasty, has no complaints of bruising or bleeding and an unremarkable history. He is receiving no medications. The most appropriate next step is to

(A) order a test of bleeding time
(B) order platelet aggregation studies
(C) perform a bone marrow examination
(D) review the peripheral blood smear
(E) begin treatment with prednisone

3. A 25-year-old policeman is admitted to the hospital because of axillary thrombophlebitis. The history reveals that 2 years earlier he was admitted to a hospital for right femoral vein thrombosis, which required massive doses of heparin to achieve any prolongation of the partial thromboplastin time (PTT). He currently is receiving warfarin. The patient's older sister had one episode of deep venous thrombosis during her first pregnancy, and his younger brother had a mesenteric vein thrombosis at age 20. Which of the following tests would be most useful in assessing this patient's current thrombotic event?

(A) Protein C level
(B) Protein S level
(C) AT III level
(D) Prothrombin time (PT)
(E) Partial thromboplastin time (PTT)

4. A 75-year-old, previously healthy woman is admitted to the hospital because of gross hematuria. The patient says she began to notice spontaneous bruising over her arms, legs, and chest about 2 weeks earlier. Two years ago, she underwent cataract surgery, prior to which prothrombin time (PT) and partial thromboplastin time (PTT) tests were normal. Laboratory studies now reveal that PT, thrombin time (TT), fibrinogen level, bleeding time, and platelet count all are within normal limits but that PTT is markedly prolonged. Which of the following tests should be ordered?

(A) Mixing study
(B) Factor XII assay
(C) Factor XIII screen
(D) Platelet aggregation study
(E) Test for fibrin split products (FSPs)

5. Vitamin K deficiency most commonly shows up as an abnormality on which of the following screening tests?

(A) Platelet count
(B) Prothrombin time (PT)
(C) Partial thromboplastin time (PTT)
(D) Thrombin time (TT)
(E) Bleeding time

Directions: The item below contains four suggested answers, of which **one or more** is correct. Choose the answer

A if **1, 2, and 3** are correct
B if **1 and 3** are correct
C if **2 and 4** are correct
D if **4** is correct
E if **1, 2, 3, and 4** are correct

6. A patient with end-stage liver disease is admitted to the intensive care unit with bleeding from esophageal varices. Coagulation screening of this patient is likely to reveal

(1) prolonged prothrombin time (PT)
(2) prolonged partial thromboplastin time (PTT)
(3) prolonged thrombin time (TT)
(4) decreased platelet count

ANSWERS AND EXPLANATIONS

1. The answer is D *[I D 1 c; Figure 16-2].*
Hemophilia is associated with a prolonged partial thromboplastin time (PTT) and not with a prolonged bleeding time. Hemophilia is an inherited deficiency of factor VIII or factor IX; these deficiencies do not interfere with platelet function. Conditions that do prolong bleeding time include uremia, thrombocytopenia, multiple myeloma, and von Willebrand's disease.

2. The answer is D *[I D 1 a (1)].*
Thrombocytopenia (decreased platelet count) always should be confirmed by evaluation of the peripheral blood smear. In addition to providing information about the other cellular elements of the blood, which may clue to a diagnosis, a peripheral smear reveals clumped platelets that may have been inappropriately counted in an automated counter (so-called pseudothrombocytopenia) and, thus, eliminates the need for further evaluation. Bone marrow examination, for example, would not be necessary if the platelet count was not truly low, and treatment with prednisone would only be instituted if immunologic destruction of platelets was causing true thrombocytopenia. Bleeding time and platelet aggregation studies are most helpful in evaluating platelet function rather than number.

3. The answer is C *[Ch 15 II A 1; Ch 16 II A 1, C 2 a].*
This patient's history is highly suggestive of antithrombin III (AT III) deficiency, particularly the heparin resistance experienced during treatment of the first thrombotic episode. A reduced AT III level would strongly support this diagnosis. Measurement of protein C and protein S levels might give misleading results; both of these proteins are vitamin K–dependent and, thus, would be reduced while the patient is receiving warfarin (a vitamin K antagonist). Neither prothrombin time (PT) nor partial thromboplastin time (PTT) is affected by abnormalities of the naturally occurring anticoagulants.

4. The answer is A *[Ch 14 IV C 2; Ch 16 I C 2 b, c; D 2 a].*
This patient's history and clinical presentation suggest the development of a clotting factor inhibitor; to document or exclude this diagnosis, a mixing study should be performed to determine whether the addition of normal plasma corrects the prolonged partial thromboplastin time (PTT). An uncorrected PTT indicates the presence of an inhibitor, whose specificity should then be determined. Specific clotting factor levels may be helpful, but the choice of which factors to measure is based on statistical likelihood after the mixing study results confirm the presence of an inhibitor. Abnormal platelet function, deficiency of factor XIII, or the presence of fibrin split products (FSPs) would not be expected to cause isolated prolongation of the PTT.

5. The answer is B *[I D 3 a].*
Vitamin K deficiency results in the production of ineffective vitamin K–dependent coagulation factors (i.e., II, VII, IX, and X) and, therefore, may be associated with a prolongation of both prothrombin time (PT) and partial thromboplastin time (PTT). However, factor VII deficiency occurs first because of this factor's short half-life; thus, PT is the screening test most commonly affected by vitamin K deficiency. Platelet number and function are not affected by vitamin K deficiency, and fibrinogen levels remain normal, thus maintaining a normal thrombin time (TT).

6. The answer is E (all) *[I D 3 c].*
Most coagulation factors are produced in the liver. End-stage liver disease causes a decrease in factor production, resulting in prolonged prothrombin time (PT) [due to factor VII deficiency] and prolonged partial thromboplastin time (PTT) [due to deficiencies of factor IX, factor X, prothrombin, and others]. The thrombin time (TT) is prolonged in liver disease as a result of decreased and sometimes functionally abnormal fibrinogen. The platelet count often is decreased as a result of associated hypersplenism.

17
Clinical Aspects of Transfusion Therapy

Leigh C. Jefferies

I. BLOOD PRODUCTS FOR TRANSFUSION THERAPY

A. Blood product preparation

1. **Blood for donation**
   a. Donors must meet specific requirements of age, weight, medical history, and physical examination.
   b. The **usual donation** is 450 ml of whole blood, which may be maintained as such or separated into components.
   c. In special circumstances **hemapheresis** may be used to collect particular components (e.g., platelets, plasma, granulocytes) in larger quantities by processing a greater volume of blood from a single donor. This procedure involves removal of whole blood by phlebotomy, with separation of the desired component (e.g., platelets) and return of other components (e.g., plasma, red cells, leukocytes) to the donor.

2. **Laboratory tests**
   a. The following tests are performed on the blood of each donor at the time of collection to reduce the possibility of transmission of **infectious disease**. If any of these tests are positive, the blood is not transfused.
      (1) **Hepatitis B surface antigen (HB_sAg)** to detect hepatitis B virus
      (2) **Antibodies against human immunodeficiency virus type I and II (anti–HIV-I-II)** to detect antibody to HIV-I retrovirus
      (3) **Antibodies against human T cell lymphotropic virus type I and II (anti–HTLV-I-II)**
      (4) **Antibody to hepatitis C (anti-HCV)**
      (5) **Antibody to hepatitis B core antigen (anti-HB_c)** and **elevated alanine aminotransferase (ALT)** as surrogate markers for non-A, non-B hepatitis, and **rapid plasma reagent (RPR),** the serologic test for syphilis
   b. **ABO group** and **Rh(D) type** are also determined and are important in the selection of blood for transfusion (see II B–C).

3. **Separation of whole blood into components**
   a. Components available for transfusion therapy are obtained by a series of centrifugation steps (Figure 17-1).
   b. **Plasma** separated from the cellular components may be frozen [fresh frozen plasma (FFP)] or, alternatively, may be fractionated by more complex procedures into a number of products.

4. **Anticoagulant–preservative solutions.** These substances are added to the blood collection system to prevent clotting and provide the proper nutrients for continued metabolism of cellular products during storage. Examples include **CPD** (citrate, phosphate, dextrose) and **CPDA-1** [CPD supplemented with adenine as a substrate for adenosine triphosphate (ATP) synthesis]. Citrate serves as the anticoagulant by binding calcium.

5. **Storage conditions and shelf life.** These depend on the individual blood products.
   a. **Whole blood** and **red blood cells** are maintained at 1°–6° C for up to 21–42 days, depending on the preservative solution used.
   b. **Platelets** are stored at room temperature (20°–24° C) for up to 5 days.
   c. **FFP** and **cryoprecipitate** are stored at − 18° C for up to 12 months.
   d. **Granulocytes** may be maintained for only 24 hours at room temperature before transfusion.

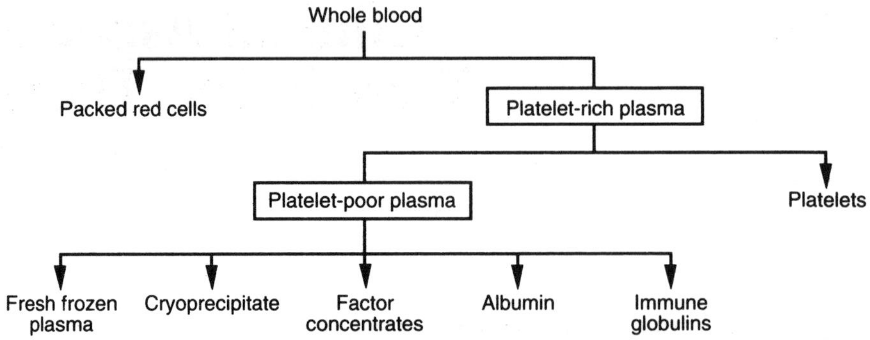

Figure 17-1. Separation of single-donor whole blood into components available for transfusion therapy. Blood products shown in *boxes* are further refined into products that are appropriate for transfusion therapy.

6. **Biochemical changes in stored blood ("storage lesion")**
   a. Blood stored at 1°–6° C undergoes measurable biochemical changes, including decreases in plasma pH, red cell adenosine triphosphate (ATP), and red cell 2,3-diphosphoglycerate (DPG), and increases in plasma potassium, sodium, and hemoglobin. With the exception of decreased DPG, these changes are usually of little clinical significance, unless a severely compromised patient is given massive quantities of stored blood (see III C).
   b. The **oxygen dissociation curve** (see Figure 9-2) is affected by changes in red cell DPG (as well as by pH). **Decreased levels of DPG** cause a greater affinity of hemoglobin for oxygen at a given Po_2, and, therefore, less oxygen is released to the tissues.
      (1) This is of practical significance when a recipient with small intravascular volume requires large amounts of blood. For example, neonates undergoing exchange transfusion receive blood (red cells) that has not been stored longer than 7 days to ensure adequate DPG levels.
      (2) This is not of practical significance for adults because the transfusion of red cells usually represents a small fraction of total blood volume, and red cell DPG regenerates within hours of transfusion.

B. **Individual blood products available for transfusion therapy.** In general, the appropriate uses and the doses and responses discussed below are relevant for transfusion in adults. These may be different for the pediatric population, particularly neonates.

1. **Whole blood**
   a. **Description**
      (1) One unit of whole blood contains approximately 450 ml of blood plus 63 ml of anticoagulant preservative.
      (2) Whole blood has had no blood constituents physically removed and, therefore, contains **red cells** (hematocrit ranging from 34% to 44%), **plasma, platelets,** and **leukocytes.**
         (a) The plasma contains albumin, immunoglobulins, and other plasma proteins, including coagulation factors; however, levels of the labile coagulation factors V and VIII are significantly decreased during storage.
         (b) Platelets and granulocytes lose viability in whole blood stored longer than 24 hours.
   b. **Appropriate uses**
      (1) Because whole blood provides both oxygen-carrying capacity (red blood cells) and volume expansion (plasma), the primary indication is for patients who are **actively bleeding** and have sustained a **loss of total blood volume greater than 35%–40%**. Examples include trauma patients and patients undergoing surgery with massive blood loss who are at risk of hemorrhagic shock.
      (2) Whole blood may also be used for **exchange transfusion** in patients with **sickle cell disease**.
   c. **Dosage and response.** The volume of whole blood needed will depend on the intravascular volume loss or volume of exchange. In an adult, 1 unit of whole blood will increase the hemoglobin approximately 1 g/dl.

d. Inappropriate uses

(1) Whole blood should not be used for patients with chronic anemia who are normovolemic and require only an increase in red cell mass; packed red cells should be used in these cases.

(2) Whole blood cannot be used to supply coagulation factors because it does not contain sufficient levels of labile factors V and VIII.

(3) Whole blood cannot be used to supply platelets or granulocytes.

2. Packed red blood cells

a. Description

(1) Red blood cells, prepared from whole blood by centrifugation, have a volume of 250–350 ml and a hematocrit of 50%–80%, depending on the anticoagulant–preservative solution used. A unit of red cells has the same oxygen-carrying capacity as a unit of whole blood because they each contain approximately the same number of red cells.

(2) Packed red blood cells do not contain functional platelets or granulocytes or significant levels of coagulation factors.

b. Appropriate uses. Packed red blood cells are of value in patients needing **oxygen-carrying capacity** for whom volume overload may be a potential problem. These include:

(1) Patients with **chronic symptomatic anemia** who require an increase in red cell mass (oxygen-carrying capacity) but do not require volume replacement

(2) Patients who are **actively bleeding** (e.g., from trauma, surgery, spontaneous hemorrhage), resulting in a loss of total blood volume greater than 25% (whole blood may be given to patients with significantly greater losses)

c. Dosage and response

(1) Transfusion requirements should be based primarily on the patient's clinical status, not on a predetermined hemoglobin or hematocrit value. Factors to consider include the patient's age, the degree and duration of anemia, the intravascular volume, and the presence of underlying cardiac, pulmonary, or vascular disease.

(2) Adequate oxygen-carrying capacity can be met in an adult by a hemoglobin concentration of 7 g/dl to maintain cardiopulmonary function when the intravascular volume is adequate for perfusion. One unit of packed red cells will increase the hemoglobin concentration about 1 g/dl in an adult.

d. Inappropriate uses

(1) Red blood cells cannot be used to supply platelets, granulocytes, or coagulation factors.

(2) Red blood cells are not indicated when total blood volume loss may be safely restored by the use of crystalloid (electrolyte) solutions alone. A general guideline is to use such solutions initially for losses of up to 25% of the total blood volume.

3. Random-donor platelet concentrates

a. Description. Platelets are separated from single units of whole blood and suspended in small amounts of plasma. Each bag should contain at least 5.5×10^{10} platelets in 50–70 ml plasma.

b. Appropriate uses. Platelet transfusions are of value in the following situations:

(1) Prophylactically in nonbleeding patients with a platelet count of $15–20 \times 10^3/\mu l$ or lower

(a) These are usually patients with bone marrow hypoplasia that is the result of chemotherapy, tumor invasion, or primary aplasia.

(b) Although platelet counts below $15–20 \times 10^3/\mu l$ are frequently tolerated, severely low platelet counts may predispose patients to petechiae, ecchymosis, epistaxis, or more serious bleeding such as central nervous system (CNS) or gastrointestinal hemorrhage.

(2) Prophylactically before surgery or invasive procedures (such as spinal tap or insertion of a central line) in patients with a platelet count below $50–60 \times 10^3/\mu l$

(3) For documented bleeding in patients with a platelet count below $50–60 \times 10^3/\mu l$

(4) For patients with documented abnormal platelet function before invasive procedures or to treat bleeding

c. Dosage and response. Generally, multiple units of platelets (6–8) are pooled before transfusion. Generally, one unit of platelets will increase the platelet count in a 70-kg adult by $5 \times 10^3/\mu l$ ($5 \times 10^9/L$).

d. Inappropriate uses

(1) Prophylactic platelet transfusion for thrombocytopenia is generally not indicated in cases of accelerated platelet destruction [idiopathic thrombocytopenic purpura (ITP) or thrombotic thrombocytopenic purpura (TTP)].

(2) Platelet transfusion is generally not indicated in cases of platelet function disorders that are the result of extrinsic causes such as uremia, von Willebrand's disease, or hyperglobulinemia.

4. Human leukocyte antigens (HLA)–matched platelets

a. Description

(1) HLA-matched platelets are collected by hemapheresis from an individual donor. One unit (or bag) of single-donor platelets usually contains 3×10^{11} platelets, which is equal to 6–8 units of random-donor platelet concentrate. The volume of plasma in the product varies from 200 to 400 ml.

(2) HLA typing is performed on donor and recipient lymphocytes. The best available HLA match between the donor and recipient at the A and B loci depends on the donor pool.

b. Appropriate uses. HLA-matched platelets are indicated for patients who require platelet transfusions but are refractory to platelet transfusions because of **HLA alloimmunization;** that is, the emergence of antibodies against HLA antigens on platelets. (Alloimmunization against non-HLA platelet-specific antigens can also occur; however, matching for these other antigens is not practical at this time.)

(1) Refractoriness is defined by the lack of expected rise in platelet count after transfusion and may be due to alloimmunization or other causes, including fever, infection, sepsis, bleeding, disseminated intravascular coagulation (DIC), or splenomegaly.

(2) Calculation of the **post-transfusion platelet count increment (CI)** is useful in assessing refractoriness:

$$\text{CI} = \frac{\text{post-transfusion platelet count} - \text{pretransfusion platelet count}}{\text{Platelets transfused} \times 10^{11}} \times \text{BSA}$$

where BSA = body surface area in square meters.

(a) A CI higher than $7.5–10 \times 10^9$/L from a sample drawn from 10 minutes to 1 hour after transfusion, or a CI higher than 4.5×10^9/L from a sample drawn 8–24 hours after transfusion, is considered acceptable (i.e., **not refractory**).

(b) The 1-hour count may be helpful in distinguishing alloimmunization from other, nonimmunologic, causes of refractoriness to platelet transfusion. In alloimmunization, both 1-hour and 24-hour post-transfusion counts are typically low, whereas the 1-hour count may be acceptable with other causes of refractoriness [I B 4 b (1)].

c. Dosage and response. The dosage necessary depends on the patient's pretransfusion platelet count and the desired CI. The response depends in part on the HLA match between the donor and recipient and ideally provides an acceptable CI. Refractoriness, however, is not always overcome by the use of HLA-matched platelets.

d. Inappropriate uses. HLA-matched platelets are not indicated in patients who are refractory to platelet transfusions for reasons other than HLA alloimmunization. In such patients, HLA-matched platelets would not survive any longer in vivo than would random-donor platelet concentrates.

5. Granulocyte concentrates

a. Description. Granulocyte concentrates are usually prepared by **leukapheresis** (hemapheresis with selective removal of leukocytes) from a single donor. Each unit contains more than 10×10^{10} granulocytes, and some lymphocytes, platelets, and red blood cells, in 200–300 ml of plasma. Because of rapid loss of function during storage, granulocytes are infused within 24 hours of collection.

b. Appropriate uses

(1) Patients with **profound neutropenia** (absolute granulocyte count below 0.5×10^9/ml) that is due to myeloid hypoplasia of bone marrow with documented **infection unresponsive to antibiotics** and a likely **chance for recovery of bone marrow function** may be candidates for granulocyte transfusion.

(2) Septic neonates and patients with **severe granulocyte dysfunction syndromes** (e.g., chronic granulomatous disease) may also benefit from granulocyte transfusion.

c. **Dosage and response.** At least 4–6 days of granulocyte therapy (i.e., 1 unit/day) are necessary to demonstrate a beneficial effect. Response is usually monitored by response to anti-infective therapy, since transfusions do not measurably increase peripheral blood levels of granulocytes.
d. **Inappropriate uses.** The prophylactic use of granulocytes is of questionable value.

6. **Fresh frozen plasma (FFP)**
   a. **Description**
      (1) FFP is prepared from whole blood by separating and freezing the plasma within 6 hours of phlebotomy.
      (2) Along with water and electrolytes, plasma contains albumin, globulins, coagulation factors, and other proteins. Plasma maintained in the frozen state will contain both labile coagulation factors (V and VIII) and stable factors (I, II, VII, IX, X, XI, XII, XIII, and others). In general, 1 ml of plasma contains one unit of coagulation factor activity.
      (3) The volume of a single unit of FFP will range from 200 to 250 ml.
   b. **Appropriate uses**
      (1) FFP may be indicated in cases of **multiple coagulation factor deficiencies** [as evidenced by prolonged prothrombin time (PT) or partial thromboplastin time (PTT)] **when the patient is bleeding or at risk of bleeding**. Examples include:
         (a) Patients with liver disease who are bleeding or are at risk of bleeding from a planned invasive procedure
         (b) Patients with DIC
      (2) FFP may be indicated in **massive transfusion** (i.e., the administration of a volume of blood and blood components equal to or greater than the patient's estimated blood volume within a 24-hour period).
         (a) Deficiencies in coagulation factors (and in platelets) are seen in some patients during and after massive transfusion for hemorrhagic shock. Resuscitation with fluid and blood components deficient in coagulation factors may possibly contribute to a "dilutional coagulopathy." Bleeding seen in this setting may also be related to the degree of tissue injury and development of DIC.
         (b) Because there is no direct correlation between the volume of blood transfused and the development of abnormal coagulation parameters or bleeding, formulas (e.g., transfuse FFP after every 8–10 units of packed red blood cells) may be used only as general guidelines; the need for FFP should be determined by monitoring the PT or PTT and evidence of bleeding.
      (3) FFP may be used to reverse the **effect of warfarin** when the reversal effected by administration of vitamin K would not be fast enough.
         (a) It may be necessary to reverse the effect of warfarin anticoagulants before surgery or an invasive procedure to ensure adequate coagulation or in cases of warfarin overdosage.
         (b) Vitamin K is used whenever possible to reverse the effect of warfarin on the vitamin K–dependent coagulation factors. Because this may take up to 24 hours (with oral administration of vitamin K), emergencies may warrant the use of FFP to provide coagulation factors.
      (4) FFP may be used to correct a **specific coagulation factor deficiency,** such as antithrombin III, factor II, V, VII, IX, X, or XI, or protein C or S, when a specific factor concentrate (such as factor VIII) is not available.
      (5) FFP is used to replace the plasma in patients with **TTP** by plasma exchange (plasmapheresis). Simple infusion of FFP may be of some benefit if plasma exchange is not possible. The component in FFP that exerts the apparent therapeutic effect in this disease has not been identified.
   c. **Dosage and response.** The amount of FFP needed will depend on the clinical situation and the underlying disease process; for initial therapy, 15 ml/kg (4–6 units) are often required. The PT and PTT (see Ch 14 II) provide useful guides to additional therapy. These screening tests reach normal values when coagulation factors are at or above 30% of normal.
   d. **Inappropriate uses**
      (1) FFP should not be used as a volume expander or as a nutritional supplement.
      (2) FFP should not be used to treat bleeding alone or prolonged PT or PTT alone.
      (3) FFP should not be given by standing orders or orders by formula.
      (4) FFP is not a suitable source for immunoglobulins; purified immunoglobulin G (IgG) is available for intravenous administration for specific indications.

7. **Cryoprecipitate**
   a. **Description.** Cryoprecipitate is prepared by thawing one unit of FFP at 4° C. The cold, insoluble precipitate, resuspended in 10–15 ml of plasma, contains approximately 80–120 units of **factor VIII:C** (the coagulant property of factor VIII), 200 mg of **fibrinogen,** 40%–70% of the **von Willebrand factor (VIII:vWF)** present in the initial unit of FFP, and 20%–30% of the **factor XIII** present in the initial unit.
   b. **Appropriate uses**
      (1) Because it is rich in both factors VIII:C and VIII:vWF, cryoprecipitate is used to treat **von Willebrand's disease,** in which there is a partial deficiency of factor VIII:C as well as defective or decreased VIII:vWF. [A trial with desmopressin (1-desamino-8-D-arginine vasopressin; DDAVP) is recommended for von Willebrand's disease type I and may eliminate the need for cryoprecipitate in some patients.]
      (2) Cryoprecipitate is used to treat **hypofibrinogenemia,** which may be acquired as a part of the DIC syndrome or may occur as a rare isolated inherited deficiency. The use of cryoprecipitate is generally not indicated unless the fibrinogen level is below 100–120 mg/dl and there is evidence of active bleeding.
      (3) Cryoprecipitate may be used to treat bleeding or for prophylaxis in **hemophilia A (factor VIII:C deficiency)** as an alternative to lyophilized factor VIII (see I B 11).
      (4) Cryoprecipitate may be used to treat **factor XIII deficiency**.
      (5) Cryoprecipitate can be used to treat **bleeding related to renal failure;** the reason for cessation of bleeding in some patients is not known.
   c. **Dosage and response**
      (1) The precise quantity of **factor VIII:vWF** present in cryoprecipitate is not routinely determined, and the amount of cryoprecipitate required to treat bleeding episodes or to prepare for surgery varies greatly among patients with **von Willebrand's disease**. A general recommended dose is one bag of cryoprecipitate per 6 kg body weight.
      (2) For the replacement of **factor VIII:C,** the number of bags needed may be calculated using the following formula:

$$\frac{\text{Plasma volume} \times [\text{desired factor level in U/ml} - \text{initial factor level in U/ml}]}{\text{80 U factor VIII:C/bag of cryoprecipitate}} = \text{number of bags}$$

where plasma volume (in ml) = [weight (in kg) × 70 ml/kg] × (1 − Hct). This formula does not take into account factor VIII in the extravascular space, which is estimated at 1.5 times the amount in the intravascular space. Dose response may be lower than expected, depending upon saturation of the extravascular space. Responses should be monitored with periodic plasma VIII:C assays. The desired level of VIII:C varies with the clinical situation (e.g., bleeding versus surgery) and requires maintenance dosing.
      (3) Factor VIII:C levels may be reported as percent of normal (e.g., 50% = 0.5 U/ml).
      (4) The number of bags necessary to achieve a desired **fibrinogen** level may be calculated, using a formula similar to that described for factor VIII:C, substituting 200 mg fibrinogen/bag, and expressing desired and initial fibrinogen levels in mg/ml. In an emergency situation, 10 bags can be given to provide approximately 2 g of fibrinogen, which is usually sufficient to achieve adequate levels for hemostasis. The measurement of fibrinogen blood levels is important to guide therapy.
      (5) Transfusion of 2–3 ml of plasma per kilogram of body weight affects hemostasis in patients with factor XIII deficiency for up to 4 weeks. Alternatively, cryoprecipitate, which has two to four times more factor XIII per volume than plasma, may be used.
   d. **Inappropriate uses.** Cryoprecipitate is not appropriate for patients with deficiencies of factors other than VIII:C, VIII:vWF, XIII, or fibrinogen.

8. **Albumin**
   a. **Description.** Serum albumin, prepared from plasma, is available in concentrations of 50 or 250 g/L.
   b. **Appropriate uses.** Albumin solutions bring about volume expansion and are used to treat hypovolemia or decreased colloid oncotic pressure. Appropriate indications for albumin therapy include:
      (1) **Acute volume expansion** in
         (a) Patients with **chronic albumin depletion** (for example, protein-losing enteropathy with edema that is resistant to diuretics, or in liver failure with concomitant hypotension.)

(b) Patients with **hypovolemia in shock** when the serum albumin level may be low (crystalloids are frequently used as first-line treatment, but colloids such as albumin may also be appropriate)

(2) **Long-term replacement,** as in extensive **burns**

(3) **Acute hemodilution,** as in **cardiopulmonary bypass priming** or replacement of removed plasma in therapeutic **plasmapheresis**

c. **Dosage and response.** The dose will depend on the patient's underlying condition, plasma volume, and desired circulating plasma level (e.g., 5.0 g/dl).

d. **Inappropriate uses.** Albumin is not indicated for nutritional support or wound healing.

9. **Immune serum globulin**

a. **Description**

(1) Immune serum globulin may be concentrated from plasma as a sterile lyophilized preparation or as solutions for intravenous or for intramuscular use. Over 90% of the protein is IgG, with trace amounts of IgA and IgM.

(2) The half-lives of intravenous and intramuscular preparations have been reported to vary from 18 to 32 days.

b. **Appropriate uses**

(1) Immune serum globulin can be used as replacement therapy for **primary immunodeficiency states** such as congenital agammaglobulinemias, common variable immunodeficiency, Wiskott-Aldrich syndrome, and severe combined immunodeficiency disorder (SCID).

(2) Intravenous immune serum globulin has been used to treat **autoimmune disorders,** most notably acute and chronic **ITP,** and **acquired immune deficiency syndrome–related (AIDS-related) thrombocytopenia**.

c. **Dosage and response.** Vials of immune serum globulin indicate the amount of protein present (0.5–10.0 g). The dose depends on the reason for administration and on whether an intramuscular or intravenous preparation is used.

d. **Inappropriate uses.** In general, individuals with a history of IgA deficiency who have anti-IgA antibody may show severe anaphylactic reactions to plasma products and, therefore, should not receive immune serum globulins.

10. **Rh(D)* immune globulin**

a. **Description.** Rh(D) immune globulin is a concentrated solution of anti-Rh(D) IgG antibodies prepared from the plasma of individuals immunized to the Rh(D) antigen. A 1-ml full-dose vial or syringe (known as a **300-μg dose**) is sufficient to counteract the immunizing effects of 15 ml of Rh(D)-positive red cells (or 30 ml of whole blood).

b. **Appropriate uses**

(1) Rh(D) immune globulin is indicated to prevent Rh(D) immunization in Rh(D)-negative women exposed to Rh(D)-positive red cells by **fetomaternal hemorrhage**. Rh(D) immune globulin is given:

(a) Postpartum to unsensitized Rh(D)-negative women delivering Rh(D)-positive infants

(b) Antepartum to unsensitized Rh(D)-negative women at 28 weeks gestation

(c) After other possible causes of fetomaternal hemorrhage: abortion, miscarriage, vaginal hemorrhage, ectopic pregnancy, abdominal trauma, or amniocentesis

(2) Rh(D) immune globulin should also be considered to prevent Rh(D) immunization in unsensitized Rh(D)-negative women of childbearing age who have been exposed to **Rh(D)-positive blood products** (red cells or platelets or granulocytes containing red cells). Considerations include the age of the patient, the quantity of blood product transfused, and the consequences of Rh(D) immunization on future transfusions or pregnancies. Many vials via intramuscular injection may be problematic, particularly in a patient with severe thrombocytopenia.

c. **Dosage and response**

(1) Antepartum or postpartum a full (300-μg) dose is given within 72 hours of exposure to Rh(D)-positive red cells. Postpartum, or after suspected fetomaternal hemorrhage, maternal blood is screened to determine if unexpectedly large fetomaternal hemorrhage has occurred, requiring additional Rh(D) immune globulin.

---

*The Fisher-Race nomenclature system is used here; in the Wiener system, the D antigen is called Rh_0.

(2) Larger doses may be necessary if Rh(D) immune globulin is used to prevent immunization following the transfusion of Rh(D)-positive blood products.

d. Inappropriate uses

(1) Rh(D)-negative women who deliver Rh(D)-negative infants are not candidates for Rh(D) immune globulin.

(2) Rh(D)-negative women who are known to be sensitized (i.e., have already developed anti-D antibodies because of exposure during a previous pregnancy or transfusion) and will not benefit from Rh(D) immune globulin.

(3) Rh(D)-positive women are not candidates for Rh(D) immune globulin.

11. Factor VIII concentrate

a. Description

(1) Factor VIII (antihemophilic factor; factor VIII:C) concentrate is prepared by the fractionation of pooled plasma. The quantity of factor VIII is expressed in international units (IU): 1 IU is the amount of factor VIII activity present in 1 ml of normal plasma.

(2) A half-life range of 12–18 hours has been reported.

(3) Several types of lyophilized concentrates are available, differing in the degree of purity and the method of treatment used to inactivate viruses.

b. Appropriate uses. Factor VIII concentrate is used to prevent or control hemorrhage in:

(1) Patients with **hemophilia A** who have moderate to severe congenital factor VIII deficiency

(2) Patients with a **low level of factor VIII inhibitors** [patients with levels over 10 Bethesda units/ml of plasma are given anti-inhibitor coagulation complex (see I B 13)]

c. Dosage and response

(1) The dose of lyophilized factor VIII required to achieve the desired in vivo levels may be calculated by using a formula similar to that described for cryoprecipitate:

$$\frac{\text{Plasma volume} \times [\text{desired IU/ml} - \text{initial IU/ml}]}{\text{IU/bottle of factor VIII}} = \text{number of bottles}$$

(2) When factor VIII is used to treat patients with factor VIII inhibitors, the effectiveness of therapy should be monitored by assaying both the patient's factor VIII levels and inhibitor titers.

d. Inappropriate uses. In general, Factor VIII concentrate alone should not be used for the treatment of von Willebrand's disease since most concentrates lack the factor VIII:vWF needed for normal platelet function. [Some concentrates, e.g., Humate P, do preserve vWF activity and may be efficacious in controlling hemorrhage (see Ch 14 III B 4 c)].

12. Factor IX concentrate (prothrombin complex concentrate)

a. Description. Factor IX concentrate is prepared by the fractionation of plasma and contains coagulation factor IX along with traces of factors II (prothrombin), VII, and X. Factor IX concentrates are available either as prothrombin complex concentrates with significant levels of vitamin K-dependent coagulation factors, which were introduced in the 1960s, or as more purified factor IX concentrates, which were introduced recently. Specific activity (U/mg) of factor IX varies among the commercial products.

b. Appropriate uses

(1) Factor IX concentrate is used to treat patients with **factor IX deficiency (hemophilia B or Christmas disease).**

(2) Preparations of factor IX concentrate produced in earlier years contain significant amounts of factors VII and X and may be used to treat patients with congenital deficiencies of **factors VII and X.**

(3) Prothrombin concentrates may also be used to treat patients with hemophilia A who have inhibitors to factor VIII.

c. Inappropriate uses. Factor IX concentrate should not be used for patients with liver disease; FFP can be used to provide labile and stable coagulation factors (see I B 6). Thrombosis and DIC may be associated with the use of factor IX concentrate, although newly developed factor IX products appear to be less thrombogenic than the older preparations.

13. Anti-inhibitor coagulation complex

a. Description. Anti-inhibitor coagulation complex is prepared by fractionation of pooled human plasma and is a stable, sterile product containing properties that bypass inhibitors of factor VIII activity. It consists of activator and precursor vitamin K coagulation factors, including activated factor VII and factor X.

b. Appropriate uses

(1) Anti-inhibitor coagulation complex is indicated for hemophilic and nonhemophilic patients with a **high titer of factor VIII inhibitors** (> 10 Bethesda units/ml). (Patients with titers below 10 Bethesda units/ml are given factor VIII concentrate.)

(2) Patients with factor IX inhibitors who have serious bleeding episodes may also benefit from anti-inhibitor coagulation complex.

c. Dosage and response. The dosage depends on the severity of the patient's condition. The risk of thrombosis and DIC are high, and patients receiving this product should be monitored for these complications.

d. Inappropriate uses

(1) Anti-inhibitor coagulation complex should not be administered to patients with liver disease. FFP is available to supply all stable and labile coagulation factors for patients with multiple coagulation factor deficiency (e.g., liver disease).

(2) Patients with a low level of factor VIII inhibitors are treated with factor VIII concentrates.

14. **Other products.** Blood proteins under investigation for potential clinical usefulness include **antithrombin III, protein S, protein C,** and **fibronectin**.

II. COMPATIBILITY (PRETRANSFUSION) TESTING

A. Overview. Compatibility testing represents a series of tests on the patient's (recipient's) blood and the donor blood to ensure proper selection of blood components for safe transfusion.

1. First, **ABO group** and **Rh(D) type** are determined on the patient's red blood cells, and the patient's serum is screened for clinically significant **alloantibodies against red blood cells**. These tests are performed on donor blood at the time of collection.
2. Next, a **crossmatch** is performed between the patient's serum and the donor's red blood cells. In some cases, a **direct antiglobulin test** may also be an important part of pretransfusion testing.
3. In vitro detection of antigen–antibody interaction may be accomplished by a variety of laboratory methods [e.g., radioimmunoassay (RIA), enzyme-linked immunosorbent assay (ELISA)]. For routine evaluation, the endpoint for pretransfusion testing is **agglutination,** or clumping of red cells. Agglutination occurs when antibodies against a particular red cell antigen form bridges between the red cells expressing that antigen.

B. Determination of the patient's (recipient's) ABO group

1. **Introduction.** The ABO blood group system is the most important blood group system to be considered in transfusion practice and is the only blood group system in which reciprocal antibodies are consistently present in the serum of normal individuals when their red blood cells lack the corresponding antigens (Table 17-1). The ABO group of a patient is determined by testing the patient's red blood cells and serum with commercial antisera (anti-A and anti-B) and cells (A, B, and O), respectively, for agglutination.
2. **Biochemical basis of the ABO blood group system**

a. A blood group system consists of a group of red cell antigens produced directly or indirectly by alleles at a single gene locus or closely linked loci.

b. ABO blood group expression depends on gene-encoded glycosyltransferase enzymes that determine the terminal immunodominant sugar on the particular oligosaccharides associated with the red cell membrane glycosphingolipids. Specifically:

(1) **Group A** individuals have a gene-encoded transferase that links ***N*-acetylgalactosamine** to the precursor oligosaccharide.

Table 17-1. Antigens and Antibodies in the ABO Blood Group System

ABO Group	Red Cell Antigens Present	Red Cell Antibodies Present in Serum
A	A	Anti-B
B	B	Anti-A
AB	A and B	Neither
O	Neither	Anti-A and Anti-B

(2) **Group B** individuals have a different transferase that links **galactose** to the precursor oligosaccharide.
(3) **Group O** individuals have **neither** of these enzymes and, thus, do not express A or B red cell antigens.
(4) **Group AB** individuals have **both** of these enzymes and express both antigens.

3. Clinical significance

a. Transfusion of ABO-incompatible blood may induce an **acute hemolytic transfusion reaction** because the presence of antibody in the recipient's serum causes hemolysis of transfused red cells expressing the corresponding antigen (e.g., the transfusion of group A red blood cells or whole blood to a group B patient whose serum contains anti-A antibodies). It is usually the IgM component of the antibody that activates complement and causes red cell lysis. Group O red blood cells lack both A and B antigens and, therefore, may be transfused in an emergency to patients of unknown ABO type (see II G 2) without causing an acute hemolytic transfusion reaction.

b. **ABO hemolytic disease of the newborn** may result when maternal anti-A and anti-B antibodies of the IgG isotype cross the placenta and bind to fetal red cells expressing the corresponding antigen (see II F 2 b).

C. Determination of the patient's (recipient's) Rh(D) type

1. Introduction

a. After A and B, the D antigen is the most important red cell antigen in transfusion practice. This protein antigen is part of the Rh blood group system, a complex system that is composed of more than 40 different red cell antigens. Other important Rh antigens include C, E, c, and e.

b. In contrast to the A and B antigens, the reciprocal antibody is not normally present in the serum of Rh(D)-negative individuals unless they have been immunized by exposure to foreign Rh(D)-positive red cells during transfusion or pregnancy. Commercial anti-D antiserum is used to test the patient's red blood cells for the presence of the D antigen.

2. Clinical significance

a. The Rh(D) antigen is a potent immunogen. Over 80% of Rh(D)-negative individuals who receive a unit of Rh(D)-positive red blood cells will become immunized and produce anti-D antibodies.
(1) Once an individual is immunized, that person must receive only Rh(D)-negative red cells or whole blood to avoid a transfusion reaction.
(2) Unimmunized Rh(D)-negative individuals should receive only Rh(D)-negative cellular blood products to avoid immunization.

b. Anti-D antibody is the most common cause of severe hemolytic disease of the newborn. Therefore, it is important to transfuse only Rh(D)-negative cellular blood products to unimmunized Rh(D)-negative females until the end of the childbearing years. Once immunization occurs, future pregnancies [if the fetus is Rh(D)-positive] may be complicated by hemolytic disease of the newborn.

D. Detection of clinically significant alloantibodies in the patient's serum (antibody screen; indirect antiglobulin test)

1. Introduction

a. In addition to the ABO and Rh systems, many other blood group systems also define important red cell membrane antigens. Examples include the **Kell, Duffy,** and **Kidd** blood groups. In most cases, in contrast to the ABO system, the **alloantibodies** against these antigens are not normally present unless the individual has been immunized by pregnancy or transfusion.

b. To detect these antibodies, an **antibody screen** is performed on the patient's serum by incubation with commercial red blood cells whose surface antigen expression is known. The agglutination of reagent red blood cells is assessed under different conditions.
(1) Anti–red blood cell IgM antibodies, for example, may readily agglutinate red blood cells at room temperature.
(2) In contrast, anti–red blood cell IgG antibodies may coat red blood cells but not cause

detectable agglutination without the addition of antiglobulin reagent (rabbit anti–human IgG, the **Coombs' reagent**), which effects agglutination by crosslinking the IgG molecules on red blood cells. Therefore, the antibody screen may also be referred to as the **indirect antiglobulin test**.

2. **Clinical significance**
   a. Red cell alloantibodies are designated clinically significant if they are likely to cause immune destruction in vivo of red blood cells expressing the corresponding antigen. This is determined in part by the antibody specificity, thermal amplitude, titer, and isotype of the antibody.
   b. These alloantibodies may **cause hemolytic transfusion reactions** or **hemolytic disease of the newborn**. For a patient who has a clinically significant antibody in the serum, it is important to select blood products (red cells or whole blood) that lack expression of the corresponding antigen.

E. Crossmatch between the patient's serum and the donor's red blood cells

1. **Introduction.** The final phase of pretransfusion testing is the crossmatch between the patient's serum and red blood cells from the donated red cell or whole blood unit. (Granulocyte units are also tested owing to contaminating red blood cells.) Agglutination of donor red cells by the patient's serum indicates the presence of an antibody causing an incompatible crossmatch. When an antibody screen has identified antibodies in the patient's serum, a compatible crossmatch may be possible by choosing units that lack the corresponding antigen.

2. **Clinical significance.** For patients with multiple antibodies or with antibodies against antigens of high frequency in the donor population, it may be difficult to find compatible blood. It is necessary to find a compatible crossmatch, however, to avoid transfusion reactions and ensure the normal survival of transfused red cells.

F. Direct antiglobulin test (Coombs' test). Although not a part of routine compatibility testing, this test may be important in the evaluation of patients before transfusion and in certain other clinical settings.

1. **Introduction.** The direct antiglobulin test is used to detect IgG or complement (C3b and C3d) binding to red blood cells. Anti–human globulin (**anti–human IgG**), also referred to as **Coombs' reagent,** causes agglutination of red blood cells that have surface IgG. Anti–human complement can be used in a similar way to detect red cells that have surface complement.

2. **Clinical significance**
   a. **Suspected hemolytic transfusion reaction.** Red cells in a patient's circulation may have surface-bound IgG or surface-bound complement, which has been deposited by IgM antibodies, such as naturally occurring anti-A or anti-B antibody.
      (1) A positive direct antiglobulin test supports the diagnosis of transfusion reaction in the proper setting and may, thus, guide therapeutic considerations (see III A 1).
      (2) The identification of such antibodies is also important before the selection and transfusion of subsequent units of blood, which should lack the corresponding antigen to prevent another reaction.
   b. **Suspected hemolytic disease of the newborn.** Red cells of an affected infant may bind with maternal IgG antibody that has traversed the placenta if the mother has been immunized against a foreign antigen on the infant's red cells. Many different red cell antibodies may cause this syndrome.
      (1) Detection of these antibodies in both the mother's and the infant's serum is necessary to make the diagnosis of hemolytic disease of the newborn.
      (2) Identification of such antibodies is important before the selection of blood for the transfusion of affected infants. (Units should lack the corresponding antigen.)
   c. **Suspected autoimmune hemolytic anemia.** Red cells of affected patients usually have surface-bound IgG (and occasionally complement) in warm autoimmune hemolytic anemia and usually have surface-bound complement in cold autoimmune hemolytic anemia.
      (1) A positive direct antiglobulin test in the appropriate setting supports the diagnosis of autoimmune hemolytic anemia. Evaluation of the IgG antibody stripped from the red cells helps to determine if the anemia is due to an autoantibody, as in warm autoimmune hemolytic anemia or due to an alloantibody, as in acute or delayed hemolytic transfusion reactions.

(2) A positive direct antiglobulin test may also support the diagnosis of **drug-induced immune hemolytic anemia** in the appropriate setting.

G. Selection of blood products for transfusion

1. Routine transfusion

a. Whole blood, red cells, or granulocytes (which usually contain a significant amount of contaminating red cells)

(1) All phases of pretransfusion testing are required; crossmatch-compatible blood of the same ABO group is transfused.

(2) Rh(D)-positive individuals may receive Rh(D)-positive or Rh(D)-negative blood. Rh(D)-negative individuals, however, should receive only Rh(D)-negative red cell products to prevent immunization to the D antigen when this blood is available.

b. Platelets

(1) It is preferable to transfuse platelets of the same ABO group as the recipient, if available, in part because anti-A or anti-B antibodies may be present in the plasma in which the platelets are suspended. Such passively transfused antibodies may bind to the patient's red cells (as shown by a positive direct antiglobulin test), although evidence of hemolysis is uncommon. There is some evidence that A or B antigens present on platelets may contribute to the decreased survival of these platelets in recipients with the corresponding antibodies.

(2) Rh(D)-negative platelets are transfused to unsensitized Rh(D)-negative individuals because even a small amount of contaminating red cells in the platelets may result in immunization to the D antigen.

(3) The other phases of pretransfusion testing (antibody screen of patient serum and crossmatch) are not necessary.

c. FFP or cryoprecipitate

(1) The patient should receive products of his or her ABO group to avoid transfusion of anti-A or anti-B antibodies that could bind to his or her red cells.

(2) Because FFP and cryoprecipitate are cell-free products, they are given without regard for the Rh(D) type, and neither the antibody screen of the patient's serum nor a crossmatch is required.

2. Emergency transfusion

a. Rarely, emergency transfusion of **red blood cells** is necessary before a patient sample can be obtained and pretransfusion testing performed. (Examples include trauma or ruptured aortic aneurysm with sudden, severe intravascular volume loss.)

(1) In these cases, a life-saving transfusion of **group O red cells** may be necessary. Whole blood is not given in these circumstances to avoid the transfusion of large amounts of anti-A and anti-B antibodies. Rh(D)-negative blood should be given to females under age 50 if Rh(D) type is unknown. Alternatively, if time permits ABO and Rh(D) testing of the recipient, it may be possible to select ABO- and Rh(D)-matched red cells or whole blood.

(2) In either case, because antibody screening of the recipient serum and crossmatch have not been performed, this blood is uncrossmatched and the risk of hemolytic transfusion is of concern.

b. During the time required to determine the necessity for **platelets,** the recipient's ABO and Rh(D) type can usually be determined. Lack of availability of platelets of a specific ABO and Rh(D) type in an urgent circumstance, however, may warrant transfusion of platelets of ABO group and Rh(D) type other than that of the recipient; this is preferable to withholding platelets in patients with bleeding caused by thrombocytopenia, for example.

c. During the time required to determine the necessity for **FFP** or **cryoprecipitate** and to thaw these frozen products, the patient's ABO group can usually be determined.

III. ADVERSE EFFECTS OF TRANSFUSION

A. Immune-mediated adverse effects

1. Acute hemolytic transfusion reactions

a. Pathogenesis. Acute hemolytic transfusion reactions are usually due to transfusion of **ABO-incompatible whole blood** or **red blood cells** following a clerical error (e.g., mislabeling of a patient's sample for ABO typing) or transfusion of blood to a patient other than the intended recipient.

(1) The IgM component of naturally occurring anti-A or anti-B antibodies present in the patient's serum agglutinates transfused red cells that have the corresponding antigen, leading to complement activation and acute intravascular hemolysis.

(2) The subsequent involvement of neuroendocrine and coagulation systems may lead to shock, acute renal failure, and DIC.

b. Signs and symptoms. The onset and severity of signs and symptoms are variable, depending on the amount of blood transfused and the specific ABO mismatch, and may include fever, chills, chest pain, back pain, pain at the infusion site, nausea, dyspnea, hemoglobinuria, oliguria, bleeding, hypotension, and shock. In anesthetized patients, the only signs may be uncontrolled hypotension, hemoglobinuria, and excessive bleeding.

c. Treatment and prevention

(1) Transfusion should be immediately discontinued upon onset of suspicious symptoms, and venous access should be maintained. Initial therapy is aimed at vigorous treatment of hypotension and promotion of renal blood flow with fluids and diuretics.

(2) A postreaction blood sample along with the unit in question should be submitted for prompt evaluation and clerical checks. Hemoglobinemia and a positive direct antiglobulin test (evidence of complement or antibody on the patient's red cells) support the diagnosis. Additional tests to evaluate hemolysis include hemoglobin, hematocrit, and lactate dehydrogenase (LDH). Indirect serum bilirubin should peak 3–6 hours after an acute hemolytic episode.

(3) **Prevention** requires accurate labeling of patient samples and accurate identification of the recipient at the time of transfusion.

2. Delayed hemolytic transfusion reactions

a. Pathogenesis. Delayed reactions are due to primary or secondary immunization against **red cell alloantigens** (i.e., foreign antigens not present on the patient's red blood cells), such as Kell, Duffy, Kidd, or Rh system antigens.

(1) Primary antibody production begins 1–2 weeks following exposure. A secondary, or anamnestic, response typically occurs in the previously immunized patient whose titer has dropped below detectable levels. Following re-exposure to the red cell alloantigen, a rapid increase in antibody titer (usually IgG) is seen over the subsequent 1–5 days.

(2) The characteristics of the antibody and the number of foreign red blood cells present determines the degree of shortened red cell survival and whether clinical symptoms will be evident.

b. Signs and symptoms. Delayed reactions may be subclinical, particularly if they are due to primary alloimmunization, and manifest initially only by an unexplained fall in hemoglobin. In cases with a rapid rise in the titer of the antibody or when the antibody activates complement, the recipient may develop fever, chills, anemia, jaundice, and hemoglobinemia.

c. Treatment and prevention

(1) Patients suspected of having a delayed hemolytic transfusion reaction should be evaluated for immune-mediated hemolysis with the direct antiglobulin test (usually positive for IgG) and antibody screen (indirect antiglobulin test) to document the presence of a new circulating alloantibody, along with other laboratory tests for hemolysis.

(2) Serious sequelae are infrequent with delayed hemolytic transfusion reactions; however, patients with underlying disease may require additional treatment. For example, it may be necessary to monitor renal function in patients with renal disease.

3. Febrile nonhemolytic transfusion reaction

a. Pathogenesis. Febrile nonhemolytic transfusion reactions occur because the recipient develops **agglutinating or cytotoxic antibodies** against antigens on donor granulocytes, lymphocytes, or platelets (such antigens may be present in red blood cells, whole blood, platelets, or granulocyte products). The antibodies (often called **leukoagglutinins**) may have HLA or granulocyte antigen specificity; they are more commonly seen in multitransfused patients or multiparous women who have had repeated exposure to these antigens. Antigen–antibody interaction leads to activation of complement and release of pyrogens.

b. Signs and symptoms. Fever (i.e., a rise in temperature of 1° or more) is seen during or shortly after transfusion and may be accompanied by chills and occasionally by rigors.

c. Treatment and prevention

(1) Febrile nonhemolytic transfusion reactions are diagnosed by exclusion. The transfusion should be discontinued and a hemolytic transfusion reaction should be ruled out

by the appropriate tests. Underlying sepsis and bacterial contamination of the blood product (very rare) may also be considered. The fever and chills usually respond to antipyretics.

(2) Repeated febrile reactions warrant the use of in-line filters to remove contaminating leukocytes from packed red blood cells, whole blood, or platelets to prevent future reactions.

4. Noncardiogenic pulmonary edema

a. Pathogenesis. Noncardiogenic pulmonary edema is a rare reaction that is due to potent **leukoagglutinins** present in either the recipient or the donor. These antibodies tend to be more commonly seen in multiparous women. Antigen–antibody interaction leads to leukocyte aggregation and trapping in the pulmonary microvasculature, causing increased vascular permeability and activation of complement, with generation of anaphylatoxins.

b. Signs and symptoms. The usual presentation includes acute pulmonary edema, occasionally fulminant, without evidence of left ventricular dysfunction, and accompanied by fever and chills.

c. Treatment and prevention

(1) When such reactions are suspected, the transfusion should be discontinued and causes of pulmonary edema investigated. Acute hemolytic transfusion reaction should be ruled out. In some cases, early resolution has followed aggressive pulmonary supportive measures and the use of intravenous steroids.

(2) It may be prudent to investigate recipient and donor plasma for leukoagglutinins. Patients with such antibodies may require leukocyte-free products, and donors with such antibodies may be deferred from future donation.

5. Allergic transfusion reactions

a. Urticarial reactions

(1) **Pathogenesis.** Urticarial reactions develop as a result of transfused soluble atopens. They appear to be more common in individuals with a history of allergy, and may be seen following transfusion of plasma or cellular blood products (e.g., red cells, platelets, granulocytes), since the latter also contain significant amounts of plasma. Symptoms are mediated by histamine released from IgE- or IgG-coated mast cells.

(2) **Signs and symptoms.** Urticarial reactions are manifested by hives and pruritus, usually without fever or other symptoms.

(3) **Treatment and prevention.** The administration of antihistamine during temporary interruption of the transfusion usually abates the symptoms. Simple urticarial reactions are the only transfusion reactions in which the transfusion does not necessarily need to be permanently discontinued. Repeated urticarial reactions unresponsive to medications may warrant removal of excess plasma from cellular blood products.

b. Anaphylactic reactions

(1) **Pathogenesis.** Transfusion-associated anaphylactic reactions are relatively rare and are seen most frequently in patients who are IgA-deficient and have developed high titers of anti-IgA antibodies. Although the incidence of IgA deficiency is relatively high (1 in 700), the occurrence of anaphylactic reactions following transfusion is considerably less common. Other causes include reactions to transfused allergens [e.g., penicillin, ethylene oxide, and alloantigens (e.g., C4 albumin)].

(2) **Signs and symptoms.** Symptoms (e.g., dyspnea, bronchospasm, vomiting, diarrhea, hypotension) may occur after only a small volume has been transfused.

(3) **Treatment.** The transfusion should be stopped immediately. Therapy includes treatment of hypotension, administration of epinephrine, and prevention of hypoxia.

(4) **Prevention**

(a) Individuals with a class-specific (IgA) anti-IgA titer of 1:256 or greater and those who have experienced a previous anaphylactic transfusion reaction due to anti-IgA antibodies should receive products from donors who lack IgA.

(b) Alternatively, red blood cells may be extensively washed free of plasma, and these patients may be enrolled in autologous donor programs before elective surgery.

6. Alloimmunization. Following transfusion, individuals may become immunized against a number of different alloantigenic components in blood products, including red cell antigens, platelet-specific antigens, granulocyte-specific antigens, and HLA antigens (on leukocytes and platelets).

a. Alloimmunization to red cell antigens

(1) Pathogenesis

(a) Alloimmunization to foreign red cell antigens may occur following transfusion or pregnancy. These unexpected alloantibodies (as opposed to naturally occurring anti-A and anti-B antibodies) may be found in 0.3%–2% of the population. Primary (usually IgM) and secondary (usually IgG) immune responses may be detected by a rise in titer of red cell-specific antibodies.

(b) Whether alloimmunization occurs depends in part on the immunogenicity of the particular antigen. For example, the D antigen is strongly immunogenic: More than 80% of Rh(D)-negative individuals receiving a single unit of Rh(D)-positive blood will develop anti-D antibodies.

(2) Signs and symptoms. Under certain circumstances (e.g., transfusion of red cells expressing the respective antigen), these alloantibodies may be associated with acute or delayed hemolytic transfusion reactions (see III A 1, 2).

(3) Treatment is the same as it is for acute or delayed hemolytic reactions (see III A 1 c, 2 c).

(4) Prevention. It is important that red cell alloantibodies be detected and characterized. Clinically significant alloantibodies necessitate the selection of donor whole blood or red cell units that lack the corresponding antigen to ensure compatibility. This may be difficult for patients with multiple antibodies or antibodies against antigens of high frequency in the population. The incidence of immunization may be decreased by the judicious use of red cell transfusion.

b. Alloimmunization to platelets

(1) Pathogenesis. Alloimmunization to platelets involves the development of antibodies against platelet-associated HLA antigens or against platelet-specific antigens (e.g., $P1^{A1}$, Bak^{a}, Pen).

(a) Alloimmunization to **platelet-associated HLA antigens** results in **refractoriness to platelet transfusions** (see I B 4) and is typically seen in multiply transfused patients with leukemia, solid tumors, or aplastic anemia.

(b) Alloimmunization to **platelet-specific antigens** may cause **neonatal alloimmune thrombocytopenia (NATP)** if the mother develops antibody against fetal platelets (such as anti-$P1^{A1}$ antibody in a $P1^{A1}$-negative mother with a $P1^{A1}$-positive infant).

(c) Alloimmunization to **platelet-specific antigens** may also cause **post-transfusion purpura,** seen in a $P1^{A1}$-negative transfusion recipient who develops a platelet-specific antibody that, curiously, destroys both $P1^{A1}$-positive and $P1^{A1}$-negative platelets.

(2) Signs and symptoms

(a) Alloimmunization to platelet-associated **HLA antigens** results in refractoriness to platelet transfusions. One-hour post-transfusion platelet counts fail to show significant increases in numbers of circulating platelets. Bleeding may be a problem in severely thrombocytopenic patients.

(b) Neonates with **NATP** develop thrombocytopenia with petechiae and bleeding minutes to hours after birth. The risk for intracranial, gastrointestinal, or genitourinary hemorrhage is significant in the first 24 hours of life.

(c) Patients with **post-transfusion purpura** have a serious risk of hemorrhage from profound thrombocytopenia that occurs 5–10 days after transfusion and may last for several weeks.

(3) Treatment and prevention

(a) HLA-matched platelets are used for patients who are **refractory to platelet transfusions** (see I B 4).

(b) Therapy for **NATP** is directed at replacing the neonate's platelets with platelets that will not be destroyed by the maternal antibody (e.g., with the mother's platelets washed free of antibody-containing plasma) and treating the complications of hemorrhage. Cesarean section may be appropriate for mothers who have had children with documented NATP, to avoid hemorrhage associated with birth trauma.

(c) **Post-transfusion purpura** does not usually respond to platelet transfusion; plasmapheresis to remove the antiplatelet antibody is the therapy of choice in post-transfusion purpura. Washed red blood cells, products from $P1^{A1}$-negative donors, or autologous blood may be options for future transfusions to avoid re-exposure to the common platelet antigen $P1^{A1}$.

7. **Graft-versus-host disease (GVHD)**
   a. **Pathogenesis.** GVHD may occur when immunocompetent allogeneic lymphocytes are transfused or transplanted into a severely immunocompromised recipient (the host). The mature donor-derived T lymphocytes proliferate in response to the recipient's major and minor histocompatibility (HLA) antigens. GVHD has been observed after transfusion of whole blood, red blood cells, platelets, or granulocytes but not after the administration of FFP or cryoprecipitate.
   b. **Signs and symptoms.** GVHD is characterized by fever, liver function abnormalities, diarrhea, and an erythematous skin rash that may progress to generalized erythroderma. Pancytopenia may also be present in GVHD except when the disease follows bone marrow transplantation. In post-transfusion GVHD, symptoms begin within 30 days of transfusion. The high mortality rate is usually related to infectious disease complications.
   c. **Treatment and prevention.** Therapy has included steroids, antithymocyte globulin, methotrexate, and cyclosporine. Irradiation of all blood products (except frozen noncellular plasma products) is currently the most efficient method available for the prevention of post-transfusion GVHD. Absolute indications for product irradiation include allogeneic and autologous bone marrow transplantation, congenital immune deficiency syndromes, certain malignancies predisposed to immune suppression, intrauterine exchange transfusions, and directed donor blood from first-degree family members of recipients.

B. **Infectious disease transmission**

1. **Transfusion-transmitted viral hepatitis**
   a. **General considerations.** Viral hepatitis remains the most common serious complication of blood transfusion. Post-transfusion hepatitis can occur after transfusion of any blood component but is rarely seen with immune serum globulin, monoclonal heat-treated factor VIII, or heat-treated albumin.
   b. **Etiologic agents.** The great majority of cases are due to non-A, non-B hepatitis caused by **hepatitis C (HCV)**. Fewer than 2% of cases are attributable to **hepatitis B** virus (HBV), **hepatitis D (HDV),** and **cytomegalovirus (CMV)**. **Hepatitis A** virus (HAV), the infectious agent of epidemic hepatitis, does not cause a carrier state and is an extremely unusual cause of post-transfusion hepatitis. **Hepatitis E (HEV)** causes an epidemic form of non-A, non-B hepatitis. Other yet unidentified non-A, non-B viruses may cause a small percentage of post-transfusion hepatitis cases.
   c. **Clinical features of acute viral hepatitis.** Certain signs and symptoms and laboratory features are common to acute viral hepatitis, regardless of the particular agent.
      (1) In the majority of cases, infection is **subclinical,** manifested only by elevated serum transaminases [alanine and aspartate aminotransferase (ALT, AST)] and serologic markers.
      (2) **Anicteric hepatitis** may be observed in 20%–25% of patients, with anorexia, nausea, vomiting, diarrhea, arthralgia, myalgias, pharyngitis, and low-grade fever.
      (3) Less commonly, **icteric hepatitis** is present, with similar but more severe symptoms along with jaundice, profound weakness, acholic stools, and elevated liver enzymes.
   d. **Diagnosis** of the particular viral agent causing hepatitis relies on detection of specific serologic markers (Table 17-2).
   e. **Specific hepatotropic viruses transmitted by transfusion**
      (1) **Hepatitis C virus (HCV)**
         (a) **Virology.** Recently, the primary agent causing post-transfusion non-A, non-B hepatitis has been cloned and designated **HCV**.
         (b) **Clinical features.** This virus causes more than 95% of post-transfusion hepatitis cases and about 20% of cases of sporadic acute viral hepatitis.
            (i) The incubation period ranges from 2 to 26 weeks. Acute infection is usually subclinical; only 25% of patients develop symptoms.
            (ii) Diagnosis has traditionally been made by exclusion of other viruses. Serologic tests for HCV have recently been developed.
         (c) **Treatment and prognosis.** Treatment includes nonspecific support. The tendency to chronicity is significant; approximately 50% of those affected have biochemical evidence of **chronic liver disease,** many with cirrhosis. Interferon-α may be of value as therapy for chronic disease.
         (d) **Prevention of transfusion transmission.** Donor screening for anti-HB_c and for increased ALT levels, measured as surrogate markers for non-A, non-B hepatitis, has

Table 17-2. Serologic Diagnosis of Post-Transfusion Viral Hepatitis

	Results of Serologic Testing								
					Anti-HB_c				
Hepatitis Agent	**Anti-HDV**	**Anti-HCV**	**HB_sAg**	**Anti-HB_s**	**Total***	**IgM**	**HB_eAg**	**Anti-HB_e**	**Interpretation**
B virus			+	−	+	+	+	−	Acute HBV
			−	−	+	+	+/−	+	Early convalescence from HBV
			+	−	+	−	+/−	+/−	Chronic HB_sAg carrier
			−	+	+	−	−	+	Previous HBV in recovery
			−	+	−	−	−	−	Previous HBV or vaccination with HB_sAg
			−	−	+	−	−	−	Previous HBV
D virus	+/−								Acute HDV
	+								Previous or chronic HDV
C virus	Anti-C	+							†

HBV = hepatitis B virus; HDV = hepatitis D virus; anti-HDV = antibody to hepatitis D virus; anti-HCV = antibody to hepatitis C virus; HB_sAg = hepatitis B surface antigen; anti-HB_s = antibody to hepatitis B surface antigen; anti-HB_c = antibody to hepatitis B core antigen; HB_eAg = hepatitis B e antigen; anti-HB_e = antibody to hepatitis B e antigen; + = present; − = absent; +/− = may be present or absent.

*Total = IgG + IgM

†A repeatedly reactive test for anti-HCV by enzyme-linked immunosorbent assay (ELISA) would indicate past or present infection with HCV. Supplemental, confirmatory tests are under development. Current tests do not distinguish between acute or chronic infection or between ongoing infection and recovery.

contributed to decreased viral transmission in the past. Recently developed assays to detect antibody against the HCV are now used in donor screening and will further prevent transfusion transmission.

(2) Hepatitis B virus (HBV)

(a) Virology. HBV is a double-stranded DNA virus. The **core** contains DNA polymerase, the **core antigen (HB_cAg),** and the **e antigen (HB_eAg)**. The viral **coat** has the **HB_sAg**.

(b) Clinical features

(i) HBV causes only a small percentage of post-transfusion hepatitis. However, it causes about 60% of sporadic cases of acute viral hepatitis, representing the major cause of hepatitis in homosexuals, medical personnel, and intravenous drug users. The major mode of transmission is parenteral (percutaneous via contaminated needles or transfusion and intimate contact via saliva or semen). Vertical transmission from mother to neonate is also important.

(ii) The incubation period ranges from 6 to 11 weeks. About 60% of those with HBV have subclinical infection.

(iii) Diagnosis relies on the detection of serologic markers.

(c) Treatment and prognosis. Although 85%–90% of patients with HBV recover completely, a small percentage have fulminant hepatitis, and 1%–3% develop chronic hepatitis. HBV vaccine may be effective for pre-exposure prophylaxis in high-risk individuals. HBV immune globulin given alone or in combination with HBV vaccine may be used for postexposure prophylaxis.

(d) Prevention of transfusion transmission. Routine donor screening for HB_sAg prevents transfusion transmission.

(3) Hepatitis D virus (HDV)

(a) Virology. HDV is a defective RNA virus and **requires the presence of HBV** for infection.

(b) Clinical features. HDV spreads by parenteral transmission and may occasionally be associated with post-transfusion hepatitis. Infection may occur simultaneously as a coinfection with acute HBV or as a superinfection in a patient with chronic HBV who is exposed to HBV/HDV-positive blood. The incubation period is 2–20 weeks.

(c) **Treatment and prognosis.** Treatment consists of nonspecific support. The presence of HDV is correlated with a severe form of hepatitis and a greater frequency of cirrhosis.

(d) **Prevention of transfusion transmission.** Donors are not tested routinely for antibody to HDV. Prevention depends on screening for HBV.

2. Herpes virus transmission

a. Etiologic agents. Among herpes viruses, **CMV** and **Epstein-Barr virus (EBV)** may cause transfusion-transmitted disease.

(1) **CMV** seroconversion may be seen in 1.2%–1.5% of immunocompetent seronegative recipients following transfusion.

(2) Despite the high percentage of donors capable of transmitting **EBV** infection, few recipients become infected. This is due in part to the fact that most recipients are immune, possessing EBV-neutralizing antibodies.

b. Clinical features

(1) In **immunocompetent patients,** transmission of **CMV** is usually subclinical and without sequelae, manifested only by seroconversion. In contrast, **immunocompromised patients** (e.g., premature infants, immunosuppressed transplant recipients) may develop significant CMV infections such as mononucleosis syndrome, retinitis, hepatitis, pneumonitis, or disseminated disease.

(2) Some cases of post-transfusion infectious mononucleosis–like syndrome may be attributable to **EBV**.

c. Prevention of transfusion transmission

(1) Blood products from donors who are seronegative for **CMV** are recommended for seronegative infants born to seronegative mothers and for CMV-negative cardiac and bone marrow transplant recipients receiving CMV-negative transplants.

(2) Because very few transfusion-acquired **EBV** infections are symptomatic, there is no need to test blood products for reduced risk of EBV transmission.

3. Retrovirus transmission

a. Etiologic agents

(1) An uncommon, yet devastating, complication of transfusion is transmission of **HIV-I**. Most cases are attributable to transfusions before routine testing of donors for HIV-I. As of this writing, the risk of a unit of blood being contaminated by HIV-I after donor testing is estimated to range from 1:100,000 to 1:1,000,000.

(2) **HTLV-I** is another retrovirus, not closely related to HIV-I, that may be transmitted by transfusion. HTLV-I infection is endemic primarily in Japan, the Caribbean, and some areas of Africa. The seropositivity rate in the United States is low. (**HTLV-II** is closely related to HTLV-I; however, modes of transmission and disease associations are currently not well established.)

b. Clinical features

(1) For adult cases of transfusion-transmitted **AIDS,** the latency period between transfusion and diagnosis has ranged from less than 1 year to greater than 7 years. HIV-I may be transmitted by whole blood, cellular components, and plasma, but not by albumin or immunoglobulin because of viral inactivation during processing.

(2) **HTLV-I** has been associated with **adult T cell leukemia/lymphoma** and with the degenerative neurologic disease **tropical spastic paraparesis**. The epidemiology of this virus and the potential for transfusion transmission is currently under investigation.

(a) Transfusion-transmitted **leukemia/lymphoma** from HTLV-I has not been reported, in part because of the long latency period of this virus.

(b) Transfusion-associated **neurologic disease** has been described in Japan and rarely in the United States.

c. Prevention of transfusion transmission

(1) Elimination as donors of those individuals with high risk factors for these viruses remains important in the prevention of viral transmission. Routine screening of donors for HIV-I, HTLV-I, and HTLV-II antibodies further significantly reduces the risk.

(2) Because some products are pooled from many donors (e.g., concentrates of coagulation factors VIII and IX), these products traditionally have carried increased risk of

viral transmission. The combination of heat, chemicals, and monoclonal antibody purification have made it possible to provide coagulation concentrates with greatly reduced risk of retrovirus transmission.

4. Transfusion-transmitted nonviral infections

a. Malaria

(1) Etiologic agents. Worldwide, different strains of malaria (e.g., *Plasmodium falciparum, P. malariae, P. ovale, P. vivax*) are responsible for transfusion-transmitted disease.

(2) Clinical features. Although malaria is a worldwide health problem, transfusion-associated malaria is rare in the United States. Estimates vary from fewer than 2 cases per 10 million units of blood transfused in nonendemic countries to 500 or more cases per 10 million units in some endemic countries.

(3) Treatment and prognosis. Transfusion-transmitted malaria usually responds to conventional drug therapy; however, there may be a relatively high fatality rate in nonmalarious countries because of delays in diagnosis.

(4) Prevention of transfusion transmission. The low incidence of transfusion-associated malaria in the United States is due in part to the routine deferral of both donors originating from endemic areas and donors who have travelled to endemic areas without the use of antimalarial drugs.

b. Syphilis

(1) Etiologic agent. Transfusion-transmitted syphilis, once a serious problem but now rare in the Western world, is caused by the spirochete *Treponema pallidum*.

(2) Clinical features. The incubation period for transfusion-transmitted syphilis varies from 4 weeks to 4 months (average 9–10 weeks). Patients usually exhibit a typical secondary eruption. (Venereally transmitted disease is characterized by three stages: primary, with a painless genital ulcer or chancre; secondary, with diffuse skin rash and lymphadenopathy; and tertiary, with cardiovascular and CNS involvement.)

(3) Prevention of transfusion transmission. The serologic testing that is still performed in the United States cannot prevent all cases of transfusion-transmitted syphilis because in early primary syphilis, when spirochetemia is most prominent, serologic tests are frequently negative. Prevention, thus, remains largely due to the routine practice of storing blood (with the exception of platelets and granulocytes) at low temperatures before transfusion, which effectively kills the organism.

c. Other bacterial infections

(1) Etiologic agents. Bacteria documented to have contaminated blood components include the **gram-negative bacteria:** *Pseudomonas* species, *Citrobacter freundii, Escherichia coli,* and *Yersinia enterocolitica*. In general, contamination is more likely to occur in products stored at room temperature (platelets).

(2) Clinical features. Although this potential complication of transfusion is very rare, bacterial contamination may be devastating because bacterial endotoxins may cause shock, DIC, and renal failure. Evaluation of febrile transfusion reactions may include bacterial culture of the patient and blood product. This depends on the persistence of fever and other symptoms.

(3) Prevention of transfusion transmission. Bacterial contamination is prevented primarily through adherence to sterile techniques during the collection, processing, and storage of blood components and to donor deferral policies.

d. Other infectious diseases transmissible by transfusion include **Chagas' disease** (*Trypanosoma cruzi*), **toxoplasmosis** (*Toxoplasma gondii*), **babesiosis** (*Babesia microti*), and **brucellosis** (*Brucella* species).

C. Complications related to massive transfusion. Massive transfusion is defined as the replacement of at least 1 blood volume with blood components within a 24-hour period. Massive transfusion may be necessary because of trauma, complicated vascular surgery, or liver transplantation. Massive transfusion may be associated with certain complications that are not routinely encountered with the transfusion of smaller volumes of blood components.

1. Hemostatic abnormalities

a. Clinical features. Because whole blood and red blood cells do not contain normal levels of functioning platelets or labile coagulation factors, transfusion of large quantities of these red cell products may lead to some dilution of platelets and coagulation factors in the circulation. **Coagulopathy** and **thrombocytopenia** seen with massive transfusion, however, may also be related to tissue hypoperfusion and DIC.

b. **Treatment and prevention.** Strategies for replacement of coagulation factors and platelets in massive transfusion should be based on assessment of the type and severity of bleeding and on laboratory evaluation, including PT or PTT and platelet count.

2. **Citrate toxicity**
   a. **Clinical features.** Citrate is an important component of anticoagulant solutions used for blood storage. Rapid transfusion of excessive amounts of citrate may have side effects, such as cardiac dysfunction, because of the resultant **hypocalcemia**. However, a normothermic adult with a normally functioning liver can tolerate 1 unit of whole blood every 5 minutes without needing supplemental calcium.
   b. **Treatment and prevention.** If the **critical rate of 1 unit of whole blood every 5 minutes** is exceeded, particularly in the presence of hypothermia, severe liver disease, or acute heart failure, calcium administration may be warranted in the form of calcium chloride or calcium gluconate given to the patient, not added to the blood.

3. **Hypothermia**
   a. **Clinical features.** Hypothermia may accompany the transfusion of massive volumes of refrigerated, stored blood. A decrease in body temperature may impair citrate metabolism, increase the affinity of hemoglobin for oxygen, and cause life-threatening cardiac arrhythmias.
   b. **Treatment and prevention.** The use of blood warmers is standard practice in the setting of massive transfusion (their use is unnecessary, however, with the transfusion of small volumes of blood, such as 1–3 units over several hours).

4. **Acid–base imbalance**
   a. **Clinical features. Metabolic acidosis** may be an **early finding** in massive transfusion, owing in part to tissue hypoperfusion or the immediate acid load of citrated blood. A **late finding,** however, may be **metabolic alkalosis,** resulting in part from the metabolism of citrate and lactate to bicarbonate.
   b. **Treatment and prevention.** Restoration of blood pressure and tissue perfusion may rapidly improve acidosis. Administration of bicarbonate in an attempt to correct for acid load may worsen the alkalosis after perfusion is restored.

5. **Potassium imbalance**
   a. **Clinical features**
      (1) The concentration of potassium in the plasma or red cell components increases during storage. Significant **hyperkalemia** due to massive transfusion is uncommon in **adults,** however, unless underlying hyperkalemia and acidosis are present. **Neonates** undergoing exchange transfusion routinely require fresh blood (i.e., blood that is less than 7 days old) to prevent significant hyperkalemia.
      (2) Conversely, **hypokalemia** may be seen during massive transfusion, owing to metabolic alkalosis secondary to the metabolism of citrate to bicarbonate; this is exacerbated if exogenous bicarbonate is given.
   b. **Treatment and prevention.** Potassium abnormalities may affect cardiac function, and monitoring of potassium levels may be prudent in the massively transfused patient. Washing of red blood cells may be necessary for neonatal exchange transfusion if blood less than 7 days old is not available.

6. **Mechanical trauma to red cells**
   a. **Clinical features.** Mechanical trauma to red cells may be caused by faulty blood warmers, mechanical pumps, or extracorporeal circulation. The inadvertent exposure of red cells to intravenous solutions other than isotonic saline (e.g., dextrose) or accidental administration of drugs in transfusion lines may also cause hemolysis.
   b. **Treatment and prevention.** Evidence of hemolysis during massive transfusion warrants investigation for mechanical trauma (as well as for hemolytic transfusion reaction) and correction of the cause.

D. Other nonimmunologic complications

1. **Circulatory overload**
   a. **Clinical features.** Patients with compromised cardiac or pulmonary status, chronic anemia with expanded plasma volume, or both may not tolerate increases in blood volume from transfusion and can develop symptoms of circulatory overload, such as dyspnea, orthopnea, cyanosis, and peripheral edema.

b. **Treatment and prevention.** Therapy includes discontinuing the transfusion and treatment of the volume overload (e.g., with diuretics, oxygen). Susceptible patients in need of oxygen-carrying capacity should receive red cells, not whole blood, infused slowly, perhaps in small increments (i.e., dispensed in aliquots of the desired total amount).

2. **Hemosiderosis**
   a. **Clinical features.** Because each unit of red blood cells contains approximately 200 mg of iron, chronically transfused patients, such as thalassemic patients with persistent hemolysis, may have significant iron accumulation in tissues. Hemosiderosis may cause hepatic, endocrine, or cardiac dysfunction.
   b. **Treatment and prevention.** Patients likely to require a high transfusion regimen should be monitored for serum iron and ferritin. **Deferoxamine,** an iron-chelating agent, is administered to increase the excretion of excess iron.

IV. ALTERNATIVES TO THE TRANSFUSION OF HOMOLOGOUS BLOOD

A. **Transfusion of autologous blood.** Autologous blood is any blood component donated by the intended recipient.

1. **Benefits.** Autologous blood transfusions eliminate the risks of:
   a. Infectious disease transmission
   b. Alloimmunization to foreign antigens (e.g., red blood cells, platelets, leukocytes, proteins)
   c. Hemolytic, febrile, or allergic reactions caused by alloantibodies
   d. GVHD

2. **Categories of autologous transfusion**
   a. **Autologous whole blood or red blood cells** may be obtained before, during, or after surgical procedures.
      (1) **Preoperative donation**
         (a) Autologous donations may be recommended prior to elective surgery when significant blood loss is anticipated, and, thus, the patient is likely to require transfusion of red cells.
         (b) The **donation period** may extend over several weeks, no more frequently than every 3 days, with the last phlebotomy at least 72 hours before the surgical procedure. **Iron replacement therapy** may be necessary during the period of donation, to replenish bone marrow iron reserves and to maintain adequate red cell production.
         (c) **Contraindications** to autologous donation may include bacteremia, symptomatic angina, symptomatic aortic stenosis and other valvular heart disease, recent seizures, and hematocrit less than 33%.
      (2) **Intraoperative hemodilution and short-term salvage**
         (a) **Normovolemic hemodilution** of the patient's blood volume is typically done in cardiopulmonary bypass procedures. After induction anesthesia and before surgery, 1 or more units of blood are removed and are replaced with crystalloid or colloid. After surgery, the autologous blood may be transfused, and diuretics may be used to reduce plasma volume.
         (b) The two primary **benefits** of hemodilution are improved blood flow in the microcirculation and loss of fewer red cells in a given volume of operative blood loss.
      (3) **Intraoperative blood salvage**
         (a) **Indications** include procedures in which substantial blood loss is anticipated, such as cardiac, vascular, orthopedic, neurologic, or obstetric surgery; the need for intraoperative homologous blood may be reduced by 50%–90%.
         (b) The **technique** for reclaiming intraoperative blood loss is to aspirate at the operative site, centrifuge the blood, wash the red blood cells thus obtained, and reinfuse the red blood cells during surgery or in the immediate postoperative period.
         (c) **Contraindications** include surgery involving gross contamination by bacteria or other microorganisms, as is seen with bowel surgery, or contamination by malignant tumor.
         (d) Possible **complications** include air embolus, hemolysis, DIC, sepsis, or dissemination of malignancy.

(4) **Postoperative blood salvage**
   (a) The primary **indication** for postoperative blood salvage is significant drainage from a cavity, such as chest cavity drainage after cardiothoracic surgery.
   (b) The **technique** is to collect blood during the 24- to 48-hour postoperative period, filter it, and reinfuse it within 6 hours of collection.
   (c) **Contraindications** and **complications** are similar to those associated with intra-operative salvage.

b. **Autologous FFP or cryoprecipitate** can be collected preoperatively and frozen for future use, although indications for this are very uncommon.

c. **Autologous platelets** may be collected preoperatively by hemapheresis and frozen for future use. This procedure is reserved for patients with certain malignancies in anticipation of future bone marrow suppression during chemotherapy. Autologous platelets may also be collected preoperatively and maintained unfrozen for a few days for patients undergoing cardiothoracic surgery.

d. **Autologous "fibrin glue," or concentrated fibrinogen,** may be used for its adhesive properties in a variety of surgical procedures (e.g., otologic, neurologic, vascular). This concentrated fibrinogen fraction is separated from autologous plasma.

B. Use of growth factors

1. **Erythropoietin** causes increased production of red blood cells. Use of recombinant erythropoietin in certain patients (e.g., those with chronic renal disease) may decrease the need for red blood cell transfusion.

2. **Other recombinant growth factors,** such as granulocyte–colony-stimulating factor (G-CSF) and granulocyte–macrophage colony-stimulating factor (GM-CSF), may be given to patients undergoing chemotherapy or bone marrow transplantation to stimulate hematopoiesis (see Ch 2 II B 5).

C. Use of blood substitutes

1. **Unmodified hemoglobin** has been investigated and found to be toxic (due to contamination with red cell stroma) and of limited efficacy because of its high affinity for oxygen.

2. **Chemically modified hemoglobin** and recombinant hemoglobin are currently under investigation.

3. Oxygen is highly soluble in **perfluorocarbon compounds,** and these have been used in both animal and human trials.

STUDY QUESTIONS

Directions: Each of the numbered items or incomplete statements in this section is followed by answers or by completions of the statement. Select the **one** lettered answer or completion that is **best** in each case.

1. Rh immune globulin is indicated in which of the following circumstances?

(A) Postpartum in an Rh(D)-positive mother with an Rh(D)-negative infant
(B) Postpartum in a previously sensitized Rh(D)-negative mother with an Rh(D)-positive infant
(C) Postpartum in an unsensitized Rh(D)-negative mother with an Rh(D)-positive infant
(D) Following amniocentesis in an Rh(D)-positive woman
(E) At 28 weeks gestation in an Rh(D)-positive woman

Questions 2 and 3

A 65-year-old woman is admitted for resection of a colonic carcinoma. She complains of progressive fatigue, weakness, dyspnea on exertion, and bloody stools. Her hemoglobin is 6.5 g/dl, and her hematocrit is 19%, with hypochromic, microcytic red blood cells on peripheral smear. Screening coagulation studies [prothrombin time (PT) and partial thromboplastin time (PTT)], platelet count, electrolytes, liver enzymes, blood urea nitrogen (BUN), and creatinine are all normal.

2. Which of the following blood products would be indicated before surgery?

(A) Two units of whole blood
(B) Four units of fresh frozen plasma
(C) Three units of washed red blood cells
(D) Two units of red blood cells
(E) Six units of random-donor platelets

3. It is anticipated that the patient may need intraoperative transfusion with red blood cells. Which of the following forms of red blood cells would be appropriate?

(A) Homologous red blood cells
(B) Intraoperatively salvaged red blood cells
(C) Autologous red blood cells
(D) Frozen red blood cells
(E) Leukocyte-depleted red blood cells

4. HLA-matched platelets may be indicated in which of the following situations?

(A) Before surgery in a patient with a platelet count of $30 \times 10^3/\mu l$
(B) In a patient with leukemia whose platelet count is $5 \times 10^3/\mu l$ immediately after transfusion of random-donor platelets
(C) Before surgery in a patient with idiopathic thrombocytopenic purpura (ITP)
(D) After massive transfusion in a bleeding patient with a platelet count of $25 \times 10^3/\mu l$
(E) In a patient with sepsis, disseminated intravascular coagulation (DIC), and a platelet count of $30 \times 10^3/\mu l$

5. Which of the following patients would benefit from transfusion of fresh frozen plasma? A patient

(A) with liver disease and prolonged prothrombin time (PT) and partial thromboplastin time (PTT)
(B) with gastrointestinal bleeding and normal PT and PTT
(C) scheduled for elective endoscopy with prolonged PT and PTT because of coumadin therapy
(D) with bleeding caused by thrombocytopenia
(E) with excessive postoperative bleeding and prolonged PT and PTT

1-C
2-D
3-A
4-B
5-E

Directions: Each item below contains four suggested answers of which **one or more** is correct. Choose the answer

A if **1, 2, and 3** are correct
B if **1 and 3** are correct
C if **2 and 4** are correct
D if **4** is correct
E if **1, 2, 3, and 4** are correct

6. Urticarial transfusion reactions are characterized by

(1) fever and chills
(2) hypotension
(3) back pain and pain at the infusion site
(4) local erythema, hives, and itching

7. The direct antiglobulin test is likely to be positive in which of the following cases?

(1) A patient with anemia secondary to an artificial heart valve
(2) A patient with a delayed hemolytic transfusion reaction
(3) The mother of an infant with hemolytic disease of the newborn
(4) A patient with autoimmune hemolytic anemia

8. True statements concerning transfusion transmission of viral disease include which of the following?

(1) Hepatitis B is the most common cause of acute post-transfusion viral hepatitis
(2) Human T cell lymphotropic virus type I (HTLV-I) may be transmitted by transfusion and causes acquired immune deficiency syndrome (AIDS)
(3) Cytomegalovirus (CMV) transmitted by transfusion leads to hepatitis in immunocompetent patients
(4) Transfusion-transmitted hepatitis C has a significant tendency to chronicity

9. Which of the following transfusion reactions may be due to antibodies against leukocyte antigens?

(1) Anaphylactic transfusion reaction
(2) Febrile nonhemolytic transfusion reaction
(3) Acute hemolytic transfusion reaction
(4) Noncardiogenic pulmonary edema

10. True statements regarding the ABO blood group system include which of the following?

(1) The ABO blood group system is the most important blood group system in transfusion practice
(2) Expression of carbohydrate antigen is dependent on gene-encoded glycosyltransferase enzymes
(3) ABO group determination is a routine component of pretransfusion testing
(4) Individuals who are group AB have naturally occurring anti-A and anti-B antibodies

---

6-D
7-C
8-D
9-C
10-A

ANSWERS AND EXPLANATIONS

1. The answer is C *[I B 10 b].*
Rh sensitization in an Rh(D)-negative woman can cause erythroblastosis fetalis in her Rh(D)-positive infant. Rh immune globulin is given to previously unsensitized Rh(D)-negative women (i.e., women who have not made anti-D antibody in response to previous exposure), to prevent sensitization following exposure to Rh(D)-positive red cells. Exposure may occur during transfusion or fetomaternal hemorrhage at delivery or from trauma during pregnancy (e.g., amniocentesis). During pregnancy, Rh immune globulin is also given at 28 weeks gestation to unsensitized Rh(D)-negative women even though the infant's Rh(D) type is unknown. Previously sensitized Rh(D)-negative individuals will not benefit from Rh immune globulin, and Rh(D)-positive women do not need it.

2–3. The answers are: 2-D *[I B 2],* **3-A** *[IV A].*
The patient is symptomatic from chronic anemia and should have her hemoglobin deficit corrected before undergoing major surgery. This is best achieved with red blood cells. Whole blood is indicated only when both plasma replacement and improved oxygen-carrying capacity are needed, as in massive blood transfusion or exchange transfusion. Fresh frozen plasma (FFP) is not indicated since the patient does not have evidence of a coagulopathy. Red cells should be washed only when plasma or leukocytes must be removed, as in cases of repeated allergic or febrile reactions after the transfusion of red cells. (Leukocytes can more efficiently be removed by in-line filters.)

Only homologous red cells are indicated in intraoperative transfusion. Since the patient is anemic, she is not an appropriate candidate for autologous donation. Intraoperative cell salvage is unsuitable because it is contraindicated in surgery involving the bowel to prevent bacterial contamination and is also generally contraindicated during primary resection of malignant tumors. Frozen red cells are primarily used when units with rare blood type are necessary: for example, for transfusion of patients who have antibodies to very common antigens, when only rare units (frozen for such future need) will be compatible. Leukocyte-depleted red blood cells are indicated to prevent the recurrence of febrile transfusion reactions.

4. The answer is B *[I B 4 b].*
Platelets matched for histocompatibility locus antigens (HLA)-matched platelets are indicated in patients who are refractory to platelet transfusions because of suspected alloimmunization to HLA antigens. This condition may be seen in patients who have been transfused many times and is best documented by a low 1-hour post-transfusion platelet count. Other causes of refractoriness, such as sepsis, splenomegaly, and disseminated intravascular coagulation (DIC), must be ruled out. Platelet transfusion is generally not indicated in patients with idiopathic thrombocytopenic purpura (ITP); however, before surgery (e.g., splenectomy), platelet transfusion may be warranted. For these patients, however, there is no advantage to using HLA-matched platelets.

5. The answer is E *[I B 6 b].*
Fresh frozen plasma (FFP) contains all labile and stable coagulation factors. It is given to patients with a deficiency of multiple coagulation factors [as evidenced by a prolonged prothrombin time (PT) or partial thromboplastin time (PTT)] who are bleeding or at risk of bleeding. It is not appropriate to use FFP to treat a prolonged PT or PTT when bleeding is not present or imminent or when bleeding is probably due to other causes. Vitamin K should be used rather than FFP to reverse the effect of coumadin when time permits.

6. The answer is D (4) *[III A 5 a].*
Urticarial reactions are typically characterized by erythema, hives, and itching, without fever or other symptoms. These limited cutaneous reactions may be due to allergy to a soluble product in donor plasma. Fever, chills, hypotension, and pain may be associated with acute hemolytic transfusion reaction.

7. The answer is C (2, 4) *[II F].*
The direct antiglobulin test detects IgG antibody or complement bound to red blood cells in vivo and may be used to evaluate the suspected immune-mediated destruction of red blood cells. In acute and delayed hemolytic transfusion reactions, alloantibody, complement, or both are usually detected on transfused red blood cells in the patient. In autoimmune hemolytic anemia, autoantibody, complement, or both are usually detected on the patient's own red blood cells. In hemolytic disease of the newborn, the infant usually has a positive antiglobulin test for IgG antibody. The mother will not be expected to have a positive direct antiglobulin test.

8. The answer is D (4) *[III B 1–3].*
Hepatitis C (HCV), not B (HBV), is the most common cause of post-transfusion viral hepatitis. A significant percentage of HCV patients have biochemical evidence of chronicity and histologic evidence of cirrhosis. Human T cell lymphotropic virus type I (HTLV-I) can be transmitted by transfusion; however, it is not associated with severe immune deficiency. HTLV-I is associated with adult T cell leukemia and lymphoma and tropical spastic paraparesis, but the transmission of these diseases by transfusion may be rare. Transmission of cytomegalovirus (CMV) is of concern in the immunosuppressed patient and may cause mononucleosis, retinitis, hepatitis, or disseminated disease.

9. The answer is C (2, 4) *[III A 3, 4].*
Antibodies against leukocyte antigens (leukoagglutinins) may cause febrile nonhemolytic transfusion reactions and noncardiogenic pulmonary edema. These antibodies may recognize granulocyte-specific antigens or human leukocyte (HLA) antigens and are seen more commonly among multiply transfused patients or multiparous women. Acute hemolytic transfusion reactions are caused by antibodies to red blood cell antigens, usually anti-A and anti-B antibodies. Anaphylactic transfusion reactions may be due to a high titer of antibodies against IgA.

10. The answer is A (1, 2, 3) *[II B].*
The ABO blood group system is the most important blood group system to be considered in transfusion practice. It is the only blood group system in which naturally occurring antibodies (e.g., anti-A, anti-B) are predictably present when the corresponding antigen is absent on the red blood cell. Individuals who are group AB do not have anti-A or anti-B antibodies.

Comprehensive Exam

QUESTIONS

Directions: Each of the numbered items or incomplete statements in this section is followed by answers or by completions of the statement. Select the **one** lettered answer or completion that is **best** in each case.

1. Hematopoiesis in a 10-year-old patient with sickle cell anemia and hemolysis proceeds in the

(A) liver
(B) red pulp of the spleen
(C) marrow of the axial skeleton
(D) cortex of the thymus
(E) marrow of the skull, sternum, and iliac crest

2. All of the following clinical conditions are associated with decreased levels of erythropoietin EXCEPT

(A) anemia of renal disease
(B) autoimmune hemolytic anemia
(C) polycythemia vera (PV)
(D) anemia of hypothyroidism
(E) anemia in starvation

3. A 23-year-old woman with four children was found to have severe iron deficiency, probably due to her multiple pregnancies. Her physician started her on oral ferrous sulfate, at 300 mg every 8 hours. Her hemoglobin 1 month later was only slightly higher than the previous level, and the patient insists that she is taking her medication diligently. Examination showed brown stools to be negative for occult blood on the guaiac slide test. Which of the following reasons is the most likely explanation for the patient's poor response to treatment?

(A) Malabsorption of iron
(B) Continued intermittent blood loss
(C) Inflammatory bowel condition
(D) Poor compliance
(E) Poor release of iron from the preparation

4. The primary site of folate absorption is the

(A) terminal ileum
(B) proximal jejunum
(C) both
(D) neither

5. An asymptomatic 36-year-old black male is referred to a hematologist after a routine blood examination reveals a low mean corpuscular volume (MCV). He has no history of lead exposure, and there is no family history of anemia except for a grandfather who had a vague history of low blood counts. The patient is not taking any medications and does not drink alcohol. His stool is negative for occult blood, and his serum ferritin level is normal. Hemoglobin electrophoresis is normal. What is the most likely diagnosis?

(A) Early iron deficiency
(B) Anemia of chronic disease
(C) Lead poisoning
(D) Thalassemia minor
(E) Sideroblastic anemia

6. A young woman with known sickle cell disease, who has had multiple transfusions in the past, is admitted to the hospital with severe pain in her abdomen and in all four extremities, acute respiratory distress, and disseminated intravascular coagulation (DIC); she is afebrile. Her hemoglobin level was 8 g/dl, which is her baseline level; however, she was transfused to a hemoglobin level of 10 g/dl 7 days ago in preparation for an elective cholecystectomy. Her post-transfusion hemoglobin electrophoresis shows 60% hemoglobin A (Hb A) and 40% hemoglobin S (Hb S), and her repeat studies on admission show 10% Hb A and 90% Hb S, values similar to those pretransfusion. The most likely cause of her acute crisis is

(A) sickle cell crisis
(B) delayed hemolytic transfusion reaction
(C) splenic crisis
(D) acute chest syndrome
(E) sepsis

7. A 72-year-old woman is admitted to the hospital for a change in her personality and for falling. She is found to be anemic, with a hemoglobin concentration of 5 g/dl, a mean corpuscular volume (MCV) of 120 fl per red cell, a 0.5% reticulocyte count, a white blood count (WBC) of 4500/μl, and a platelet count of 125,000/μl. Her diet is normal, and she has no intestinal symptoms; her only medication is multivitamins. She has no history of surgery. Which of the following results of diagnostic tests would be most likely in this case?

(A) Low serum folate, normal B_{12}, high lactate dehydrogenase (LDH), and megaloblastic bone marrow
(B) Abnormal Schilling test, parts I, II, and III
(C) High serum folate, low B_{12}, hypersegmentation of neutrophils, positive test for antibodies to intrinsic factor, achlorhydria, abnormal part I ($<$ 8% excretion) and normal part II (10% excretion) of Schilling test
(D) Positive Coombs' test, CT scan of the head showing a cerebellar hemangioblastoma, hypoplastic bone marrow
(E) Bone marrow showing megaloblastic changes associated with increased blasts, abnormal chromosomes, and ringed sideroblasts

8. As a supplement to morphologic examination and clinical features, which of the following laboratory tests is useful in distinguishing between chronic myelogenous leukemia (CML) and reactive neutrophilia and other myeloproliferative disorders?

(A) Terminal deoxynucleotidyl transferase (TdT)
(B) Tartrate-resistant acid phosphatase (TRAP)
(C) Leukocyte alkaline phosphatase (LAP)
(D) Monoclonal surface immunoglobulin
(E) Cytochemical stains for myeloperoxidase

9. A 32-year-old man with a lifelong history of bruising is scheduled for elective hernia repair. He has had no previous surgery, but recent aggressive dental cleaning and sealing caused him to bleed for 24 hours. He has no other medical problems and is taking no medications. Bleeding time was measured on two occasions to be greater than 15 minutes, and the platelet count is 230,000/μl. All other screening coagulation tests are normal, and the peripheral smear is unremarkable. The next step in the evaluation of this patient is to

(A) measure the level of antiplatelet antibodies
(B) conduct platelet aggregation studies
(C) proceed with surgery as planned, without further studies
(D) conduct a bone marrow examination
(E) transfuse with platelets and recheck the bleeding time

10. A 65-year-old woman is seen before cataract surgery. She has had no previous surgery except for a dental extraction, after which she bled for 10 days and required transfusion of 2 units of blood. One sibling died from postoperative hemorrhage during childhood, and there is a history of bleeding in a number of relatives, both male and female. Her partial thromboplastin time (PTT) is markedly prolonged, and her bleeding time is within normal limits. The most likely diagnosis is a deficiency of

(A) factor VII
(B) factor VIII
(C) factor XI
(D) factor XII
(E) Fletcher factor (high-molecular-weight kininogen)

11. The treatment of choice for thrombotic thrombocytopenic purpura (TTP) is

(A) steroids
(B) splenectomy
(C) plasmapheresis with fresh frozen plasma replacement
(D) heparin
(E) aspirin

12. A 15-year-old girl develops massive bleeding from a wound site 36 hours after a large cyst is removed from her right thigh. Local measures to control the bleeding are unsuccessful. Prothrombin time (PT), partial thromboplastin time (PTT), thrombin time, platelet count, and bleeding time all are within normal limits. There is no family history of excessive bleeding. Which of the following tests should be ordered?

(A) Factor IX level
(B) Factor XII level
(C) Urea clot lysis test
(D) Platelet aggregation study
(E) Mixing test

13. A 55-year-old previously well man is admitted to the hospital because of pneumonia. Antibiotic therapy is administered, which lowers his temperature, although it continues to spike. A hematologist is consulted to review the admission test results, which include a hemoglobin of 13 g/dl, a white blood cell count (WBC) of 9000/μl, and a platelet count of 70,000/μl. The next step in the evaluation of this patient should be

(A) bone marrow examination
(B) bleeding time measurement
(C) peripheral blood smear examination
(D) platelet aggregation studies
(E) antiplatelet antibodies measurement

14. A 28-year-old man who was well yesterday presents in the emergency room with lobar-type pneumonia. He has a hemoglobin count of 14 g/dl and a white blood cell count (WBC) of 14,000/μl, with an increased number of polymorphonuclear cells and band forms. A few nucleated red cells and several red cells with Howell-Jolly bodies are noted. The patient has no history of a previous operation, and physical examination reveals no abdominal scars. Which of the following procedures is correct for this patient?

(A) Blood culture and oral antibiotics on an outpatient basis
(B) A sputum Gram stain and oral antibiotics on an outpatient basis
(C) Blood culture, sputum Gram stain, and hospital admission to await the test results
(D) Blood culture and intravenous antibiotics

15. Which one of the following laboratory test results indicates a hypoproliferative anemia?

(A) Normal mean corpuscular volume (MCV)
(B) Increased red cell distribution width (RDW)
(C) Low reticulocyte count
(D) Low hemoglobin level
(E) Increased serum iron

16. With hepatic storage of 2–5 mg, which vitamin deficiency will develop within 2–12 years?

(A) Vitamin B_{12}
(B) Folate
(C) Both
(D) Neither

17. In the workup of a patient with hypochromic, microcytic anemia and a positive family history of β thalassemia, which of the following tests is most helpful in establishing a diagnosis of β thalassemia?

(A) Serum iron and iron-binding capacity
(B) Bone marrow iron stains
(C) Hemoglobin electrophoresis
(D) Heinz body preparation

18. A 54-year-old obese man who chain-smokes and has a history of hypertension is called by his physician because of a blood count showing a hematocrit of 55%, a white blood cell count (WBC) of 9700/μl, and a platelet count of 450,000/μl; physical examination is normal except for an elevated diastolic pressure of 110 mm Hg. The next study or procedure in this patient should be

(A) phlebotomy to prevent a cerebrovascular accident
(B) arterial blood gases and chest x-ray
(C) carboxyhemoglobin determination
(D) red cell mass determination by chromium 51 (^{51}Cr) labeling
(E) serum erythropoietin determination

19. Disseminated intravascular coagulation (DIC) is a particularly prominent and common complication associated with which of the following conditions?

(A) Chronic lymphocytic leukemia (CLL)
(B) Chronic myelogenous leukemia (CML)
(C) Multiple myeloma
(D) Acute promyelocytic leukemia (FAB M3 subtype)
(E) Hodgkin's disease

20. Aspirin has which of the following effects on platelets? It

(A) shortens platelet life span
(B) results in abnormal platelet aggregation
(C) decreases platelet production
(D) prolongs the bleeding time

21. The likelihood that the daughter of a patient with severe hemophilia B will be a carrier of hemophilia is

(A) 0%
(B) 25%
(C) 50%
(D) 75%
(E) 100%

22. A 29-year-old woman presents with severe thrombocytopenia. She was well until 3 days ago, when she developed fever and noted blood in her urine. She also noted a "rash" on her legs, which is actually petechiae. This morning she was mildly confused, and her family brought her to the hospital. On physical examination, the only findings are mild disorientation to time and place and petechiae over the lower extremities. Hemoglobin is 7 g/dl, white blood cell count (WBC) is 11,000/μl with a normal differential, and platelet count is 10,000/μl. Examination of the peripheral blood smear confirms severe thrombocytopenia, and there are numerous schistocytes. White cells are unremarkable. The most likely diagnosis is

(A) idiopathic thrombocytopenic purpura (ITP)
(B) systemic lupus erythematosus (SLE)
(C) thrombotic thrombocytopenic purpura (TTP)
(D) sepsis
(E) drug-induced thrombocytopenia

Questions 23–25

A 22-year-old male college student presents at the student health service complaining of extreme fatigue, sore throat, difficulty concentrating, and a temperature of 38°–39° C over the last week. Physical examination is unremarkable except for mild lymph node enlargement in axillary, cervical, and inguinal regions and a palpable spleen tip. A blood count shows hemoglobin of 10 g/dl, platelets of 105,000/μl, and white blood cell (WBC) count of 22,000/μl with 60% lymphoid cells. The laboratory blood profile also shows an absolute red cell count of 2.3×10^6/μl, mean corpuscular volume (MCV) of 125 fl, and mean cell hemoglobin concentration of 43 g/dl.

23. What is the most likely diagnosis for this patient?

(A) Infectious lymphocytosis
(B) *Bordetella pertussis* infection
(C) Cytomegalovirus (CMV) mononucleosis syndrome
(D) Mononucleosis secondary to Epstein-Barr virus (EBV) infection (infectious mononucleosis)
(E) Mononucleosis secondary to *Toxoplasma gondii* infection

24. Which of the following is the most likely etiology for anemia [hemoglobin (Hb) 10 g/dl] in this patient?

(A) An immune-mediated mechanism
(B) Compromise of erythroid production secondary to EBV infection of bone marrow precursors
(C) Virus-associated hemophagocytic syndrome
(D) Slow gastrointestinal blood loss since the start of illness owing to thrombocytopenia
(E) Disseminated intravascular coagulation (DIC)

25. Which of the following is the cause of the abnormal blood profile values?

(A) Pronounced reticulocytosis
(B) Release of nucleated red cells from the bone marrow
(C) Red cell agglutination
(D) Rouleaux formation secondary to elevation of acute phase serum proteins
(E) Malfunctioning laboratory blood counter

26. Five days after beginning warfarin therapy for atrial fibrillation, a 60-year-old man returns to his physician complaining of large patches of discolored skin over his flanks and legs, some of which have formed open sores. This complication is most likely the result of

(A) AT III deficiency
(B) bleeding secondary to excessive anticoagulation
(C) drug allergy
(D) protein C deficiency
(E) drug-induced thrombocytopenia

27. In a patient with poorly defined megaloblastic anemia, it is prudent to give a therapeutic trial using

(A) hydroxycobalamin
(B) folic acid
(C) both
(D) neither

28. An 18-year-old Italian tourist visiting relatives in the United States presents to the emergency room with dark urine, headache, fatigue, and back pain. He has a history of similar episodes, and he has an uncle who has had the same symptoms. He had eaten an Italian bean dish several hours before becoming sick. His hemoglobin is 10 g/dl with a reticulocyte count of 13%, and results of the urine test are positive for occult blood. Which test should be ordered next?

(A) Hemoglobin electrophoresis
(B) Cholecystography for bile stones
(C) Heinz bodies test
(D) Ham and sugar water tests
(E) Coombs' test

29. At which of these blood neutrophil levels do patients acquire a significant risk of opportunistic infection?

(A) $< 1000/\mu l$
(B) $1000–1500/\mu l$
(C) $1500–2000/\mu l$
(D) $2000–2500/\mu l$
(E) $2500–3000/\mu l$

30. A 56-year-old woman with a history of ovarian cancer treated by chemotherapy several years ago presents to the clinic with complaints of fatigue and the recent development of small hemorrhages on her arms. She has the following laboratory values: hemoglobin: 9.6 g/dl; white blood cell count (WBC): $2900/\mu l$; platelets: $56{,}000/\mu l$. A bone marrow aspirate is hypercellular and contains approximately 10% blasts (normal < 5%), with megaloblastic morphologic changes in the red cell precursors and megakaryocytes with abnormal nuclei. Cytogenetic analysis reveals a clone with a deletion of the long arm of chromosome 7. What diagnosis best fits this patient's condition?

(A) Preleukemia (myelodysplastic syndrome)
(B) Megaloblastic anemia
(C) Acute lymphocytic leukemia (ALL)
(D) Acute nonlymphocytic (myelogenous) leukemia (ANLL)
(E) Chronic myelogenous leukemia (CML)

31. The metabolism of which of the following compounds plays the major role in the response of granulocytes and monocytes to inflammatory stimuli?

(A) Arachidonic acid
(B) Glycogen
(C) Hydrogen peroxide
(D) Glutamate
(E) Deoxyuridine

32. A patient was diagnosed by lymph node biopsy and chest x-ray as having Hodgkin's lymphoma with an enlarged mediastinal mass. Which test should be performed first before proceeding with therapy?

(A) Lymphangiography
(B) CT scan of the chest, abdomen, and pelvis
(C) Bilateral bone marrow biopsy
(D) Staging laparotomy

33. In a 5-year-old girl with de novo acute leukemia, is the distinction between acute lymphocytic leukemia (ALL) and acute myelogenous leukemia (AML) important clinically, and why?

(A) Yes, very different therapeutic regimens are used, even though both diseases are equally curable in children
(B) No, both are about equally curable with a common therapeutic approach
(C) Yes, acute lymphocytic leukemia (ALL) has a higher 5-year survival rate than acute myelogenous leukemia (AML), and both are treated with different therapeutic regimens
(D) No, even though different therapeutic regimens are used, the 5-year survival rate is comparable in both classes of leukemia
(E) Yes, patients with AML are more likely to have central nervous system (CNS) involvement

34. A previously well 27-year-old woman presents with a petechial rash. She has had no recent bleeding nor any recent illnesses. Hemoglobin, hematocrit, and white blood cell count (WBC) are normal. Examination of the peripheral blood smear reveals normal red and white cells, and the smear is remarkable only for a paucity of platelets. The most likely diagnosis in this patient is

(A) aleukemic leukemia
(B) idiopathic thrombocytopenic purpura (ITP)
(C) amegakaryocytic thrombocytopenia
(D) Glanzmann's thrombasthenia
(E) drug-induced thrombocytopenia

35. Which of the following characteristics are common to B and T lymphocytes?

(A) Monoclonal surface membrane immunoglobulin
(B) Leukocyte alkaline phosphatase (LAP)
(C) Membrane antigen CD8
(D) Membrane antigen CD19
(E) Variable (V), diversity (D), joining (J), and constant (C) gene segments

Questions 36–37

A 19-year-old man is evaluated prior to elective hernia repair because of a family history of bleeding. The patient, who has no siblings, says that neither of his parents has experienced extraordinary bleeding and both have undergone surgery. One maternal uncle died as a child due to bleeding after trauma, and the patient's maternal grandfather died at age 45 due to bleeding after an appendectomy. Three maternal aunts are alive and asymptomatic, but one of them has a young son who bled excessively after a minor accident. There are no cases of excessive bleeding among members of the patient's father's family.

36. Which of the following screening tests is most likely to be abnormal in this patient?

(A) Platelet count
(B) Prothrombin time (PT)
(C) Partial thromboplastin time (PTT)
(D) Thrombin time
(E) Bleeding time

37. In the event that all screening tests are normal, what is the best course of action to be taken next?

(A) Proceed with surgery
(B) Perform platelet aggregation studies
(C) Perform a mixing study
(D) Perform specific factor assays
(E) Perform screening tests on the patient's mother

38. Which one of the following statements is true?

(A) Acute leukemias are predominantly an expansion of mature bone marrow cells that function ineffectively, leading to patient death by infection or bleeding
(B) Despite their name, it is common for chronic leukemias to kill the patient within the first 12 months of disease
(C) The neutrophil leukocyte alkaline phosphatase (LAP) reaction is often useful in distinguishing among chronic myelogenous leukemia (CML), reactive neutrophilia, and other myeloproliferative disorders
(D) Surgical debulking of leukemic tissue is often useful before administering chemotherapy
(E) Leukemia is the most common cancer in adults

39. A physician is asked to examine a 40-year-old patient with a platelet count of 550,000/μl, who has been in the intensive care unit for 7 days because of multiple trauma from a motorcycle accident. After multiple transfusions, his hemoglobin is now 12 g/dl and white blood cell count (WBC) is 9000/μl, with a normal differential count. Which of the following statements is true in this situation?

(A) The thrombocytosis is probably the result of the transfusions
(B) The patient probably has essential thrombocythemia and will require chemotherapy
(C) The thrombocytosis is probably drug-induced
(D) The thrombocytosis is probably reactive and will require no treatment
(E) The patient probably has polycythemia vera (PV) and will require chemotherapy

40. A hematologist is consulted regarding a 67-year-old woman in the coronary care unit who has a slight prolongation of her partial thromboplastin time (PTT). The thrombin time also is prolonged, but the prothrombin time (PT), platelet count, and quantitative fibrinogen are all normal. The patient's coagulation profile on admission was normal. The patient is asymptomatic, and the referring physician says that the patient is receiving no medications except occasional nitroglycerin. The most likely cause of these findings is

(A) dysfibrinogenemia
(B) factor XIII deficiency
(C) lupus anticoagulant
(D) heparin
(E) artifact

41. A young, previously healthy woman is admitted to the intensive care unit with thrombocytopenia and intermittent confusion. Laboratory studies reveal a hemoglobin of 6 g/dl, a white blood cell count (WBC) of 7000/μl with a normal differential, a platelet count of 6000/μl, and prothrombin time (PT) and partial thromboplastin time (PTT) within normal limits. Peripheral blood smear reveals many schistocytes and helmet cells. The patient has a temperature of 100° F and, except for petechiae, appears normal on physical examination. The most likely diagnosis is

(A) disseminated intravascular coagulation (DIC)
(B) thrombotic thrombocytopenic purpura (TTP)
(C) drug-induced thrombocytopenia
(D) acute leukemia
(E) idiopathic thrombocytopenic purpura (ITP)

42. Urticaria pigmentosa is associated with which of the following leukocyte types?

(A) Basophil
(B) Neutrophil
(C) Monocyte
(D) Lymphocyte
(E) Mast cell

43. All of the following are major regions of T lymphocyte distribution in the body EXCEPT

(A) Lymph nodes
(B) Thymus
(C) Spleen
(D) Gastrointestinal tract
(E) Peripheral blood

44. Which of the following features is most characteristic of histiocytosis X?

(A) Proliferation of Langerhans' cells
(B) Cytogenetic abnormalities of the X chromosome in association with tissue histiocytosis
(C) Cytoplasmic accumulation of sphingomyelin
(D) β-Glucosidase deficiency

45. A patient with known polycythemia vera (PV) managed with phlebotomy alone is admitted to the hospital because of sudden onset of left-sided weakness. Physical examination reveals scattered bruises and ecchymoses, and CT scan reveals a small intracranial bleed. Laboratory findings include a hematocrit of 45%, normal prothrombin time (PT) and partial thromboplastin time (PTT) results, and a platelet count of 2,000,000/μl. Which of the following tests is most likely to be abnormal in this patient?

(A) Bleeding time
(B) Thrombin time
(C) Fibrinogen level
(D) Factor VIII screen

46. The etiology of the anemia seen with thrombotic thrombocytopenia (TTP) is believed to be

(A) antibody-mediated
(B) secondary to hypersplenism
(C) the result of infection
(D) the result of bleeding
(E) the result of the formation of platelet plugs in small vessels

47. The cytoplasm of mature neutrophils contains

(A) primary (azurophilic) granules
(B) secondary (specific) granules
(C) both
(D) neither

48. A 24-year-old black woman is admitted to the hospital with a severe macrocytic anemia, low white blood cell count (WBC), and mild thrombocytopenia. Her bone marrow is hypercellular, with marked megaloblastic changes. Her serum vitamin B_{12} level is extremely low, and her Schilling test shows an abnormal part I and a normal part II. Which of the following tests is LEAST helpful in the establishment of the diagnosis?

(A) Serum folate level
(B) Anti–intrinsic factor antibody
(C) Gastric hydrochloric acid for achlorhydria
(D) Anti–parietal cell antibody
(E) Part III of the Schilling test

49. Drug-induced bone marrow aplasia initiated through exposure to chloramphenicol is the result of a

(A) dose-dependent marrow cell suppression
(B) idiosyncratic mechanism
(C) both
(D) neither

50. All of the following complications are a result of the immune status of the recipient during the post-transplantation period EXCEPT

(A) fungal infections
(B) graft rejection
(C) herpes zoster
(D) graft-versus-host disease (GVHD)
(E) interstitial pneumonia

51. Anemia in chronic renal failure can be attributed to all of the following factors EXCEPT

(A) low erythropoietin levels
(B) shortened red cell survival
(C) direct marrow suppression
(D) decreased plasma volume
(E) bleeding from platelet dysfunction

52. An asymptomatic 45-year-old man was found to have a mild hypochromic, microcytic anemia and to be iron-deficient. He has no family history of anemia and does not drink alcohol. All of the following tests are indicated for this patient EXCEPT

(A) hemoglobin electrophoresis
(B) upper GI series
(C) barium enema
(D) stool guaiac slide test
(E) urinalysis for hematuria or hemoglobinuria

53. All of the following clinical manifestations associated with megaloblastic anemia are reversible with replacement therapy EXCEPT

(A) spinal cord damage
(B) anemia
(C) neutropenia
(D) peripheral neuropathy
(E) thrombocytopenia

54. A young man with sickle cell disease has had a cough and fever for a few days. He presented to the physician with multiple nonspecific pains in his chest, abdomen, and extremities. His chest x-ray shows a left lower lobe infiltrate. All of the following conditions are possible in this patient EXCEPT

(A) acute chest syndrome
(B) sickle cell crisis
(C) pneumococcal pneumonia
(D) hand–foot syndrome

55. All of the following statements are true regarding the workup of an undefined anemia EXCEPT

(A) common causes should be sought first, such as anemia due to obvious or occult blood loss by a history of bleeding in the gastrointestinal tract, genitourinary tract, and respiratory system
(B) the ability of the bone marrow to respond to the anemia should be determined by measuring the reticulocyte count, white blood cell count, and platelet count
(C) a bone marrow study is required eventually to establish the diagnosis in all forms of anemia
(D) hemolysis is detected by measuring lactate dehydrogenase (LDH) and free haptoglobin, free hemoglobin, and indirect bilirubin in the serum
(E) the peripheral blood smear is examined to help define the anemia

56. All of the following statements about chronic leukemias are true EXCEPT

(A) the indolent and low-grade quality of most chronic leukemias allows time to achieve cures with appropriate therapy
(B) many cases exhibit specific chromosome abnormalities
(C) chronic myelogenous leukemia (CML) almost always progresses to an acute leukemia
(D) chronic lymphocytic leukemia (CLL) is generally a neoplasm of B lymphocytes
(E) chronic leukemias are proliferations or accumulations of mature or differentiated cells

57. Bernard-Soulier syndrome, a congenital deficiency of glycoprotein Ib (GP Ib), is associated with all of the following abnormalities EXCEPT

(A) prolonged bleeding time
(B) large platelets on peripheral smear
(C) impaired platelet aggregation with adenosine diphosphate (ADP)
(D) decreased binding of von Willebrand factor (vWF)
(E) propensity to bruise easily

58. A 36-year-old woman with a history of excessive menstrual bleeding was referred to the hematologist for hypochromic, microcytic anemia. All of the following procedures are appropriate for this patient EXCEPT

(A) tests to measure serum iron, iron-binding capacity, and percent saturation
(B) pelvic examination
(C) test to measure serum ferritin
(D) oral ferrous sulfate
(E) bone marrow study for iron stores

59. All of the following endocrinopathies can lead to a hypoproliferative anemia EXCEPT

(A) diabetes mellitus
(B) hypothyroidism
(C) hypopituitarism
(D) hyperparathyroidism
(E) hypogonadism

60. A 38-year-old man was discovered to have diabetes mellitus. He was noted on examination to have a "bronze" complexion, with a serum iron level of 200 μg/dl, 90% saturation, and a serum ferritin level of 1450 μg/dl. The following procedures are indicated in this patient EXCEPT

(A) chelation therapy with desferoxamine
(B) phlebotomy if the patient is not anemic
(C) ferritin levels of immediate family members
(D) liver biopsy
(E) insulin therapy only, with careful follow-up

61. Which of the following conditions is LEAST likely to be associated with eosinophilia?

(A) Hypereosinophilic syndrome
(B) Chronic myelogenous leukemia (CML)
(C) Parasitic infection
(D) *Staphylococcus aureus* infection
(E) Asthma

62. The etiologic agents implicated in chronic acquired pure red cell aplasia include all of the following EXCEPT

(A) chronic lymphocytic leukemia (CLL)
(B) Hodgkin's lymphoma
(C) non-Hodgkin's lymphoma
(D) thymoma
(E) Diamond-Blackfan syndrome

63. An 18-year-old woman with a family history of spherocytosis was found to be experiencing increasing levels of anemia; an appropriate preparation for splenectomy would include all of the following EXCEPT

(A) pneumococcal vaccination
(B) folic acid replacement
(C) iron replacement or supplementation
(D) prophylactic administration of oral penicillin

Directions: Each group of items in this section consists of lettered options followed by a set of numbered items. For each item, select the **one** lettered option that is most closely associated with it. Each lettered option may be selected once, more than once, or not at all.

Questions 64–68

For each function of plasma proteins, select the associated protein.

(A) Lipoprotein
(B) Complement
(C) Fibrinogen
(D) Transferrin
(E) None of the above

64. Fatty acid transport

65. Iron transport

66. Cholesterol transport

67. Infection resistance

68. Clot formation

Questions 69–72

Match each drug listed below with the hemolytic mechanism that it induces.

(A) Hapten-related mechanism
(B) "Innocent bystander" mechanism
(C) True autoimmune hemolytic anemia
(D) Activation of the reticuloendothelial system (RES) macrophages
(E) Allergy to a contaminant

69. Sulfonamides

70. α-Methyldopa

71. Penicillin

72. Phenacetin

Questions 73–74

Match the medical emergency experienced in sickle cell disease with the appropriate treatment modality.

(A) Bone marrow transplantation
(B) Exchange transfusions
(C) Hyperbaric oxygen
(D) Transfusion of packed red cells for supportive therapy
(E) Infusion of urea or cyanate

73. Aplastic crisis

74. Splenic crisis

Questions 75–79

For each neoplastic characteristic listed below, select the associated leukemia or lymphoma.

(A) Non-Hodgkin's lymphoma
(B) Hodgkin's disease
(C) Multiple myeloma
(D) Waldenström's macroglobulinemia

75. Orderly spread from one lymph node group to the next

76. Monoclonal IgM paraprotein

77. Monoclonal IgG paraprotein

78. Follicular pattern

79. Reed-Sternberg (RS) cells

Questions 80–83

Match each laboratory finding listed below with the most appropriate clinical condition.

(A) von Willebrand's disease
(B) Hemophilia A
(C) Both
(D) Neither

80. Prolonged bleeding time

81. Decreased factor VIII:C level

82. Decreased factor VIII:Ag level

83. Prolonged prothrombin time (PT)

Questions 84–88

Match each neutrophil disorder listed below with the characteristic most closely associated with it.

(A) Integrin
(B) Prominent cytoplasmic granules
(C) Atypical lymphocytes
(D) Döhle bodies
(E) Neutrophil nuclear segmentation

84. Chédiak-Higashi syndrome

85. Pelger-Hüet anomaly

86. Mononucleosis syndromes

87. Leukocyte adherence disorders

88. May-Hegglin anomaly

Questions 89–93

For each clinical situation listed below, select the most appropriate blood product.

(A) Cryoprecipitate
(B) Factor IX concentrate
(C) Albumin
(D) Fresh frozen plasma
(E) Intravenous immune serum globulin

89. Disseminated intravascular coagulation (DIC) with a fibrinogen level of 65 mg/ml

90. Resuscitation for hypovolemia associated with shock

91. von Willebrand's disease with bleeding

92. Congenital agammaglobulinemia

93. Hemophilia B before major surgery

ANSWERS AND EXPLANATIONS

1. The answer is C *[Ch 2 I B 1 b (2)].*
The patient younger than 20 years with hemolysis compensates for the increased red cell destruction with an increase in red cell production in medullary sites. Hematopoiesis does not extend to extramedullary sites such as the liver and spleen in order to support the demand for increased production; rather, medullary sites undergo hypertrophy (e.g., cranial bossing in the skull). After birth, the loci of hematopoiesis shift from all bone marrow cavities in the neonate to strictly the marrow cavities of the axial skeleton. However, it is not until age 20 that hematopoiesis is further limited to the skull, vertebrae, sternum, iliac bones, and proximal ends of the long bones of the extremities. The major contribution of the spleen to hematopoiesis occurs in utero; after birth, its participation is very limited. The thymus is the site of T cell maturation from progenitor cells in response to infection; it does not contribute to the creation of blood cells. In utero, the liver is the primary source of red cells from week 9 to week 24 of gestation, and its contribution may extend to 2 weeks after birth. Beyond that, however, the liver does not participate in hematopoiesis.

2. The answer is B *[Ch 4 II A, B; Table 4-1].*
Severe autoimmune hemolytic anemia can cause an acute drop in hemoglobin levels (due to renal tissue hypoxia) and is associated with high erythropoietin levels and reticulocytosis. Erythropoietin levels would be decreased in severe renal disease (as a result of damaged cortical cells, which are the source of erythropoietin), in polycythemia vera (PV) [as a result of the decreased secretion of erythropoietin caused by increased oxygen tension], in hypothyroidism (as a result of a decreased metabolic rate and tissue oxygen requirement), and in starvation (as a result of the overall decreased synthesis of proteins, including erythropoietin).

3. The answer is D *[Ch 5 IV E 5].*
The clue to poor compliance on the part of the patient is the brown stools since patients taking iron have dark or black stools from excess unabsorbed iron from the preparation. Malabsorption, intermittent blood loss, inflammatory bowel, and poor release of iron from the medication are all possible causes of the poor response to iron replacement but are unlikely in this asymptomatic patient.

4. The answer is B *[Ch 6 II A 6, B 2 b (2)].*
The proximal jejunum is the primary site of folate absorption. Vitamin B_{12} attaches to receptors on the microvilli in the distal 3–4 feet of ileum, which is the major site of vitamin B_{12} absorption.

5. The answer is D *[Ch 8 IV A 2 e].*
This patient with a low mean corpuscular volume (MCV) and no signs of anemia probably does not have any of the common causes of microcytic anemia, such as iron deficiency (ruled out by normal serum ferritin), anemia of chronic disease (without a chronic disease), lead poisoning (without an exposure history), or sideroblastic anemia (without anemia). Most patients with β thalassemia minor are asymptomatic and even have a negative family history, without demonstration of hemoglobin A_2 (Hb A_2) or hemoglobin H (Hb H) in an α thalassemia carrier by hemoglobin electrophoresis.

6. The answer is B *[Ch 9 II E 3 d (1) (e)].*
The evidence of a delayed hemolytic transfusion reaction is the acute drop in hemoglobin A (Hb A) from 60% to 10%, indicating destruction of the normal cells. Delayed hemolytic reactions to transfusion may mimic a regular sickle cell crisis, but the reactions may be severe enough to cause acute respiratory distress and disseminated intravascular coagulation (DIC). Alloimmunization to donor blood from previous transfusions is the cause of this reaction. Splenic crisis and sepsis are possible in this patient and could likely be diagnosed in that a delayed hemolytic transfusion reaction is often misdiagnosed.

7. The answer is C *[Ch 10 I D 3].*
The elderly patient under discussion most likely has pernicious anemia (PA) and, therefore, would display high levels of serum folate, low levels of vitamin B_{12}, hypersegmentation of neutrophils, achlorhydria, and an abnormal part I and normal part II Schilling test. A test for antibodies to intrinsic factor would be positive. The patient's normal diet would rule out other macrocytic anemias. The intake of multivitamins, which contain folate, aggravates the neurologic symptoms of PA. PA is not associated with abnormal chromosomes, and ringed sideroblasts are not seen in the bone marrow of PA patients. Increased folate levels are associated with vitamin B_{12} deficiency due to a lack of folate methylation and the subsequent escape of folate from within the cells into the serum.

8. The answer is C *[Ch 12 II C 2 b].*
Neutrophil leukocyte alkaline phosphatase (LAP) levels are characteristically low in chronic myelogenous leukemia (CML) but normal or elevated in reactive neutrophilia and other myeloproliferative disorders. Terminal deoxynucleotidyl transferase (TdT) is seen in immature lymphoblasts and is useful in the distinction of acute lymphocytic leukemia (ALL) and acute myelogenous leukemia (AML). Tartrate-resistant acid phosphatase (TRAP) is useful in confirming the diagnosis of hairy cell leukemia. Monoclonal surface immunoglobulin is a feature of neoplastic lymphoid proliferations; the differential diagnosis here is among granulocyte proliferations. Cytochemical stains for myeloperoxidase detect maturing granulocytes that are present in CML, reactive neutrophilia, and myeloproliferative disorders.

9. The answer is B *[Ch 13 V A 1 b (2)].*
A consistently prolonged bleeding time in a patient whose history suggests a bleeding disorder should be investigated before the patient undergoes an elective surgical procedure. The prolonged bleeding time along with this patient's normal platelet count suggests a platelet function defect, so evaluation of platelet aggregation would be an appropriate next step. Some inherited abnormalities of platelet function can result in significant surgical bleeding. Antiplatelet antibodies usually result in thrombocytopenia, and a bone marrow examination would not be very helpful in light of the normal platelet count and smear. Although transfusion with platelets might well correct the bleeding time, this trial would still not define the specific abnormality. In addition, it would be unwise to subject any patient to fresh blood products unless there is a clear therapeutic indication.

10. The answer is C *[Ch 14 II A 1; III C].*
Factor XI deficiency is autosomally transmitted and can be the cause of serious postoperative bleeding in this patient, even though it is mild enough to cause no spontaneous symptoms. Neither factor XII deficiency nor Fletcher factor deficiency results in a bleeding disorder, and inherited factor VIII deficiency occurs only in males. Factor VII deficiency would cause a prolongation of the prothrombin time (PT) but not the partial thromboplastin time (PTT).

11. The answer is C *[Ch 15 III B 5 a].*
Although steroids, splenectomy, heparin, and aspirin all have been tried in patients with thrombotic thrombocytopenic purpura (TTP), the most consistent therapeutic responses are seen in patients who receive fresh frozen plasma. Fresh frozen plasma often is given with plasmapheresis to allow replacement of a significant portion of the blood volume. Apheresis alone, or with plasma substitutes for replacement, is not effective.

12. The answer is C *[Ch 14 II A 5; Ch 16 I C 2 a (4)].*
The urea clot lysis test is required to screen for factor XIII deficiency, since factor XIII activity is not assessed by prothrombin time (PT), partial thromboplastin time (PTT), or thrombin time. The delayed onset of bleeding in this patient (i.e., 36 hours after surgery) and normal results on coagulation screening make factor XIII deficiency a consideration. Factor XII deficiency, which is detectable by screening, is not associated with bleeding. Factor IX deficiency also would likely have been picked up on screening. Given the normal bleeding time, a platelet aggregation study is unnecessary. Likewise, a mixing test is not meaningful in the absence of any abnormality on screening tests.

13. The answer is C *[Ch 16 I D 1 a].*
Examination of the peripheral blood smear must never be overlooked when evaluating a patient with thrombocytopenia. Unreported abnormalities of the red cells may offer a clue to the etiology. Occasionally, there is a discrepancy between the number of platelets seen on the smear and the number found by the automated count (so-called "pseudothrombocytopenia"), in which clumping of platelets in a specific anticoagulant [usually ethylenediaminetetraacetic acid (EDTA)] results in marked underestimation of the count.

Bone marrow examination is conducted to classify the thrombocytopenia according to the likely mechanism of the low platelet count and would be unnecessary if the platelet count was not truly low. Bleeding time and platelet aggregation are measures of platelet function, not number. Antiplatelet antibodies may provide more supportive diagnostic evidence in complex situations.

14. The answer is D *[Ch 2 III C 1].*
A young patient with pneumonia-like symptoms, who has a hemoglobin count of 14 g/dl and a white blood cell count (WBC) of 14,000/μl with an increased number of polymorphonuclear cells and band forms, is displaying evidence of hyposplenism, despite the absence of splenectomy. Congenital asplenia

may occur in an individual who has not had a splenectomy or other illness associated with hyposplenism. The increased risk for fulminating pneumococcal sepsis with its high mortality rate should prompt the physician to draw appropriate cultures and to initiate antibiotic therapy immediately. The prescription of oral antibiotics in conjunction with the performance of a blood culture or a sputum Gram stain would be appropriate for a patient with community-acquired lobar pneumonia if the spleen were functioning correctly. It would not be appropriate to forgo the administration of antibiotics and have the patient await test results in the hospital because it may take several days for the results to become available.

15. The answer is C *[Ch 4 II A 2 a].*
A reticulocyte count reflects bone marrow activity in response to anemia. A low reticulocyte count, which reflects decreased bone marrow activity, is a characteristic of hypoproliferative anemia. In cases of anemia caused by extreme blood loss or hemolysis, the bone marrow compensates by producing new red blood cells, which is reflected in a high reticulocyte count.

Increased red cell distribution width (RDW) reflects a wide variation in the size and shape of red cells and does not reflect the bone marrow erythroid activity. A normal mean corpuscular volume (MCV), which indicates that red blood cells are of normal size, is not specific for any type of anemia.

Low hemoglobin levels indicate anemia but do not indicate the type of anemia or the mechanism involved in its formation. Increased levels of iron in the serum may be found in hypoproliferative anemias due to poor utilization. However, the level of serum iron may rise with an iron-rich diet, so it is not a reliable indicator of hypoproliferative anemia.

16. The answer is A *[Ch 6 II B 2 a (4)].*
Vitamin B_{12} has a large storage pool in the liver, and if no B_{12} is supplied because of diet or malabsorption, a net loss of 1–3 μg/day will take anywhere from 2 to 12 years to deplete the hepatic stores.

17. The answer is C *[Ch 8 IV A 3 b].*
The definitive diagnosis of β thalassemia is based on finding an increased proportion of hemoglobin A_2 (Hb A_2) [to $>$ 3.5%], a decreased hemoglobin A (Hb A) [the degree depends on the severity of the inherited defect], and an increased proportion of hemoglobin F (Hb F) [in hereditary persistence of fetal hemoglobin (HPFH)] on hemoglobin electrophoresis. Findings that suggest thalassemia include a hypochromic, microcytic anemia [i.e., low mean corpuscular volume (MCV)], Heinz bodies, a positive family history, and normal iron stores in the bone marrow. Hemoglobin electrophoresis is needed to establish the type of thalassemia (i.e., α or β). Other nonspecific findings in β thalassemia include poikilocytosis and fragmented dacryocytes on blood smear.

18. The answer is D *[Ch 10 II A 1; Figure 10-6].*
The first step in the workup of a patient with an elevated hematocrit is to determine if true erythrocytosis is present or if it is spurious erythrocytosis or pseudoerythrocytosis, which is commonly seen in obese, hypertensive individuals with certain types of aggressive personalities. Even though chronic heavy smokers can develop true erythrocytosis by the formation of high levels of carboxyhemoglobin, the rest of the workup is not necessary unless elevation of red cell mass is documented.

19. The answer is D *[Ch 12 II B 1 a (1) (b)].*
Disseminated intravascular coagulation (DIC) is frequently seen with the FAB M3 subtype of acute myelogenous leukemia (AML), which features a proliferation of hypergranular promyelocytes, often with prominent Auer rods, which represent aggregations of these primary neutrophilic granules. The granules contain procoagulant substances that activate the coagulation cascade. DIC may be present at diagnosis of the leukemia or may develop in association with the destruction of leukemic cells during chemotherapy. For this reason, heparin anticoagulation may be used therapeutically to interfere with the depletion of coagulation factors and the formation of fibrin thrombi.

20. The answer is D *[Ch 13 II C 2 c; V B 4 a (1)].*
Aspirin has no effect on platelet production or life span, but it does significantly affect platelet function, causing a measurable increase in the bleeding time. This effect is caused by aspirin's inhibition of platelet cyclooxygenase, the enzyme needed for the production of thromboxane. Without thromboxane, platelet aggregation does not occur. Platelet response to high doses of potent aggregating agents (e.g., thrombin) is not affected by aspirin.

21. The answer is E *[Ch 14 III A 1 a; Figure 14-4].*
The daughter of a hemophilia patient will be a carrier for the disease. Hemophilia B is the result of a deficiency of factor IX, which is coded for on the X chromosome. Every female offspring receives one X

chromosome from her mother and one from her father; if the father has hemophilia, she will be an "obligate carrier" of the gene. The daughter will not, however, have any clinical abnormalities (except in very rare instances) because the normal gene is active in 50% of her cells, resulting in the production of enough factor VIII for the purposes of hemostasis.

22. The answer is C *[Ch 13 IV A 2 b (3)].*
Severe thrombocytopenia from any cause can result in hematuria, and (if there is other blood loss) anemia. However, in this patient, these findings are combined with fever and with a peripheral smear that suggests a microangiopathic process, virtually defining the clinical entity of thrombotic thrombocytopenic purpura (TTP). Idiopathic thrombocytopenic purpura (ITP) is a likely diagnosis in a young woman, but neither ITP nor drug-induced thrombocytopenia would explain the microangiopathic hemolytic process. Systemic lupus erythematosus (SLE) with lupus cerebritis, renal disease, vasculitis, and immune thrombocytopenia would explain the findings, but this constellation of problems would be unlikely as an initial presentation, and this patient has no previous history to suggest lupus. Sepsis with disseminated intravascular coagulation (DIC) could possibly explain the findings, but again there is no suggestive history, and the prothrombin time (PT) and partial thromboplastin time (PTT) are normal, making DIC unlikely.

23–25. The answers are: 23-D, 24-A, 25-C *[Ch 11 III F 2 a].*
This patient presents the classic picture of infectious mononucleosis resulting from Epstein-Barr virus (EBV) infection. Extreme fatigue, difficulty concentrating, and fever are generalized systemic symptoms. Pharyngitis reflects the local immunologic response by T lymphocytes reactive against viral antigens on infected tonsillar B lymphocytes. Splenomegaly is also a consequence of the immunologic response to EBV. Morphologic examination of the lymphocytosis in the peripheral blood should reveal "atypical lymphocytes," which are activated T cells with increased cytoplasm and less mature nuclear chromatin. Lymphocytes of infectious lymphocytosis and pertussis are morphologically normal but increased in number; pertussis is also a disease of younger children. Serum from this patient should yield a positive monospot test for heterophile antibodies. The combination of pharyngitis and lymphadenopathy are characteristic of EBV-associated mononucleosis. CMV mononucleosis lacks both these features. Toxoplasmosis, a rare cause of mononucleosis, may have associated lymphadenopathy but not pharyngitis.

A relatively common feature of infectious mononucleosis with EBV-mediated expansion of B cells is the development of antibodies to red cells, usually directed against the I antigen. Most antibodies of this type are cold agglutinins; that is, they react with erythrocytes at temperatures below 37° C. Cold agglutinins are usually of the IgM class, and Coombs' tests may or may not be positive. The virus-associated hemophagocytic syndrome has been seen in patients with EBV infections, although the setting is usually an immunocompromised patient. Direct infection of erythroid precursors is not a feature of EBV infection. Disseminated intravascular coagulation (DIC) is a rare occurrence in infectious mononucleosis, and thrombocytopenia may cause petechiae but not hemorrhagic blood loss.

There is nothing wrong with the blood counter; the cold agglutinins in this patient are the reason for the very abnormal values. Cell counters evaluate individual erythrocytes for size as they pass through the analysis window or chamber. As the blood sample cools to room temperature (~25° C) during transport to the laboratory, antibody-mediated agglutination of red cells occurs. The agglutinates, which can be seen on peripheral blood smears prepared from the sample, are thus analyzed as a single large particle by the cell counter. That is why the mean corpuscular volume (MCV) and the mean cell hemoglobin concentration are markedly elevated and why the red cell count is inappropriately low for the hemoglobin level, which is unaffected by agglutination. Moreover, the MCV is inappropriately high for even a significant reticulocytosis. Rouleaux are red cell aggregates that form because of charge shielding by elevated concentrations of asymmetric plasma proteins (immunoglobulins and fibrinogen) and are not a problem for cell counters since they disperse in isotonic dilution of the blood in preparation for counting.

26. The answer is D *[Ch 15 II A 2 a (2)].*
Warfarin-induced necrosis is a rare complication of therapy in some patients with protein C deficiency. The onset usually is early in the course of therapy, presumably due to further decreases in protein C in response to the vitamin K antagonist action of the drug. Thrombi in the small vessels of the skin result in necrosis, which characteristically involves skin overlying fatty areas (e.g., breasts, thighs, abdomen). Skin lesions secondary to allergy, excessive anticoagulation, or thrombocytopenia would not have a selective distribution and would not be associated with necrosis. Antithrombin III (AT III) is not vitamin K-dependent; thus, AT III deficiency would not be expected to respond to warfarin therapy in this manner.

27. The answer is C *[Ch 6 III D 3 e (2) (b)].*
In a patient with an undefined megaloblastic anemia, who urgently needs therapy but in whom the spe-

cific vitamin deficiency has not yet been characterized, both folic acid and vitamin B_{12} should be given. If the patient receives folate for what is actually a vitamin B_{12} deficiency, neurologic abnormalities may be precipitated or may worsen.

28. The answer is C *[Ch 10 I E 1 b (2)].*
Symptoms as occurred in the Italian tourist suggest a diagnosis of glucose-6-phosphate dehydrogenase (G6PD) deficiency of the Mediterranean type (class II). An enzyme deficiency of less than 10% results in episodic symptoms brought about by the ingestion of an oxidative agent found in fava beans, which causes denaturation and precipitation of the patient's hemoglobin and is shown in the Heinz bodies test. Class I (< 5%) G6PD deficiency is severe, with chronic hemolysis; it is called congenital nonspherocytic hemolytic anemia. Measurement of the level of G6PD in the red cells in the class III variant is not helpful since the enzyme levels increase with reticulocytosis; in the severe class I and class II forms, the enzyme levels are not elevated in the reticulocytes and would remain low during the hemolytic process.

29. The answer is A *[Ch 11 III B 1].*
Neutropenia is defined as an absolute neutrophil count below 1500/μl. Although there is a modest risk of acquired infection with a count of 1500/μl, patients with neutrophil counts below 1000/μl for any length of time are at significant risk of acquired infection, and patients with counts below 500/μl are at extreme risk. The peripheral blood differential counts are of limited value. They must be multiplied by the total white blood cell count (WBC) to arrive at absolute numbers of circulating granulocytes, monocytes, and lymphocytes. Leukocyte percentages determined by a 100-cell manual differential count have extremely broad (95%) confidence intervals that may yield broad apparent shifts in absolute numbers. New cell counters that provide a machine analysis of neutrophil, monocyte, and lymphocyte (and even eosinophil and basophil) percentages offer better estimates of absolute number.

30. The answer is A *[Ch 3 IV; Ch 12 II B 1 a (3)].*
Clinically persistent and unexplained cytopenias associated with morphologically abnormal differentiation in bone marrow precursors define preleukemia, often referred to as the myelodysplastic syndromes. Many of these patients have bone marrow blast percentages of less than 5% and suffer from complications of bone marrow failure such as bleeding, infection, and anemia. Others show an increase in bone marrow blasts between 5% and 30% and have a higher likelihood of developing frank acute myelogenous leukemia (AML), particularly at the higher pecentages. A bone marrow blast percentage above 30% defines acute leukemia. Cytogenetic changes, if present in myelodysplastic syndromes, are similar to those observed in AML, such as an extra chromosome 8. Despite megaloblastoid morphologic changes, preleukemic syndromes do not resolve with treatment for megaloblastic anemia. It is rare for chronic myelogenous leukemia (CML) to present with low white cell and platelet counts and bone marrow dyspoiesis.

31. The answer is A *[Ch 11 I B 2 a (1) (b), 3 c; Figure 11-2].*
Of the compounds listed, the metabolism of arachidonic acid by cyclooxygenase and lipoxygenase generates derivatives with powerful effects on the inflammatory response and neutrophil function. Cyclooxygenase produces a series of prostaglandins, including PGE_2, and thromboxanes, such as A_2 and B_2, with vasoactive, vasopermeable, and chemotactic properties. 5-Lipoxygenase oxidizes arachidonate to 5-hydroperoxyarachidonate (5-HPETE), which subsequently forms a series of leukotrienes that catalyze chemotaxis, vascular permeability, release of neutrophil granule contents, and other effects. The complex (and likely interdependent) relationships of arachidonate metabolites to neutrophil function is today a subject of active investigation. Glycogen is important as an energy source for neutrophils in regions of low oxygen tension, and hydrogen peroxide is important for intracellular killing of phagocytized microorganisms.

32. The answer is C *[Ch 2 V A 2].*
A patient presenting with Hodgkin's lymphoma and an enlarged mediastinal mass should first undergo bilateral bone marrow biopsy: A positive result will identify the disease as stage IV. Bone marrow studies are very important in the staging of lymphomas; positive results obviate the need for lymphangiograms or staging laparotomies. Computed tomography (CT) may still be performed to evaluate the response to therapy but is not needed to stage the disease once the bone marrow has been examined.

33. The answer is C *[Ch 12 II B 1, 3].*
Well over half of children with acute lymphocytic leukemia (ALL) survive more than 5 years, and most of the survivors remain persistently disease-free to the point of "cure." By contrast, currently about one-

third of children with acute myelogenous leukemia (AML) show long-term survival beyond 5 years. Despite the fact that the overall survival rate of AML is poorer, AML chemotherapy includes anthracyclines and alkylating agents, which are significantly more toxic compared with the induction and maintenance regimens based on vincristine and prednisone for ALL. Somewhat more aggressive therapies are used for older children or children with poorer-risk ALL, also with generally excellent long-term survival. Central nervous system (CNS) involvement is more likely in ALL.

34. The answer is B *[Ch 13 IV A 2 b (1)].*
Idiopathic thrombocytopenic purpura (ITP) is most common in young women, and the usual presentation is of isolated thrombocytopenia without associated illness. Amegakaryocytic thrombocytopenia can occur but is much less common, especially in this age-group. Drug-induced thrombocytopenia is also possible but unlikely in a healthy woman who is taking no medications. Patients with thrombasthenia are not thrombocytopenic, and "aleukemic leukemia" is unlikely in the absence of other cytopenias.

35. The answer is E *[Ch 11 II D 1 b (1), 2 a–b, E 3 a–b; Table 11-2].*
Both monoclonal surface immunoglobulin, characteristic of B lymphocytes, and T cell antigen receptors, characteristic of T lymphocytes, are formed from variable (V), diversity (D), joining (J), and constant (C) segments of immunoglobulin and T cell antigen receptor genes. The combinatorial joining of V, D, and J regions is what permits enormous immunologic diversity from a relatively small number of gene segments. Membrane surface antigen appears early in differentiation and is specific for B lymphocytes. CD8 is found on the surface of a subset of mature T cells (suppressor cells). CD19 is a surface membrane antigen of B lymphocytes. Leukocyte alkaline phosphatase (LAP) is a cytoplasmic enzyme that is most prominent in neutrophils and is useful in the differential diagnosis of leukemoid reaction versus myeloproliferative disorders.

36–37. The answers are: 36-C, 37-D *[Ch 14 II A 1; Ch 16 I A 1 a (2) (a), D 2 a; Figure 16-3].*
Prolonged partial thromboplastin time (PTT) is the most likely finding. This patient's family history suggests an X-linked inherited bleeding disorder. Mild hemophilia A or B is a strong possibility in this patient, which would show up as a prolonged PTT caused by a deficiency of either factor VIII or factor IX. The platelet count, prothrombin time (PT), thrombin time, and bleeding time would likely be normal in this patient.

The best step to be taken next is to perform specific factor assays. In a rare patient with very mild hemophilia, factor levels are not low enough to prolong the PTT but significant bleeding occurs after surgery. Assuming that this patient's maternal grandfather had mild hemophilia, the patient's mother, then, is an obligatory carrier and the patient has a 50% chance of having hemophilia. Since it is not known whether PTT was prolonged in other family members, it is prudent to perform factor assays before proceeding with elective surgery. Screening tests of the patient's mother would likely be normal because hemophilia carriers usually have high enough levels of the affected factor to result in normal screens. Platelet aggregation studies would not be helpful in view of the normal bleeding time and apparent X-linked inheritance pattern. A mixing study generally is performed in acquired disorders to determine if the addition of normal plasma corrects an abnormal screening test and, therefore, is not helpful if the screening test is already normal.

38. The answer is C *[Ch 12 II C 1].*
The leukocyte alkaline phosphatase (LAP) reaction in neutrophils is usually low in chronic myelogenous leukemia (CML) but is normal or high in reactive neutrophilia and myeloproliferative disorders. Acute leukemias are expansions of immature bone marrow–derived cells in either the lymphoid or myeloid lineages. Chronic leukemias generally do not cause death within 1 year of diagnosis; overall mean survival rates vary from 4–8 years for chronic myelogenous and lymphocytic leukemias. Since leukemic cells are primarily located in the blood and bone marrow throughout the body, surgery has no role in tumor reduction. Leukemia is the most common cancer in children but accounts for only about 5% of adult cancers.

39. The answer is D *[Ch 13 IV B 2].*
Given the setting, it is most likely that the patient's thrombocytosis is a result of his injuries. Secondary (reactive) thrombocytosis is common after trauma, and if this patient's spleen was ruptured in the motorcycle accident, thrombocytosis could be predicted to occur after a splenectomy. Secondary thrombocytosis is a self-limiting disorder and does not require specific treatment. No drugs given in this setting are likely to cause thrombocytosis. The patient probably received transfusions of red cells alone, which would not be expected to raise the platelet count. Essential thrombocythemia is not a common disorder and is not likely with a platelet count below 600,000/μl. The same is true of polycythemia vera (PV), especially in view of the normal white blood cell count (WBC), which is usually elevated in PV.

40. The answer is D *[Ch 14 II A 1 a].*
Although dysfibrinogenemia or the lupus anticoagulant could cause the patient's laboratory findings, heparin is so frequently used to keep venous and arterial lines open that heparin is the most likely cause of this combination of laboratory findings. Because in this setting heparin is not being used therapeutically but only to flush the venous lines, it often is overlooked as a medication. Clues that heparin is the cause in this case include the setting (patients in intensive or coronary care units often have access lines kept open with heparin flushes) and the fact that the coagulation screen was normal on admission. Isolated prolongation of the thrombin time may also be noted in this situation. Careful review of the patient's medications should confirm the suspicion of heparin-induced thrombocytopenia.

41. The answer is B *[Ch 15 III B 3 a, 4].*
This patient presents with the typical features of thrombotic thrombocytopenic purpura (TTP), a rare clinical syndrome that occurs most often in young women. Patients experience an acute onset of thrombocytopenia, microangiopathic hemolytic anemia, and fluctuating neurologic abnormalities, often accompanied by fever and renal dysfunction. Disseminated intravascular coagulation (DIC) is an unlikely diagnosis, given the normal prothrombin time (PT) and partial thromboplastin time (PTT) and the absence of a precipitating cause. There is no drug history; therefore, drug-induced thrombocytopenia is an unlikely explanation for the microangiopathic changes seen on peripheral blood smear. Leukemia is unlikely with a normal white cell differential. Red cell morphology should be normal in idiopathic thrombocytopenic purpura (ITP).

42. The answer is E *[Ch 11 III D 4 a].*
Urticaria pigmentosa is primarily a childhood disorder associated with skin accumulations of mast cells appearing as brown papules, which can cause pronounced itching owing to degranulation and histamine release. Although most cases resolve spontaneously, some patients develop more generalized involvement of visceral organs, including the bone marrow, known as systemic mastocytosis, in association with dermatographism and systemic symptoms such as flushing, diarrhea, and palpitations resulting from histamine release.

43. The answer is D *[Ch 11 II C 2].*
The gastrointestinal tract is not a major region of T cell distribution. T lymphocytes occupy specific anatomic and functional regions of the lymph nodes, thymus, and spleen. Moreover, they comprise more than 80% of circulating peripheral blood lymphocytes. In lymph nodes, they populate the paracortex between B cell–dependent follicular regions. In the spleen, T lymphocytes ensheath the periarteriolar trabecular vessels as part of the splenic white pulp. Virtually the entire thymus consists of T cells in association with thymic epithelial cells and monocyte–macrophage cells; it is here that precursor T cells progress through functional differentiation into mature CD3/CD4 (helper) or CD3/CD8 (suppressor–cytotoxic) cells. Some T lymphocytes are found in association with predominantly B lymphoid regions, such as the tonsils and Peyer's patches, but these are not thought to be major functional sites.

44. The answer is A *[Ch 11 III E 4; Table 11-6].*
Histiocytosis X (more commonly referred to as Langerhans' cell histiocytosis) is a general term that encompasses a diversity of proliferations of Langerhans' cells, which probably play a role in the immunologic presentation of antigen. Characteristics of Langerhans' cells include racquet-shaped Birbeck's granules on electron microscopy and surface CD1 antigen expression. Sphingomyelin accumulation is a feature of congenitally inherited Niemann-Pick disease, whereas β-glucosidase is the enzyme lacking in patients with Gaucher's disease.

45. The answer is A *[Ch 3 III A; Ch 16 I D 1 b (2) (b)].*
Platelet function abnormalities are common in myeloproliferative disorders. Patients with thrombocytosis due to polycythemia vera (PV) or essential thrombocythemia may have either thrombotic or hemorrhagic events, the latter as a result of the platelet dysfunction. Thrombin time, fibrinogen level, and factor VIII activity would be expected to be normal in PV.

46. The answer is E *[Ch 15 III B 2 b].*
Although the etiology of thrombotic thrombocytopenia (TTP) is unknown, there is no known inciting infection and no evidence of autoimmune hemolysis. Although there may be an element of blood loss, this does not explain the microangiopathic red cell changes characteristically seen on peripheral smear. Indeed, these changes are an integral diagnostic element in this condition and are believed to reflect intravascular trauma to red cells resulting from the cells passing through platelet thrombi, which can be seen on biopsy to obstruct small vessels. Splenomegaly is not part of the syndrome, and there is no evidence for functional hypersplenism in this condition.

47. The answer is C *[Ch 11 I B 1 b (1)].*
Mature neutrophils contain both primary and secondary granules and use their constituents for physiologic functions. The azurophilic to polychrome stain of primary granules present in promyelocytes is gradually lost during the myelocyte stage of maturation and is normally not seen in mature circulating neutrophils. Toxic granulation of neutrophils reflects an increased tendency for these primary granules to stain, although with less azurophilia (purple–red) than in earlier precursors.

48. The answer is E *[Ch 6 III D 3 d (4) (c)].*
Part III of the Schilling test is performed only if part II is abnormal. The other tests listed are important in establishing a diagnosis of pernicious anemia (PA) in this young woman. Folic acid deficiency is common in this age-group, and PA is closely related to an autoimmune mechanism that can be confirmed by the detection of antibodies to intrinsic factor, parietal gastric cells, and achlorhydria.

49. The answer is C *[Ch 3 II A b (1)].*
Both dose-dependent marrow cell suppression and an idiosyncratic mechanism have been observed with exposure to chloramphenicol, the drug most commonly implicated in aplastic anemia. The dose-dependent drug effect involves the formation of erythroblasts with vacuolated cytoplasms, indicating direct toxicity and suppression, which usually are reversible upon discontinuation of the drug. The idiosyncratic mechanism usually occurs several weeks later and results in a prolonged and serious form of aplastic anemia.

50. The answer is D *[Ch 3 V C 2–5].*
The complications of viral or fungal infections or parasitic infestations presenting as interstitial pneumonia or graft rejection are all dependent on the immune status of the host or recipient. However, graft-versus-host disease (GVHD) is due to the immune status of the grafted cells, which then reject the patient or host.

51. The answer is D *[Ch 4 II A 1 a–b].*
In chronic renal failure, the plasma volume is usually increased from fluid retention, which contributes to the general lowering of hemoglobin levels. The anemia of chronic renal disease is multifactorial, including a decrease in erythropoietin production, shortened red cell survival from uremia by metabolic or mechanical mechanisms, a direct marrow suppression from uremic toxins, and, finally, chronic bleeding from platelet dysfunction.

52. The answer is A *[Ch 5 IV E 1].*
The patient in question is iron-deficient and asymptomatic. There is no family history to suggest thalassemia; therefore, hemoglobin electrophoresis is not indicated. It is most important to determine the cause of iron deficiency in this patient, and the most common cause in this age-group is an occult gastrointestinal malignancy. The guaiac test for occult blood, the upper GI series, the barium enema, and urinalysis (for hematuria) are indicated.

53. The answer is A *[Ch 6 III D 3 c, d (1), f].*
The spinal cord damage in vitamin B_{12} deficiency is irreversible. The peripheral neuropathy and the pancytopenia improve with vitamin replacement therapy.

54. The answer is D *[Ch 9 II E 3 a (2)].*
The hand–foot syndrome is commonly seen in children. It is characterized by localized pain in the hand and feet specifically secondary to infarction of bone epiphyses; sequelae of this in the adult are shortened fingers and toes. Acute chest syndrome, sickle cell crisis, and pneumococcal pneumonia are all possible diagnoses in this case. Often, the differentiation of pulmonary infarction from a pneumonia is difficult. Patients with sickle cell disease should be treated for pneumococcal infection since they are asplenic; this form of infection can be fulminant in sickle cell disease, resulting in death.

55. The answer is C *[Ch 10 I; Figure 10-1].*
Several anemias do not require a bone marrow study for their diagnosis, such as the hemoglobinopathies in sickle cell disease and other forms of hemolytic anemia. A number of these disorders [e.g., hemoglobin SS (Hb SS), hemoglobin SC (Hb SC), and hereditary spherocytosis] have such characteristic peripheral blood smears that other tests can be eliminated. Early examination of the blood smear will help reduce the costs of the anemia workup.

56. The answer is A *[Ch 12 II C 1, 2 b, d, 3 b].*
Although chronic leukemias of both lymphoid and myeloid types may follow an indolent course, like-

lihood of a "cure" is thought to be remote. This may reflect a relatively low percentage in chronic leukemias of neoplastic precursor cells in active replication, which are thus sensitive to cell-cycle chemotherapeutic agents. Median survival for chronic lymphocytic leukemia (CLL) varies with the clinical stage (extent) of disease, but for all stages there is a more or less straight-line decline in survival. Chronic myelogenous leukemia (CML) may follow a relatively indolent course for 3–5 years, whereupon blast crisis develops in most survivors.

57. The answer is C *[Ch 13 V A 1 a].*
The normal ability of a platelet to adhere to damaged vascular subendothelium and to form a plug is dependent on platelet interaction with von Willebrand factor (vWF). A specific measure of this interaction is ristocetin-induced aggregation: vWF must bind to its receptor, glycoprotein Ib (GP Ib), for this aggregation to occur. In GP Ib deficiency (i.e., Bernard-Soulier syndrome), vWF cannot bind to platelets in response to ristocetin and thus platelet aggregation does not occur. vWF is not required for platelet aggregation in response to adenosine diphosphate (ADP), collagen, or epinephrine. Bernard-Soulier syndrome is a congenital defect of platelet adhesion that is characterized by mild thrombocytopenia, prolonged bleeding time, and a propensity to bruise easily; transfusion or surgery can cause significant bleeding.

58. The answer is E *[Ch 2 V A 1].*
Serum tests to measure iron, iron-binding capacity, percent saturation, and ferritin are adequate for the diagnosis of iron deficiency in a 36-year-old woman with a history of excessive menstrual bleeding. The examination of iron stores in the bone marrow is not indicated since this test would not add any useful information but would increase patient costs and add to the patient's discomfort. A pelvic examination is more appropriate in this case so that the underlying cause of her hypermenorrhea is not missed. Upon establishing that the patient is iron-deficient, replacement therapy should be initiated.

59. The answer is A *[Ch 4 II B 1 b, 2 b, 3].*
Diabetes mellitus does not directly cause anemia. However, people with diabetes often have infections, which may lead to anemia associated with the chronic disease. Endocrinopathies can lead directly to anemia.

Hypothyroidism decreases the oxygen requirement of tissues, and thus decreases erythropoietin production, which leads to anemia.

In hypopituitarism, a decrease in growth hormone can lead to hypocellular bone marrow and, thus, anemia. Hypopituitarism can also decrease thyroid function, androgen levels, and levels of adrenal cortical hormones, all of which can also lead to anemia.

In hyperparathyroidism, increased levels of calcium or parathyroid hormone can damage the kidneys (e.g., renal calcifications) or the bone marrow (e.g., sclerosis), thus suppressing erythropoiesis and causing anemia.

Androgens increase the formation of erythropoietin and make the bone marrow more responsive to it, which increases erythropoiesis. Hypogonadism, or low levels of androgen, thus has an adverse effect on erythropoiesis, which can lead to anemia.

60. The answer is E *[Ch 5 V].*
Hereditary hemochromatosis manifests as diabetes due to damage of the pancreatic islets; increased melanin in the skin gives a bronze tinge to the complexion. Diagnosis is confirmed by measurement of serum ferritin level, iron studies, and a liver biopsy. Insulin therapy alone will treat the diabetes but will not prevent further tissue damage by the iron accumulation. Since this tissue damage is preventable if diagnosed early, it is incumbent upon the physician to screen the immediate family members for the disease.

61. The answer is D *[Ch 11 III C 2].*
Eosinophilia, defined usually as a circulating absolute eosinophil count above 500/μl, is not usually a feature of acute bacterial infection. It is a frequent accompaniment to the myeloproliferative disorders, including chronic myelogenous leukemia (CML), as well as other neoplasms. Probably the most common cause of peripheral eosinophilia in a routine clinical laboratory is asthma or another allergic condition. Parasitic infections that invade tissue are a classic cause of peripheral eosinophilia. The definition of the hypereosinophilic syndrome is a persistent eosinophil count above 1500/μl. Tissue accumulations of eosinophils may be seen in this condition associated with Charçot-Leyden crystals.

62. The answer is E *[Ch 4 II C 2 a].*
Diamond-Blackfan syndrome, which manifests in childhood, is an inherited form of pure red cell aplasia

that may be caused by a defective stem cell. Chronic lymphocytic leukemia (CLL), Hodgkin's lymphoma, non-Hodgkin's lymphoma, and thymoma are acquired adult forms of pure red cell aplasia. As part of the disease process, these forms produce an abnormal antibody to the red cell precursor that comes from a malignant or a monoclonal lymphocyte.

63. The answer is D *[Ch 2 III C 1 c; Ch 7 V C 1 d].*
A young woman with a family history of spherocytosis who presents with worsening symptoms of anemia should be prepared for splenectomy by ruling out causes of anemia other than hypersplenism. Folate deficiency can be due to the increased utilization of folate as a result of the high turnover rate caused by hemolysis. Young women may experience iron deficiency as a result of menstruation. If splenectomy is required, pneumococcal vaccine should be given before removal of the spleen, since the patient's immune response does not provide sufficient protection after splenectomy. The administration of oral prophylactic antibiotics is not necessary once the pneumococcal vaccine has been given.

64–68. The answers are: 64-E *[Ch 1 I B 3],* **65-D** *[Ch 1 I B 3 c],* **66-A** *[Ch 1 I B 3 c (3)],* **67-B** *[Ch 1 I B 3 b],* **68-C** *[Ch 1 I B 3 a].*
Fibrinogen makes an important contribution to the clotting of blood by forming fibrin. Transferrin binds and transports iron to the bone marrow for production of red blood cells. Complement aids immunoglobulin in counteracting infection. Lipoproteins are important transport proteins that deliver cholesterol and other lipids to sites of utilization and degradation throughout the body.

69–72. The answers are: 69-B *[Ch 7 V A 3 c (2)],* **70-C** *[Ch 7 V A 3 c (3)],* **71-A** *[Ch 7 V A 3 c (1)],* **72-B** *[Ch 7 V A 3 c (2)].*
Both sulfonamides and phenacetin react with IgM in the serum and form immune complexes that are absorbed in the red cell membrane, where complement can be activated and cause hemolysis; the red cell is simply an "innocent bystander."
α-Methyldopa (Aldomet) is the only drug that is believed to cause true autoimmune hemolysis.
Penicillin is antigenic; its metabolites can also cause specific antidrug IgG synthesis. High doses of penicillin can be absorbed in the red cell membrane and cause hemolysis.

73–74. The answers are: 73-D *[Ch 9 II E 3 a (1) (d)],* **74-B** *[Ch 9 II E 3 d (1) (e)].*
Aplastic crisis is a self-limited episode of worsening anemia (often to life-threatening levels) that requires supportive red cell transfusion.
Splenic crisis in the young patient with sickle cell disease is also a life-threatening condition that is managed by exchange transfusions. The modalities for preventing sickling of the cells by the administration of urea and cyanates have fallen out of use because of the negative results of clinical trials and severe toxicities. Hyperbaric oxygen is now being used in efforts to treat chronic ankle and skin ulcerations. Bone marrow transplantation may be used to treat severely affected young patients.

75–79. The answers are: 75-B *[Ch 12 III B 1 b; Table 12-6],* **76-D** *[Ch 12 IV D 1, 3 c, 4],* **77-C** *[Ch 12 IV A 3 b],* **78-A** *[Ch 12 III C 1 a (3)],* **79-B** *[Ch 12 III B 2 a].*
A unique feature of Hodgkin's disease is its methodical spread along pathways of lymph node drainage.
Macroglobulinemia is often associated with signs of more widespread lymphoproliferation such as organomegaly, anemia, higher levels of IgM paraprotein, and sometimes hyperviscosity syndrome. Monoclonal IgM paraproteins may also occur in a benign setting without these clinical findings.
IgG paraproteins are associated with both benign monoclonal gammopathies and symptomatic multiple myeloma, which generally displays osteolytic bone disease, anemia, renal compromise, and other symptoms.
Non-Hodgkin's lymphomas of B lymphoid origin may display a follicular growth pattern, recapitulating the ability of these cells to form or "home in" on germinal centers. This is not to be confused with the nodules seen in nodular sclerosing Hodgkin's disease.
Reed-Sternberg (RS) cells are characteristic of Hodgkin's disease. RS-like cells also may be seen in certain non-Hodgkin's lymphomas and even reactive conditions; therefore, the histopathologic background in which they are seen is important in making the proper diagnosis. The cellular origin of the RS cell has not yet been determined clearly.

80–83. The answers are: 80-A *[Ch 14 III B 3 a; Table 14-2],* **81-C** *[Ch 14 III B 3 a; Table 14-2],* **82-A** *[Ch 14 III B 1 d (1); Table 14-2],* **83-D** *[Ch 14 II A 2].*
Bleeding time is prolonged in von Willebrand's disease but not in hemophilia A. The von Willebrand factor (vWF) is necessary to support normal platelet function. The bleeding time is a gross measure of in

vivo platelet function and is, therefore, often abnormal when vWF is decreased or functionally abnormal. Hemophilia A is a deficiency of coagulation factor VIII, which does not directly affect platelet function as measured by the bleeding time.

Levels of factor VIII:C are decreased in both von Willebrand's disease and hemophilia A. Factor VIII circulates bound to vWF, which serves to stabilize it. Consequently, deficiency or abnormalities of vWF can also result in decreased factor VIII coagulant activity.

Factor VIII:Ag represents the antigenic activity of the vWF–factor VIII complex, and the factor VIII:Ag level is primarily determined by vWF, which is much larger. Consequently, the factor VIII:Ag level is decreased in classic von Willebrand's disease but is normal in hemophilia A.

The prothrombin time (PT) measures the extrinsic and common coagulation pathways, which are not affected by abnormalities of either factor VIII or vWF. Therefore, neither hemophilia A nor von Willebrand's disease prolong the PT.

84–88. The answers are: 84-B *[Ch 11 III B 3 a (1); Table 11-5]*, **85-E** *[Ch 11 Table 11-5]*, **86-C** *[Ch 11 III F 2 a (3)]*, **87-A** *[Ch 11 III B 3 a (3); Table 11-5]*, **88-D** *[Ch 11 III B 2 c (2), 3 c; Table 11-5]*.
Chédiak-Higashi syndrome is an autosomal recessive disorder characterized by giant granules in leukocytes caused by the abnormal fusion of cytoplasmic granules. There is overall cellular dysfunction. Clinical manifestations include albinism, susceptibility to infection, and peripheral neuropathy.

Pelger-Hüet anomaly is an inherited disorder associated with abnormal nuclear lobulation of neutrophils.

Mononucleosis syndromes are characterized by atypical lymphocytes, which are reactive peripheral blood T cells. These syndromes are the most common cause of benign lymphocytosis.

Leukocyte adherence disorders can be congenital, and they are caused by deficiencies in the integrins, a group of three families of adhesive proteins. The various families include receptors for fibroblast fibronectin, blood platelets and matrix components, and also receptors found on white blood cells, including lymphocyte function associated (LFA-1) receptors and Mac-1 receptors, which are found on macrophages. People with leukocyte adherence disorders do not have these receptors, which are important in neutrophil adherence for fighting bacterial infections.

May-Hegglin anomaly does not have any clinical effects, but is a morphologic disorder of granulocytes. Morphologic changes include the appearance of Döhle bodies, which are light blue cytoplasmic inclusions in neutrophils that represent aggregates of polyribosomes. The blue color is due to staining of the ribosomal RNA.

89–93. The answers are: 89-A *[Ch 17 I B 7 b (2)]*, **90-C** *[Ch 17 I B 8]*, **91-A** *[Ch 17 I B 7 b, c (1)]*, **92-E** *[Ch 17 I B 9 b (1)]*, **93-B** *[Ch 17 I B 12 b]*.
Cryoprecipitate contains high concentrations of factor VIII:C, fibrinogen, von Willebrand factor (vWF), and factor XIII. Therefore, cryoprecipitate is the product of choice for fibrinogen replacement, which may be necessary in some cases of disseminated intravascular coagulation (DIC), and for the treatment of von Willebrand's disease, in which there is both a partial deficiency of factor VIII:C and defective or decreased vWF.

Although crystalloids are frequently used first for the resuscitation of hypovolemia, colloids such as albumin may also be appropriate.

Immune serum globulin can be used as replacement therapy for primary immunodeficiency states such as congenital agammaglobulinemia.

Factor IX concentrate may be used for the treatment of patients with factor IX deficiency. Although fresh frozen plasma also contains factor IX, 1 unit of fresh frozen plasma (200 ml) will increase the circulating factor IX level about 3% in a 70-kg adult. For major surgery, factor IX hemostatic levels should be increased to 60%–80%. The use of factor IX concentrate will accomplish this more effectively.

Index

Note: Page numbers in *italic* denote illustrations; those followed by (t) denote tables; those followed by Q denote questions; and those followed by E denote explanations.

C

H

I

J

K

L

N

O

P

U

V